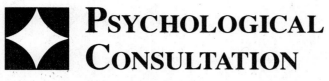

PSYCHOLOGICAL
CONSULTATION

Perspectives and Applications

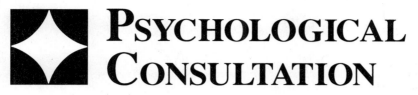

PSYCHOLOGICAL CONSULTATION
Perspectives and Applications

William A. Wallace
Marshall University
Emeritus

Donald L. Hall
Marshall University

Brooks/Cole Publishing Company

I(T)P™ An International Thomson Publishing Company

Pacific Grove • Albany • Bonn • Boston • Cincinnati • Detroit • London • Madrid • Melborne
Mexico City • New York • Paris • San Francisco • Singapore • Tokyo • Toronto • Washington

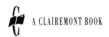
A CLAIREMONT BOOK

Sponsoring Editor: *Claire Verduin*
Art Coordinator: *Kathy Joneson*
Editorial Associate: *Patricia Vienneau*
Indexer: *Do Mi Stauber*
Production Editor: *Penelope Sky*
Advertising: *Romy Fineroff*
Manuscript Editor: *Elizabeth Judd*
Marketing: *Connie Jirovsky*

Permissions Editor: *May Clark*
Typesetting: *TBH/Typecast, Inc.*
Interior Design: *Lisa Thompson*
Interior Illustration: *Kathy Joneson*
Cover Design: *Terri Wright*
Printing and Binding: *Quebecor/Fairfield*
Cover Printing: *Phoenix Color Corporation, Inc.*

For more information, contact:

BROOKS/COLE PUBLISHING COMPANY
511 Forest Lodge Road
Pacific Grove, CA 93950
USA

International Thomson Publishing Europe
Berkshire House 168-173
High Holborn
London, WC1V 7AA, England

Thomas Nelson Australia
102 Dodds Street
South Melbourne, 3205
Victoria, Australia

Nelson Canada
1120 Birchmount Road
Scarborough, Ontario
Canada M1K 5G4
International Thomson Editores

Campos Eliseos 385, Piso 7
Col. Polanco
11560 México D.F. México

International Thomson Publishing GmbH
Königswinterer Strasse 418
53227 Bonn
Germany

International Thomson Publishing Asia
221 Henderson Road
#05-10 Henderson Building
Singapore 0315

International Thomson Publishing Japan
Hirakawacho Kyowa Building, 3F
2-2-1 Hirakawacho
Chiyoda-ku, Tokyo 102, Japan

Printed in the United States of America

10 9 8 7 6 5 4 3 2 1

Library of Congress Cataloging-in-Publication Data

Wallace, William A.
    Psychological consultation : perspectives and applications /
William A. Wallace, Donald L. Hall.
        p.   cm.
    Includes bibliographical references and index.
    ISBN 0-534-23094-6
    1. Psychological consultation.   I. Hall, Donald L.
II. Title.
BF637.C56W35   1995
158'.3—dc20   95-38967
                                                        CIP

To our wives
Lois and Jeanne

And to our children
Blake and Bill Wallace
Evan and Casey Hall

◆ CONTENTS

CHAPTER SEVEN
Consultation in Child Development Settings   164

CHAPTER EIGHT
Consultation in Health Care Settings   190

CHAPTER NINE
Consultation in Business and Industrial Settings   210

PART THREE
Issues and Concepts   235

CHAPTER TEN
Special Consultation Applications   237

CHAPTER ELEVEN
Ethical and Legal Dilemmas in Consultation   267

PART FOUR
Looking Ahead   293

◆ PREFACE

We had four main reasons for writing this book.

First, we wanted to convey the exciting potential of psychological consultation; this growing field is a relatively new frontier, and well-trained professionals can contribute to its growth and development.

Second, we are convinced that graduate-level consulting courses do not prepare students to meet the demands that await them. Many students report to us that, despite their limited training and inadequate experience, they have already assumed consultive roles as adjunct requirements of their work. Consultation should never be practiced in a trivial, unplanned, or unethical manner. The skills and insights of effective consultants are highly specialized and can be acquired only through comprehensive study and experience.

Third (and most motivating for us), is that existing texts frustrate our students. They want a book that relates theories, processes, and current research to specific skills and applications, so they can learn to integrate consultation into their internships and later careers.

Fourth, many readers of this book are professionals in various psychological disciplines (including psychology, counseling, social work, and their sub-specialties) who want a centralized source of knowledge about consultation.

Although traditional theories and current concepts are an integral part of this book, what makes it unique are the practical and extended applications in place of absolute instructions. We portray consultation as a practice that follows basic rules but is also flexible and open to alternate views; indeed, it is often shaped by the circumstances of the settings in which it is applied, and blends theoretical, conditional, and intuitive dynamics. Consequently, we discuss the many consultation methods and strategies without attaching them specifically to any one psychological discipline, citing different specialties in the many case examples.

Features

Each chapter contains an overview and a brief introduction. Key terms are set in bold-face type and defined in the text. Graphic illustrations emphasize, clarify, or supplement the discussion. Chapter glossaries may be used for quick reference and in preparing for examinations. Each chapter concludes with an annotated bibliography and a list of references and suggested readings. A cumulative glossary at the end of the book combines all the terms cited in the chapter glossaries.

Organization

Psychological Consultation: Perspectives and Applications follows a structure that was designed to be most useful to readers. We introduce the subject in the early chapters, move to more advanced technical discussions, and finally consider how consultation will develop in the future.

In Part One, "All about Consultation" (Chapters 1 through 5), we describe consultation as a distinct professional practice, distinguishing it from related human service functions. We identify the stages and processes of consultation, review theoretical approaches, emphasize evaluation, and discuss resistance to consultation.

In Part Two, "Consultation Settings" (Chapters 6 through 9), we highlight the role of consultation in specific settings, including education, child development, health care, business, and industry.

In Part Three, "Professional Issues and Concepts" (Chapters 10 and 11), we emphasize the special issues, demands, and standards that consultants confront as they work. We discuss applications that are often required by consultation roles, as well as the ethical and legal dilemmas practitioners may encounter.

In Part Four, "Looking Ahead" (Chapters 12 and 13), we discuss the many practical issues that beginners face in establishing themselves as professional consultants, and identify the trends and issues that are likely to influence consultants in the future.

Acknowledgments

Many deserving individuals contributed in some way to the development of this book. Without their inspiration, ideas, critical reading, and cooperation, *Psychological Consultation* might still be a vision rather than a reality.

We acknowledge Antoni Hardy, who was involved with the book in its formative stages and whose ideas influenced our early planning. We are grateful to Pam Stockbridge and Tara Gilman, who spent considerable time collecting information and critically reading several chapters. These two research assistants provided valuable insights. In addition, we recognize all the graduate students who participated in the classroom testing of the book and let us know what kinds of approaches they prefer. Special recognition is due to Dr. Stuart Thomas, who interrupted his busy schedule to read and critique Chapter 4.

We also thank the staff at Brooks/Cole. We owe much to our publisher, Claire Verduin, who was most gracious and supportive during the development of this project. We especially appreciate the efforts of our production editor, Penelope Sky. In addition, we acknowledge Kelly Shoemaker, Kathy Joneson, and Elaine Jones.

The following reviewers read selected chapters and suggested changes, and we appreciate their commitment and expertise: Linda A. Barnier, Idaho State University; David Botwin, University of Pittsburgh; and Ron Partin, Bowling Green State University.

We give special recognition to our wives, Lois Wallace and Jeanne Hall, who provided much inspiration. Their patience and understanding are priceless contributions.

William A. Wallace
Donald L. Hall

PART ONE

All About Consultation

In approaching the study of psychological consultation, you should not be put off by the ambiguity of the term *consultation*. Providing consultation holds different meanings for the multidisciplinary groups that take part in the consultive process. In addition, the field is plagued by the often-strong disagreements generated by consultants who apply their own specialty orientations—rather than a centralized theory of consultation—in carrying out consultive roles. Add the variation created by unique problems, settings, and relational dynamics and there is little doubt why even experienced professionals often misunderstand consultation.

Amidst overlapping concepts and double meanings, students and beginning consultants must have a clear definition of psychological consultation. Thus, the five chapters in Part I develop a somewhat generic description of what psychological consultation is and is not. Recognizing the many practical and conceptual obstacles to definitional clarity, we provide a knowledge base in the early chapters that distinguishes consultation as a professional service model. Cumulatively, the introductory chapters define consultation, identify consultive processes, and otherwise provide a foundation for later chapters. Further, the chapters in Part I are arranged in a sequence that will help you acquire basic knowledge and then proceed to more technical and advanced information. A brief overview of each chapter follows.

CHAPTER ONE
Introduction to Consultation

Chapter 1 offers an introduction to the practice of psychological consultation. It addresses the definition of consultation, makes comparisons with related psychological or human service activities, and provides a summary of the psychological, sociological, economic, and political forces that have contributed to consultation's development as a specialty area. The chapter concludes with a brief discussion of the viability of consultation, summarizing relevant empirical studies that point to consultation's effectiveness.

CHAPTER TWO
Stages of Consultation

Chapter 2 introduces readers to consultation as a process. The chapter emphasizes the elements of consultation that give potential consultants much-needed structure with respect to the consultation process. By adhering to a series of interrelated stages and dynamics, consultants avoid errors produced by omission or misdirection. We describe seven generic and developmentally ordered stages that consultants should consider as they initiate consultation and follow through with comprehensive problem solving. For each general stage, we include information about important tasks and dynamics that guide consultants through the entire process.

CHAPTER THREE
Consultation Models and Approaches

Chapter 3 continues our effort to define consultation by addressing the various approaches and models that consultants often apply in their work. A key point is that consultants should avoid whimsical or serendipitous strategies in their practices. Consultation should be grounded in substantive theoretical ideologies, predicated on reliable techniques or strategies, and tailored to the specific needs of consumers. We summarize three popular and enduring models: mental health consultation, organizational consultation, and behavioral consultation. We also provide practical guidelines that will help you interpret and apply these models.

CHAPTER FOUR
Measuring Consultation Efficacy

Chapter 4 discusses ways of evaluating consultation's efficacy as a professional service model. A range of issues that consultants must consider as they assess the effectiveness of their work are presented. Of particular significance is the discussion of the barriers and myths that make it difficult for consultants to carry out evaluation. In addition, the chapter emphasizes many of the practical issues surrounding consultation evaluation.

CHAPTER FIVE
Resistance and Reactance to the Consultation Process

Consultation is often delivered across multiple settings and in collaboration with diverse groups and individuals. Consultants must brace themselves for the widely varying reactions of others. In this chapter, we emphasize the sources of resistance and reactance and theoretical and practical strategies consultants use to manage problematic reactions. Consultants must learn to recognize resistance and reactance and to develop strategies for overcoming these obstacles.

CHAPTER ONE

Introduction to Consultation

Glossary

Annotated Bibliography

References and Suggested Readings

The complex living, runaway technology, and tendency toward specialization that characterize our society keep us endlessly searching for innovative solutions to human and organizational problems. This trend is particularly conspicuous in the human service arenas, as more and more consumers depend on mental health and psychological resources to meet their needs. Herman Holtz (1993), perhaps stirred by this reality, speculates that more than in any other historical period, "individuals in all walks of life find it increasingly difficult to cope with modern complexities without the help of various experts" (p. 1). Psychological consultation is one professional service model that appears to be benefiting inadvertently from a "help-seeking" mentality. Often referred to in this book simply as "consultation," *psychological consultation* is a broad helping approach that has received steady emphasis among the psychological professions.

Escalating numbers of consultants, greater demands for their services, and greater professional commitment to consultation point to its popularity. When asked about their attraction to this growing field, consultants offer various explanations. Some believe, for example, that consultation provides a challenging professional frontier that offers exciting options, variety, and innovative technologies. Others relish the chance to confront unique problems and develop innovative solutions in unfamiliar settings. To some consultants, the satisfaction that stems from their "expert" status as contracted or paid specialists is rewarding. Consultants, as a group, appear inspired by their altruistic desire to contribute to the psychological well-being of others or to organizational success. Many professionals find consultive roles appealing because they offer part-time opportunities that augment their daily jobs as educators, therapists, or managers. Whatever the attraction or motivation, all will find consultation stimulating and rewarding, especially the self-directed and often pioneering professionals who wish to add a career specialization.

As a group, psychological consultants represent an array of professional specialties, and of all the traits that distinguish consultation, none is more apparent than its cross-disciplinary status. Thus, throughout this book, we take a comprehensive approach to defining *psychological consultants*. A roster of psychological consultants might include, among others, professionals in psychology, counseling, and social work, including the subspecialties of each of these broad disciplines.

The Broad Concept of Consultation

The decades since World War II have brought various theoretical and practical breakthroughs that, combined with the escalating psychological demands of society, account for consultation's emergence as a professional service model (Brown, Pryzwansky, & Schulte, 1991). At first glance, one may even predict that consultation is on the brink of maturity as a formal psychological profession. Despite these accolades and hopes, however, consultation's status appears somewhat tenuous. Various growing pains imperil the future of the field. Heading the list are several issues involving consultation's theoretical shortcomings and the complications of its multidisciplinary status.

Several noted authors express apprehension about the absence of unifying theoretical ideologies. Gallessich (1985), for example, points out that the lack of cogent formulations creates an "atheoretical" status in which consultants rely more on the orientations of their respective disciplines and less on sound theories (p. 336). Bardon (1985) agrees with Gallessich that "consultation may well be at a point of developmental crisis, conceptually at an impasse, and, in general, adrift" (p. 355). Others write about the apparent lack of consistent research evidence to support consultation's claims of efficacy (Froehle & Rominger, 1993). Still others depict consultation as a "conceptually fragmented" practice in need of a cogent theoretical foundation (Brack, Jones, Smith, White, & Brack, 1993, p. 619). Holtz's (1993) concern that consultation is often misunderstood by its own practitioners is perhaps the most glaring symptom of conceptual imperfections. Bardon (1985) summarizes the situation somewhat cynically:

> What is all the fuss about? We all know what consultation is. It is whatever we do when we want a prestigious designation for professional activities different from our more routine diagnostic and intervention services performed as part of our daily work. (p. 355)

Efforts to clarify consultation are hampered by the tendency of theoretically separate specialists to define the field according to the convictions, values, and technical guidelines of their respective disciplines. Though cross-fertilization of thought among the psychological disciplines generates an abundance of ideas and information about consultation, it also brings many unanswered questions and strong disagreements. The consequence is that consultation has different meanings for different professional groups. Imagine counselors, psychologists, and social workers, for example, coming together to formulate a universal definition of therapy. Standardization of consultation concepts and principles is no less difficult.

Conceptual barriers create confusion for students and other newcomers to the field when they first begin to learn about consultation. Out of puzzlement, some may ask: "What is psychological consultation and how is it different from other professional service models?" Novice consultants may paint too dramatic a picture, assuming that consultants are valiant mental health pioneers who take charge of problems in times of human crisis or organizational chaos. Others may mistakenly expect consultants to wield unique technologies to achieve spectacular solutions. Even experienced consultants often misperceive their work as a spontaneous process that requires little planning, preparation, or organization. The need to resolve these questions and misperceptions should motivate you to thoroughly understand consultation.

Case Examples

Despite conceptual uncertainties, you should rest assured that a useful knowledge base is within your grasp. By reviewing existing theoretical and practical ideologies, and by considering practical application examples and guidelines, you will acquire an understanding that helps you distinguish myth from fact. To begin this learning process, however, you must become aware of the distinctive features of consultation. The following case examples illustrate many of the key features that we will be discussing throughout the book:

- A fourth-grade teacher asks a school counselor to help resolve complicated behavioral problems in the classroom.
- A psychologist-specialist in the treatment of eating disorders conducts a small group inservice for therapists at a local mental health center.
- A counselor enters an agreement with a small child development program to conduct parent training programs for single parents.
- The director of a general hospital asks a psychiatrist to train hospital staff in the dynamics of an innovative treatment strategy.
- A private practice counselor joins a community task force working to prevent child abuse and neglect.
- A mental health specialist responds to a request by a mental health center to design a new intake procedure.
- A drug and alcohol counselor helps the personnel manager of a federal organization implement an employee wellness program.
- A psychologist in a community agency testifies in court as an expert witness regarding theories of memory and perception.
- A residential agency for the treatment of emotional disorders in youth requires a psychologist to supervise its behavioral modification program.
- An elementary school counselor is asked by the school principal to design and carry out a drug abuse prevention program.
- A counselor specializing in organizational theory and structure accepts a manager's request to study employee stress and low morale.
- A mental health worker is asked by the program supervisor to visit the family of an agency client to discuss the dynamics of a specific mental disorder.

These examples contain numerous clues about the characteristics and dynamics of psychological consultation. Consultation can assume various shapes, depending on the problems, settings, and constituents that comprise a particular situation. Although requests for consultation are prompted by psychologically laden issues of individual or organizational origin, each consultant must address unique problems, needs, and solutions. From the examples you can see that psychological specialists who help with problems have a common commitment to psychological theory and practice, yet their specific disciplines and orientations vary. You may notice that every case example identifies several individuals, each with a unique vantage point.

Definitional Perspectives and Core Characteristics

Despite the variation generated by different settings, problems, and practitioners, the consultation process usually has several discernible features and conditions. As you learn the "core characteristics" of consultation, you will become aware of the generic

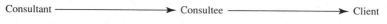

FIGURE 1.1
The linear version of the tripartite relationship in consultation

elements of the process. A review of several core characteristics is included in the discussion that follows.

Consultation Parties   The consultation process typically involves three individuals or parties and, as consultation unfolds in a particular setting, each has a significant role and contribution. In general, one party is asked to help a second party resolve a mental health issue, problem, or condition that in some way affects a third party for whom the second party is in some way formally responsible. Participants are identified respectively as the consultant, consultee, and client.

1. **The consultant**   The consultant is a **psychological professional** who helps others resolve work-related problems. Like other professionals, consultants must have the appropriate knowledge, skills, or behavioral competencies. Training, preparation, and experience are also essential to success in the field.

2. **The consultee**   The second party—the individual to whom consultation is extended—is the consultee. Though consultants may work with many individuals during a consultation assignment, the consultee is usually the person who initiates contact and who, as a result, is most invested in the processes and outcomes. The consultee requests the consultation because of a need for direction, special information, added competencies, or creative problem solving.

3. **The client**   A third participant in most cases is the client. Clients are individuals with whom consultees engage in some type of formal helping relationship. The consultee typically has some responsibility for correcting whatever deficits or conditions prompt consultation. Successful consultation results in improved client functioning or the reduction of work-related problems, along with a greater understanding of the relevant issues on the part of the consultee. Further, the clients in some consultation settings are by groups representing client systems or even organizations and programs (Caplan, 1970; Werner, 1978). In some consultation situations, the clients are not existing individuals or groups but are parties anticipated by consultees. Thus, present interventions serve a futuristic purpose by preparing consultees in advance.

Triadic Interactions   Consultants, consultees, and clients have a triadic or **tripartite relationship**. Despite all the changes in the field over the years, the triadic relationship among these three parties has remained relatively constant (Kurpius & Fuqua, 1993a). Through this helping arrangement, consultants and consultees can engage in professional dialogue and problem solving to meet the needs of a third party. This relational structure appears to be linear in the sense that the consultant works exclusively with the consultee, who in turn interacts with the client (Figure 1.1).

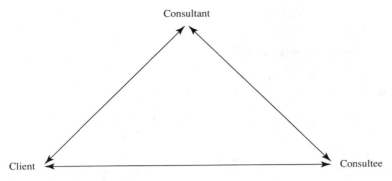

FIGURE 1.2
The non-linear version of the tripartite relationship in consultation

Despite the standard triadic structure, we would be oversimplifying if we said that exceptions do not exist. Bardon (1985), for example, writes of "instances better defined as diadic" in which the identity of the client is blurred or obscured (p. 357). Further, as we hinted earlier, some consultation relationships classify the client as a program, organization, or system, not a person. It is misleading to assume that the triadic relationship is always linear in the sense that the consultant meets with the consultee who in turn addresses the needs of the client (Kurpius & Fuqua, 1993a). In some settings the tripartite relationship contains elements of reciprocity in which each of the three parties must interact with the other parties at various points during the consultation process. In these cases, consultants observe clients, confirm diagnostic impressions through consultant-client interviews, or implement interventions in the direct presence of clients. Other roles require direct-service elements in which consultants address clients in face-to-face interventions. Thus, as a rule, consultants should acknowledge that the nature of tripartite interactions differs from one setting to another and should anticipate interactions with both parties as they take on consultation roles (Figure 1.2).

Consultees' Status   At consultation's point of entry into the human service spotlight, Caplan (1970) described the consultant-consultee relationship as an exchange that should be restricted to professionals. Caplan points out that both parties should have professional status so that consultive dialogue and relationships do not become hierarchical or create the dynamics of a supervisory situation. While Caplan's professional-status view receives support from later writers and consultants (Caplan, 1970; Conoley, Conoley, Ivey, & Scheel, 1991; Gallessich, 1982), an alternate interpretation stresses the role of nonprofessionals as consultees (Altrocchi, 1972; Conoley, 1981; Hansen, Himes, & Meier, 1990; Lippitt & Lippitt, 1978). Only a cursory review of today's complex human service and mental health delivery system should be enough to highlight the many paraprofessional or nonprofessional groups performing viable human service and mental health functions. As community agencies and programs respond to the needs of more and more consumers, staffing patterns must rely on mental health aides or technicians, teacher associates, family service specialists, community volunteers, staff assistants, and students.

Many consultants have expertise outside the domain of mental health and human services and serve consultees beyond the human service arena (Brown, Kurpius, & Morris, 1988; Dougherty, 1990; Hollway, 1991; Kurpius & Robinson, 1978). Consultees often include business and government leaders resorting to consultation to resolve the employee problems generated by a range of organizational or mental health issues. In these settings, organizational consultees bring a vast range of experiences, titles, and positions to the process.

Voluntary and Egalitarian Relationships As recognized or highly sought specialists, consultants are often touted as professionals who bring special insight to the consultation process. Some describe consultants as "experts" employed by consultees to impart unique information or render much-needed organizational diagnoses (Schein, 1978, p. 339). Though high-visibility experts are essential in certain situations, their special status should not lead to authoritarianism or consultee passivity. Consultants who rely on professional preeminence and not collegial exchange to gain consultees' support risk outcomes that have little true commitment from those who have to live with them (Schein, 1987). As an alternative, some writers urge consultants to base relationships with consultees on **egalitarian** principles (Blake & Mouton, 1976; Brown et al., 1991; Dougherty, 1990). Egalitarian relationships lack the hierarchical and intimidating dimensions that can lead to resistance. These relationships also benefit from the voluntary, rather than coerced, participation of consultees. Consultees are more likely to adopt and implement solutions when they are free to accept or reject a consultant's ideas (Blake & Mouton, 1976; Caplan, 1970; Conoley & Conoley, 1991; Dougherty, 1990; Gallessich, 1982).

Multicultural Issues Multicultural awareness should be a professional norm that guides the work of psychological consultants in all their work, especially in relationships that include consultees from diverse cultural or ethnic backgrounds and experiences. As Jackson and Hayes (1993) note,

> The integration of multicultural concerns into consultation is necessary to ensure that organizations that reflect and embrace ethnic diversity will have their needs, goals, and missions achieved. Consultants need to be aware that organizations and their respective employees may reflect ethnic cultures and may have issues relating to their cultures that warrant consideration. (p. 144)

As a rule, consultants appreciate diversity and reflect sensitivity to and respect for multicultural issues. To do otherwise not only risks unsuccessful consultation but can raise serious ethical questions or even legal liabilities (Gibbs, 1980).

Collaboration A turning point occurred during the late 1950s when consultees, previously considered passive recipients of the consultant's wisdom, began to be recognized as integral participants in the consultation process (Kurpius & Robinson, 1978). They were encouraged to contribute their insight, propose solutions, and pursue a course

of interaction and mutual commitment. This trend has evolved into the current prefer-
ence of many mental health professionals and business leaders for a collaborative style
in the workplace. **Collaboration** in consultation refers to a partnership between consultants and consultees, with each group having equal responsibility for most of the tasks
that make up the process (Conoley & Conoley, 1991; Conoley et al., 1991; Kurpius &
Brubaker, 1976; Kurpius & Robinson, 1978; Pryzwansky, 1974; Pryzwansky & White,
1983; Wenger, 1979).

Process   Consultation is recognized as a **process** that requires planning, coordinating, and organizing (Brown et al., 1991; Caplan, 1970; Dougherty, 1990; Kurpius,
Fuqua, & Rozecki, 1993). That is, consultation requires more than "fly-by-the-seat-of-
your-pants" activities in which consultants rely on spontaneous or whimsical problem
solving. Some writers contend that consultants who lack sufficient process skills may be
doomed to failure (Kurpius et al., 1993). Viewing consultation as a process-oriented activity encourages consultants to plan and organize actions according to the specific
characteristics and needs of the organization.

Pursuing consultation assignments according to a process perspective allows consultants to divide the entire operation into a distinct beginning and end, with an ensemble of interconnected stages in between (see Chapter 2). Each consultation stage
integrates processes and dynamics that have important implications for the success or
failure of the total consultation experience. The stages of consultation often overlap,
since the dynamics of one stage are systematically connected to developments in other
stages. Anticipating and managing the various stages are key responsibilities of
consultants.

Definition of Consultation

In the preceding pages, we have discussed the main features of consultation. We are
now in a position to provide a basic definition. The definition we offer is necessarily
broad; it reflects the need to generalize across the various psychological groups that do
consultation. **Psychological consultation** involves *a broad helping approach in which
qualified psychological consultants help consultees (1) resolve work-related issues
pertaining to individuals, clients, or programs that they are responsible for, (2) become
active agents in achieving solutions to problems, or (3) strengthen consultees' work-
related competencies to address similar issues in the future.* This definition should provide a guide as you study later sections of this book.

History and Major Developments

As we have noted, consultation cuts across various disciplines. Thus, its origins are difficult to trace. Some believe the history of consultation parallels the history of psychology and other areas of the social sciences. As a pioneer psychiatrist, for example,
Sigmund Freud may have inadvertently given a boost to the field of consultation

through his collaborative exchanges with French neurologist Jean-Martin Charcot and Austrian physician and physiologist Josef Breuer. Freud's work with Hermann Nothnagel, a medical professor for whom he "gave his first paid consultations," was among the earliest examples of consultation (Wallace, 1986, p. 23).

More specific developments can be traced to the American post–World War II era, in which a range of psychological, sociological, economic, and even political events have advanced consultation as a distinct area of concentration. Though a complete survey is beyond the scope of this book, a few major developments merit discussion.

Evolution of Consultation

Consultants have had a range of purposes and functions and, over time, their duties have been shaped by diverse views and ideologies. During the formative years of the 1940s and 1950s, for example, consultation in mental health settings assumed a "direct-service" approach where therapy or counseling was integrated with the consultant's other responsibilities (Kurpius & Robinson, 1978). Mental health agencies, confronted by unknown or perplexing mental disorders, often turned to specialists for help (MacLennan, Quinn, & Schroeder, 1971; Susselman, 1950). This use of consultants underscores their importance as "troubleshooters" who were called on during times of crisis and uncertainty.

Gallessich (1985) and Brown et al. (1991) contend that mental health consultation has its roots in the clinical consultation model. In the early 19th century, physicians were required to seek advice from more expert medical professionals to diagnose patients and prescribe treatment goals and methodologies. Few would dispute the notion that the clinical model left an indelible mark on the consultation field. Today, remnants of this early approach are highly visible among psychiatrists and other mental health professionals as methods for treating mental health patients (Brown et al., 1991).

The convergence of organizational philosophies and consultants' problem-solving strategies in the 1950s powered a lasting movement that would give consultants a new role. As organizational specialists or advisers, consultants were asked to help supervisors and managers resolve barriers to organizational inefficiency (Kurpius & Robinson, 1978). The emergence of organizational development in the mid-20th century was a direct result of this novel role for consultants. Over the years, these once-innovative roles have evolved into such well-known specialties as organizational consultation and work psychology (Hollway, 1991).

Caplanian Influences

Gerald Caplan (1970), a psychiatrist and influential author of a popular model of consultation, was the first to provide an in-depth, formal approach to mental health consultation. Caplan devised a novel approach to treatment in which consultants address clients' mental health problems by focusing more on the skill deficits, biases, and emotional deficiencies of the deliverers of services. Caplan's early efforts have had a major influence on modern consultation practices, and any understanding of consultation is incomplete without a study of Caplanian strategies and methodologies. We present a detailed review of his approach to consultation in Chapter 3.

Social Roles

Gallessich (1982) discusses the development of consultation within the context of social history. She points out that, as new social forces have emerged, they have prescribed how mental health services are delivered. She gives a vivid example in which, more than a century ago, strong and determined families were able to satisfy their educational, health, and socialization needs. In the aftermath of industrialization and automation, however, the demands of daily living were eased, and weak and dependent families that were more community-reliant than ever before began to meet their needs through a new culture of convenience. Thus, according to Gallessich, an interesting paradox emerged in which automation, having made life easier on the one hand, eventually created weaker families and eroded community solidarity on the other. Families had to depend more and more on social agencies and institutions for support. A logical outcome was that social agencies were forced to employ specialists for advice and technical assistance in order to cope with expanding caseloads.

Community Mental Health Center Act

The Community Mental Health Center Act of 1963 provided an early impetus for the development of consultation (Kurpius & Robinson, 1978). This landmark legislation, enacted in a mental health–minded political climate, provided specific guidelines for the integration of consultation services into community mental health services. For the first time, consultation received federal legislative emphasis as a valid way of addressing mental health needs. Innovative consultation activities were to be delivered primarily within the framework of prevention. Thus, mental health centers entered a new era of prevention-mindedness in which "consultants" extended mental health philosophies into previously underserved settings. Schools, child development programs, families, community groups, and business and industry were soon viable targets for consultation, education, and prevention programs.

Formal Literature Contributions

The attention paid to consultation in the formal literature of the various psychological disciplines also requires emphasis. An array of written testimonials and prescriptions have established consultation as a viable intervention (Brown et al., 1991). The earliest major contributions began in the 1970s (Bergan & Tombari, 1976; Kurpius & Robinson, 1978; Randolph & Graun, 1988). Beginning with the theory-building ideologies of Caplan in his now-classic book, *The Theory and Practice of Mental Health Consulta-*

tion (1970), the field gained momentum through Gallessich's comprehensive book, *The Profession and Practice of Consultation: A Handbook for Consultants, Trainers of Consultants, and Consumers of Consultation Services* (1982). A third major work, *Developing Consultation Skills* (1984), was written by Parsons and Meyers. This trend continued into the 1990s with the publication of several comprehensive books. Examples are Dougherty (1995); Brown, Pryzwansky, and Schulte (1995); Conoley and Conoley (1991); and Hansen et al. (1990).

In addition to major book contributions, some professional journals have featured consultation as a special service model. The first issue of the *Elementary School Guidance and Counseling* journal, for example, includes two articles that encourage elementary school counselors to be active consultants in the school system (Dinkmeyer, 1967). A dramatic development emerged during the late 1970s when the *Personnel and Guidance Journal,* published by the American Personnel and Guidance Association (now the American Counseling Association), devoted two special issues to the field (Sue, 1978a, 1978b). Later the *Journal of Counseling and Development* also devoted two issues to special articles that update consultation concepts (Kurpius & Fuqua, 1993a; Kurpius et al., 1993). Adding to the field's momentum in the 1980s was a special issue of *Counseling Psychologist* that includes articles written by various major contributors and practitioners (Brown & Kurpius, 1985).

Formal Training in Consultation

Since Caplan's (1970) early formulations, professional groups have embraced consultation to the extent that it is currently an important academic component of many formal training programs (Knoff, 1988). In counselor education programs, for example, accreditation standards developed by the Council for the Accreditation of Counselor and Related Educational Programs (CACREP) require graduate counseling programs to include substantive coursework and internship experiences in consultation. Standards published by the American Psychological Association (APA) and the Council for Social Work Education (CSWE) include similar discipline-driven courses in consultation training.

Though consultation has not thus far evolved into a distinct academic discipline and a sizable gap exists between consultation demands and preparation opportunities (Conyne & O'Neal, 1992), the various training programs have devoted more and more attention to consultation. In a survey of counseling psychology programs, for example, Brown (1985) found that over 95% of respondents include coursework in consultation topics. As early as 1984, approximately two-thirds of the APA's accredited predoctoral programs include a self-contained, organized consultation course (Gallessich & Watterson, 1984).

Mental Health Dilemmas

The number of people with mental health problems appears greater now than in earlier periods. In addition, recent decades have witnessed new and more severe psychological conditions, which challenge professionals to expand their expertise and problem-solving tactics. Mental health practitioners are overwhelmed, also, by rapidly developing treatment issues that emerge before training programs have incorporated research findings and treatment information into their curricula. Thus, graduates of the various psychological training programs often confront client mental disorders for which they are unprepared. To cope more effectively, the mental health delivery system must tap all the available resources. Consultants represent one important service option. Through case consultation, workshops, staff development programs, and professional collaboration, consultants can help consultees streamline their services and create other needed reforms.

Consultation and Related Professional Activities

As psychological consultants try to help consultees solve work problems, they integrate multiple roles and functions. At times these activities may appear to overlap with other human service activities (Caplan, 1970). But despite some duplication, consultation does have a recognizable identity. Clarifying this identity is the goal of this section.

Consultation and Therapy

Although consultation and **therapy** share similar elements (McGehearty, 1969; Schmidt & Osbourne, 1981), the two should not be confused (Rogawski, 1978). Even a cursory investigation turns up some obvious differences. For example, with the exception of couple or group formats, therapy is most often delivered in a diadic, rather than triadic, relationship. Further, therapy concentrates on clients' immediate personal needs or intrapsychic qualities. In contrast, consultation focuses more on consultees' professional insights and skills and rarely addresses personal issues (Caplan, 1970). Moreover, though consultation, like therapy, is encompassed by a milieu of trust and support, the purpose is to facilitate organizational or practitioner problem solving, not personal growth. Other differences stem from the fact that conventional therapist-client relationships rarely, if ever, involve peers or colleagues, while consultation is often carried out in precisely these circumstances. The therapist possesses considerable formal responsibility for the welfare of the client, while the consultee in consultation situations retains a substantial degree of autonomy.

Consultation and Supervision

Although consultation and supervision share some features and goals, they differ in several key respects. **Supervision** refers to a relatively long-term process in which authority figures monitor the work behaviors of subordinates according to prescribed policies and performance criteria. Supervisory assignments and relationships are imposed and sanctioned by the organization (Bernard & Goodyear, 1992). In contrast, consultation relationships are almost always temporary, are usually voluntary, and are not authoritarian. Moreover, consultees often have substantial input into decisions about hiring consultants. As a boss, the supervisor is primarily responsible for monitoring and evaluating employee performance (Knoff, 1988). As a helper and colleague, the consultant is charged with creating a relationship marked by collaboration and a problem-solving orientation. Moreover, supervisors address poorly performing supervisees in vastly different ways than do consultants. A supervisor may legitimately discipline a consistently tardy employee with suspension, remedial training, or firing. Consultants, in contrast, collaborate with skill-deficient consultees to assess weaknesses and strengthen skills.

Consultation and Training

Although consultation and training have the mutual purpose of enhancing consultees' skills and knowledge, there are important distinctions between the two processes. Trainers are authorities or experts who have supervisory relationships with trainees or students. They often present information in a formal, didactic way within an evaluative climate. In contrast, consultation involves egalitarian interactions and relationships and benefits from a collaborative and nonevaluative atmosphere. Though consultants may rely on formal instructional methods to address problems, training is usually restricted in scope, is time-limited, and lacks the depth or process characteristics of consultation activities.

Consultation and Advocacy

Consultants often serve as advocates for clients and consultees. In a broad sense, in fact, all consultants represent the interest of consultees as they work toward problem resolution. They are also advocates as they promote the mental health or general well-being of clients and consultees. Despite these similarities, their purpose is fundamentally different from that of advocates. **Advocacy** is the act of promoting, lobbying, or negotiating for the cause of others who are unable to plead their own case (Kurpius & Rozecki, 1992). While advocates seek to bring support to those in need, consultants are more interested in empowering consultees and clients so they can meet their own needs. By enhancing consultees' skills, consultants help consultees to become self-sufficient to the point where they no longer rely on consultive help. Finally, it is not unusual for advocates to work in voluntary, self-directed capacities, while psychological consultants often fulfill a paid or contracted role.

Consultation and Organizational Development

Consultation is closely related to the process of **organizational development (OD)**, which has been defined as the "application of behavioral-science knowledge to enhance an organization's effectiveness and efficiency" (Huse, 1978, p. 403). Though consultation is one method or strategy OD specialists may utilize (Brown et al., 1991), OD emphasizes the application of scientific research to organizational problems. Thus, unlike most psychological consultants, OD specialists require formal training in organizational theory and practice.

The focus of OD is the efficiency and productivity of the organization. Though OD specialists, like psychological consultants, may emphasize the importance of employee well-being, OD professionals do so to benefit the organization and its goals. In psychological consultation, people are generally the major targets of change. In situations where consultation addresses organizations or programs, the underlying purpose is to satisfy the psychological needs of the clients or consultees.

Consultation Functions

As we have repeated several times in this chapter, psychological consultation is a broad field involving an array of professional functions delivered across multiple settings. The consultant resembles a chameleon that assumes many appearances in adapting to various settings. For example, in some cases psychological consultants perform assessment and diagnostic procedures, formulate recommendations, and then limit themselves to a monitoring role while consultees implement the planned interventions (Bergan, 1977). In other situations, consultants are active throughout the entire process as they actually assist clients with interventions such as team building, conflict resolution, and training. Thus, on any consultation assignment, the consultant's role is defined situationally to meet the needs of the particular consultee and organization (Brown et al., 1991; Kurpius & Brubaker, 1976; Pryzwansky & White, 1983).

Though the details of each may vary, at times substantially, two broad roles dominate most consultation situations—those of the content expert and the process facilitator (Schein, 1978). The consultant is a **content expert** when the consultation assignment requires attention to specific tasks or problems. Highly technical or intricate problems that require specialized knowledge indicate the need for content-oriented consultants and rather passive consultees. In contrast, a **process facilitator** emphasizes the processes necessary to achieve solutions to problems and focuses on *how* problems are resolved. The process consultant is most interested in the active involvement of consultees in any problem-solving efforts.

Kurpius (1978, p. 335) presents an alternate model in which consultant roles are delineated according to the modality of intervention. *Modality* denotes the type of consultation activities that prevail in a given setting. According to Kurpius, consultants are in a *provision* mode when their expertise is needed to resolve client issues or generate sound solutions. In this modality, the consultant provides interventions that address client needs. In the *prescription* mode, consultants are experts who help consultees meet the needs of clients by resolving problems. This mode, similar to a doctor-patient relationship, requires the consultant to address unusual or special needs of clients that consultees do not understand. This form of consultation challenges consultants to prescribe help strategies that add to the consultee's already-in-motion treatment plan. Consultants pursue a *collaboration* mode when they serve as catalysts who encourage consultees to move in the directions necessary to resolve problems. As collaborators, consultants work to create an environment in which consultees rely on self-direction and personal initiative to implement interventions. The final modality is the *mediation* mode, in which the consultant serves an autonomous function in recognizing special problems, forming intervention plans, and calling together responsible parties to plan for change. Although at first glance the mediation mode does not seem like consultation because the consultant, not the consultee, initiates problem solving, a true consultation framework evolves as consultees respond to this call for action.

Consultation Effectiveness

Consumers, writers, and practitioners generally agree that consultation is a worthwhile and needed practice whose popularity is justified. Interestingly, these attitudes appear widespread despite the sparsity of empirical information about the usefulness of consultation. As Froehle and Rominger (1993) point out, "Existing consultation research is largely episodic and seldom rigorous, with threats to external or internal validity often limiting its applicability" (p. 693).

The lack of formal evaluative research appears to continue a trend that began earlier in the history of the field. That is, consultation practices during the 20 years following the passage of the Community Mental Health Center Act of 1963 failed to promote relevant research (Gallessich, 1982). In this period, mental health agencies often received federal dollars to provide consultation services without being held accountable for the effectiveness of their programs. This was because there were few follow-up studies. Regrettably, as Lippitt and Lippitt (1978) contend, not much has changed in the years since:

> Virtually every kind of business, government, and service organization has been involved in consultation to some extent. Judgments of the success of such consultation usually have been based on expressions of faith in the general value of consulting, but consultation has received little critical evaluation based on research findings. (p. 81)

Some deficits are attributable to the complexities of consultation activities. Researching the effectiveness of consultation is challenging in the sense that standard research methods often do not match the nature of the consultation process (Bergan & Tombari, 1976; Brown, 1985; Hershenson & Power, 1987). This mismatch occurs, for example, in consultation situations that require flexibility and innovation. As consultants solve problems by applying diverse techniques, they inadvertently compromise the conditions required by carefully controlled experimental designs (Froehle & Rominger, 1993). Other barriers stem from practical constraints. The consultant's research-based examination of outcomes, for instance, is often hampered by contractual limits, time barriers, or resistant consultees who are more interested in problem solving than research.

Despite these difficulties, a few studies have examined the effectiveness of consultation by exploring the specific elements or dynamics of the process. Though a detailed treatment is not feasible within the scope of this chapter, a few representative studies are worth discussing. Some studies have attempted to isolate factors contributing to successful versus unsuccessful consultation. Some investigators suggest, for example, that effective consultation outcomes are related to conscientious planning and organization (Bundy & Poppen, 1986; Kurpius, 1985; Schmidt & Medl, 1983). Others argue that

successful consultation requires a sound theoretical foundation (Bardon, 1985; Gallessich, 1985; Knoff, 1984; Mathias, 1992). Effective consultation also seems to depend
on certain consultant characteristics (Bergan & Tombari, 1976; Dougherty, 1990; Fine,
Grantham, & Wright, 1979; Levinson, 1985). A few researchers have looked at the importance of effective relationships between consultants and consultees (Brown & Horton, 1990; Conoley et al., 1991; Dougherty, 1990; Maitland, Fine & Tracy, 1985).

Despite the obstacles to empirical examination, some authors have applied experimental methods in evaluating consultation within mental health settings. Positive outcomes in the form of increased consultee efficiency and client growth, for instance,
have been discovered in some studies (Brunell & Avella, 1986; Herrera & Lawson,
1987; Pollock, 1979; Robinson & Wilson, 1987; Taintor, Strain, & Lazar, 1984;
Tourigny, Marie, & Drury, 1987).

Despite some encouraging findings, questions and criticisms about the effectiveness of consultation continue to arise. On the basis of extensive reviews of consultation
studies and outcomes, for example, several authors point to the weaknesses in the in-
vestigative methodologies used by consultation experimenters (Dustin & Blocher,
1984; Medway, 1979). They argue that weak methods yield weak results. Others are
alarmed by the widespread and rapidly expanding use of consultation in view of the
lack of supporting research (Dustin, 1985; Froehle & Rominger, 1993). Still others predict a bleak future for consultation as long as it remains theoretically weak (Bardon,
1985; Gallessich, 1985).

Whatever one's position, a safe assumption is that consultants cannot take their effectiveness for granted. As a group, they must isolate the particular methods that work
from those that do not by closely inspecting their successes and failures. To help novice
consultants, Froehle and Rominger (1993) offer this advice:

> As we work to define ourselves as consultants, we need to capitalize on our scientific
> inclinations, seek paradigms to help explain the realities we confront and provide guid-
> ance for our actions, ask questions about the processes in which we are engaged, and
> reflect on ourselves and our own engagement in those processes. (p. 698)

SUMMARY

The field of consultation has grown considerably since World War II and has won widespread acceptance. New roles, challenges, and rewards for consultants are emerging
all the time. This positive assessment, however, must be somewhat tentative and
guarded. Although the field has gained momentum and continues to offer an exciting
future for would-be consultants, it is not without its detractors who call for more evaluative research.

In this introductory chapter, we have devoted considerable space to the definition
and clarification of psychological consultation. In addition, we have highlighted various
historical developments shaping consultation as a viable and distinctive practice. The
discussion has also distinguished consultation procedures from other human service or
psychological activities. The chapter concluded with a brief discussion of the effectiveness of consultation.

Hopefully, this first chapter has challenged certain myths or stereotypes that you may have about what consultation is and is not. Your immediate goal is to develop a solid understanding so that as you move through the remainder of the book, you will proceed with a firm knowledge base rather than speculation. Through your learning so far, you have taken an introductory step on the path to becoming a psychological consultant.

GLOSSARY

Advocacy An activity in which one individual supports or speaks on behalf of another. Advocates assume the role of supporters to help those who cannot help themselves.

Client An individual, program, or system in the care of the consultee. Clients and consultees usually have direct, formal relationships.

Collaboration Cooperation between consultant and consultee in working toward consultation goals.

Consultant An individual—usually a psychological professional—who provides consultation to consultees. The consultant is assumed to have the expertise and methodological understanding necessary to help consultees resolve psychological concerns of their clients or others.

Consultee An individual, such as a human service provider, business manager, or supervisor, who requests help from a consultant. The consultee has a work-related concern regarding a client or client-related program or system.

Content expert A consultant who primarily shares expertise or provides information in the problem-solving process. In this role, the problems of consultees stem more from the need for specialized information and less from deficient organizational or human processes.

Egalitarian A term used to describe consultation relationships in which the consultant and consultee are considered equals. Egalitarian relationships are commonly described as "person-to-person" relationships; they are nonhierarchical.

Organizational development (OD) The application of knowledge from the behavioral sciences to organizational problems.

Process In consultation, an organized and planned approach that proceeds through a series of action steps or stages. The consultation process proceeds from a beginning point to an end point. The process nature of consultation implies a systems approach in which success during one stage can affect success in other stages.

Process facilitator A consultant who engages in process-oriented problem solving. The consultant, as a process-minded professional, helps consultees identify and correct deficient processes or activities that create organizational problems.

Psychological consultation A broad helping approach in which qualified psychological consultants help consultees (1) resolve work-related issues pertaining to individuals, clients, or programs that they are responsible for, (2) become active agents in achieving solutions to problems, or (3) strengthen consultees' work-related competencies to address similar issues in the future.

Psychological professional   A psychological or mental health provider who has formal training, background, and related experience in the psychological sciences.

Supervision   The process in which supervisors, with specialized training and experience, have authority over the work of others. Supervision implies a hierarchy of power in a relationship along with the evaluation and monitoring of supervisee performance.

Therapy   A formalized, psychological helping process, usually involving two parties. The therapist is a psychological professional who helps a client resolve direct, personal issues. Client issues usually involve behavioral or emotional disorders that inhibit growth and adaptation.

Tripartite relationship   A triadic or three-party relationship consisting of the consultant, consultee, and client. The tripartite relationship is a reciprocal relationship in which the interaction among the three parties varies with each consultation situation.

ANNOTATED BIBLIOGRAPHY

Readers who wish to review an early formal account of mental health consultation should read Gerald Caplan's 1970 book, *The Theory and Practice of Mental Health Consultation*. This book was a major catalyst in the evolution of consultation. Although somewhat dated and differing from modern-day conceptualizations in several areas, Caplan's study is an essential resource.

Two special issues of the *Personnel and Guidance Journal* (Sue, 1978a, 1978b) provide an alternate source of early consultation information. Although dated, these issues will give you a glimpse of the earliest consultation perspectives. A later issue of another journal, *Counseling Psychologist* (Brown & Kurpius, 1985), also devotes much attention to consultation issues and perspectives. Presented by educators, practitioners, and theorists, this volume provides theoretical and practical information about the status of consultation, its problems, and exciting trends. Two 1993 issues of the *Journal of Counseling and Development* focus on consultation as a paradigm for helping. Volume 71, number 6, is a special issue that includes various articles exploring the fundamental concepts and dimensions of consultation (Kurpius & Fuqua, 1993b). Volume 72, number 2, of the same journal provides articles that examine consultation from a prevention and preparation perspective (Kurpius & Fuqua, 1993c).

June Gallessich's book *The Profession and Practice of Consultation: A Handbook for Consultants, Trainers of Consultants, and Consumers of Consultation Services* (1982) offers one of the most thorough accounts of consultation. The first three chapters present an in-depth discussion of the evolution and coming of age of consultation.

Two additional books offer insight into consultation from a more contemporary perspective. Chapters 1 and 2 of A. Michael Dougherty's *Consultation: Practice and Perspectives in School and Community Settings* (2nd ed., 1995) explain the basic concept of consultation and provide a brief historical perspective. The first chapter of Duane Brown, Walter Pryzwansky, and Ann Schulte's *Psychological Consultation: Introduction to Theory and Practice* (3rd ed., 1995) outlines the purpose, definition, and promise of psychological consultation. Together, these books provide a thorough survey of the consultation field and a detailed explanation of theory and practice issues.

REFERENCES AND SUGGESTED READINGS

Altrocchi, J. (1972). Mental health consultation. In S. E. Golann & S. C. Eisdorfer (Eds.), *Handbook of community mental health* (pp. 477–508). New York: Appleton-Century-Crofts.

Bardon, J. (1985). On the verge of a breakthrough. *Counseling Psychologist, 13*(3), 355–362.

Bergan, J. R. (1977). *Behavioral consultation.* Columbus, OH: Merrill.

Bergan, J. R., & Tombari, M. (1976). Consultant skill and efficiency and the implementation and outcomes of consultation. *Journal of School Psychology, 14*(1), 3–14.

Bernard, J., & Goodyear, R. (1992). *Fundamentals of clinical supervision.* Boston: Allyn & Bacon.

Blake, R., & Mouton, J. (1976). *Consultation.* Reading, MA: Addison-Wesley.

Brack, G., Jones, E., Smith, R., White, J., & Brack, C. (1993). A primer on consultation theory: Building a flexible worldview. *Journal of Counseling and Development, 71,* 619–628.

Brown, D. (1985). The preservice training and supervision of consultants. *Counseling Psychologist, 13*(3), 410–425.

Brown, D., & Horton, G. (1990). The importance of interpersonal skills in consultee-centered consultation: A review. *Journal of Counseling and Development, 68,* 423–426.

Brown, D., & Kurpius, D. (Eds.). (1985). Consultation [Special issue]. *Counseling Psychologist, 13*(3).

Brown, D., Kurpius, D., & Morris, J. (1988). *Handbook of consultation with individuals and small groups.* Association for Counselor Education and Supervision. Alexandria, VA: Author.

Brown, D., Pryzwansky, W., & Schulte, A. (1991). *Psychological consultation: Introduction to theory and practice* (2nd ed.). Boston: Allyn & Bacon.

Brown, D., Pryzwansky, W., & Schulte, A. (1995). *Psychological consultation: Introduction to theory and practice* (3rd ed.). Boston: Allyn & Bacon.

Brunell, L., & Avella, A. (1986). Consultation with the multidisciplinary team: Preparing integrated treatment plans. *Psychotherapy in Private Practice, 4*(1), 73–86.

Bundy, M., & Poppen, W. (1986, February). School counselors' effectiveness as consultants: A research review. *Elementary School Guidance and Counseling, 20,* 215–221.

Caplan, G. (1970). *The theory and practice of mental health consultation.* New York: Basic Books.

Conoley, J. C. (Ed.). (1981). *Consultation in schools: Theory, research, procedures.* New York: Academic Press.

Conoley, J. C., & Conoley, C. W. (1991). *Consultation: A guide to practice and training* (2nd ed.). New York: Pergamon Press.

Conoley, C., Conoley, J., Ivey, D., & Scheel, J. (1991). Enhancing consultation by matching the consultee's perspectives. *Journal of Counseling and Development, 69,* 546–549.

Conyne, R., & O'Neal, J. (1992). Closing the gap between consultation training and practice. In R. Conyne & J. O'Neal (Eds.), *Organizational consultation: A casebook* (pp. 1–16). Newbury Park, CA: Sage.

Dinkmeyer, D. (1967). Elementary school guidance and the classroom teacher. *Elementary School Guidance and Counseling, 1,* 15–26.

Dougherty, A. M. (1990). *Consultation: Practice and perspectives.* Pacific Grove, CA: Brooks/Cole.

Dougherty, A. M. (1995). *Consultation: Practice and perspectives in school and community settings* (2nd ed.). Pacific Grove, CA: Brooks/Cole.

Dustin, D. (1985). On Brown's training and supervision of consultants. *Counseling Psychologist, 13*(3), 436–440.

Dustin, D., & Blocher, D. (1984). Theories and models of consultation. In R. W. Lent & S. Brown (Eds.), *Handbook of counseling psychology.* New York: Wiley.

Fine, M., Grantham, V., & Wright, J. (1979). Personal variables that facilitate or impede consultation. *Psychology in the Schools, 16*(4), 533–539.

Froehle, T., & Rominger, R., III. (1993). Directions in consultation research: Bridging the gap between science and practice. *Journal of Counseling and Development, 71,* 693–699.

Gallessich, J. (1982). *The profession and practice of consultation: A handbook for consultants, trainers of consultants, and consumers of consultation services.* San Francisco: Jossey-Bass.

Gallessich, J. (1985). Toward a meta-theory of consultation. *Counseling Psychologist, 13*(3), 336–351.

Gallessich, J., & Watterson, J. (1984, August). *Consultation education and training in APA accredited settings: An overview.* Paper presented at the 92nd annual meeting of the American Psychological Association, Toronto, Canada.

Gibbs, J. (1980). The interpersonal orientation in mental health consultation: Toward a model of ethnic variations in consultation. *Journal of Community Psychology, 8,* 195–207.

Hansen, J., Himes, B., & Meier, S. (1990). *Consultation: Concepts and practices.* Englewood Cliffs, NJ: Prentice-Hall.

Herrera, J., & Lawson, W. (1987). Effects of consultation on the ward atmosphere in a state psychiatric hospital. *Psychological Reports, 60*(2), 423–428.

Hershenson, D., & Power, P. (1987). *Mental health counseling: Theory and practice.* New York: Pergamon Press.

Hollway, W. (1991). Work psychology and organizational behavior. London: Sage.

Holtz, H. (1993). *How to succeed as an independent consultant.* New York: Wiley.

Huse, E. (1978). Organizational development. *Personnel and Guidance Journal, 56*(7), 403–406.

Jackson, D. N., & Hayes, D. H. (1993). Multicultural issues in consultation. *Journal of Counseling and Development, 72,* 144–147.

Knoff, H. M. (1984). The practice of multimodal consultation: An integrating approach for consultation service delivery. *Psychology in the Schools, 21,* 83–91.

Knoff, H. M. (1988). Clinical supervision, consultation, and counseling: A comparative analysis for supervisors and other educational leaders. *Journal of Curriculum and Supervision, 3,* 240–252.

Kurpius, D. (1978). Consultation theory and practice: An integrated model. *Personnel and Guidance Journal, 56*(6), 335–338.

Kurpius, D. (1985). Consultation intervention: Successes, failures, and proposals. *Journal of Counseling Psychology, 13*(3), 368–389.

Kurpius, D., & Brubaker, J. (1976). *Psychoeducational consultation: Definitions-functions-preparation.* Bloomington: Indiana University Press.

Kurpius, D., & Fuqua, D. (1993a). Fundamental issues in defining consultation. *Journal of Counseling and Development, 71*(6), 598–600.

Kurpius, D., & Fuqua, D. (Eds.). (1993b). Consultation I: Conceptual, structural, and operational dimensions [Special issue]. *Journal of Counseling and Development, 71*(6).

Kurpius, D., & Fuqua, D. (Eds.). (1993c). Consultation II: Prevention, preparation, and key issues [Special issue]. *Journal of Counseling and Development, 72*(2).

Kurpius, D., Fuqua, D., & Rozecki, T. (1993). The consulting process: A multidimensional approach. *Journal of Counseling and Development, 71*(6), 601–606.

Kurpius, D., & Robinson, S. (1978). An overview of consultation. *Personnel and Guidance Journal, 56*(6), 321–323.

Kurpius, D., & Rozecki, T. (1992). Outreach, advocacy, and consultation: A framework for prevention and intervention. *Elementary School Guidance and Counseling, 26,* 176–189.

Levinson, J. (1985). Invited commentary: Consultation by cliche. *Consultation, 4*(2), 165–170.

Lippitt, G., & Lippitt, R. (1978). *The consulting process in action.* La Jolla, CA: University Associates.

MacLennan, B., Quinn, R., & Schroeder, D. (1971). *The scope of community mental health consultation and education* (PHS Publication No. 2169). Washington, DC: U.S. Department of Health, Education, and Welfare, National Institute of Mental Health.

Maitland, R., Fine, M., & Tracy, D. (1985). The effects of an interpersonally-based problem-solving process on consultation outcomes. *Journal of School Psychology, 23,* 337–345.

Mathias, C. (1992). Touching the lives of children: Consultative interventions that work. *Elementary School Guidance and Counseling, 26,* 190–201.

McGehearty, L. (1969). Consultation and counseling. *Elementary School Guidance and Counseling, 3,* 155–163.

Medway, F. (1979). How effective is school consultation? A review of empirical studies. *American Journal of Community Psychology, 17,* 275–282.

Parsons, R. D., & Meyers, J. (1984). *Developing consultation skills.* San Francisco: Jossey-Bass.

Pollock, D. (1979). Consultation in a public school for the severely retarded. *Education and Training of the Mentally Retarded, 18*(4), 181–186.

Pryzwansky, W. (1974). A reconsideration of the consultation model for delivery of school-based psychological services. *American Journal of Orthopsychiatry, 44,* 579–583.

Pryzwansky, W., & White, G. (1983). The influence of consultee characteristics on preferences for consultation approaches. *Professional Psychology, 14,* 457–461.

Randolph, D., & Graun, K. (1988). Resistance to consultation: A synthesis for counselor-consultants. *Journal of Counseling and Development, 67,* 182–184.

Robinson, E. H., & Wilson, E. S. (1987). Counselor-led human relations training as a consultation strategy. *Elementary School Guidance and Counseling, 22,* 124–131.

Rogawski, A. (1978). The Caplanian model. *Personnel and Guidance Journal, 56*(6), 324–327.

Schein, E. (1978). The role of the consultant: Content expert or process facilitator? *Personnel and Guidance Journal, 56*(6), 339–343.

Schein, E. (1987). *Process consultation: Lessons for managers and consultants* (Vol. 2). Reading, MA: Addison-Wesley.

Schmidt, J., & Medl, W. (1983). Six magic steps of consulting. *School Counselor, 30*(3), 212–216.

Schmidt, J., & Osbourne, W. L. (1981). Counseling and consulting: Separate processes or the same? *Personnel and Guidance Journal, 60,* 168–171.

Sue, D. W. (Ed.). (1978a). Consultation I: Definition-models-programs [Special issue]. *Personnel and Guidance Journal, 56*(6).

Sue, D. W. (Ed.). (1978b). Consultation II: Dimensions-training-bibliography [Special issue]. *Personnel and Guidance Journal, 56*(7).

Susselman, S. (1950). The role of the psychiatrist in a probation agency. *Focus, 29,* 33.

Taintor, Z., Strain, J., & Lazar, I. (1984). Evaluation of training in geriatric consultation: Development of assessment measures. *Gerontology and Geriatrics Education, 5*(1), 73–81.

Tourigny, R., Marie, F., & Drury, M. (1987). The effects of monthly psychiatric consultation in a nursing home. *Gerontologist, 27*(3), 363–366.

Wallace, W. A. (1986). *Theories of counseling and psychotherapy: A basic issues approach.* Boston: Allyn & Bacon.

Wenger, R. (1979). Teacher response in collaborative consultation. *Psychology in the Schools, 16,* 127–131.

Werner, J. (1978). Community mental health consultation with agencies. *Personnel and Guidance Journal, 56*(7), 364–368.

CHAPTER TWO

Stages of Consultation

Glossary

Annotated Bibliography

References and Suggested Readings

 Consultation unfolds through a series of stages that involve many interdependent dynamics and processes (Kurpius, Fuqua, & Rozecki, 1993). Novice or inept consultants often overlook this and resort to hasty interventions (Kurpius et al., 1993). Even on brief consultation assignments, consultants should avoid cosmetic problem solving.

Consultation often resembles a system of loosely sequenced, overlapping activities. The dynamics of one stage frequently influence those of another. The consultant's understanding of problems during the early stages of the process, for example, influences decisions about later, action-oriented interventions (Bergan & Tombari, 1976). Conversely, the developments and discoveries of later consultation stages may force consultants to retrace their steps to correct mistakes and oversights of previous stages.

A **consultation stage** represents an identifiable interval in the consultation process. Each stage consists of dynamics and processes that consultants should address, at least partially, before moving ahead to other stages. But consultation stages often lack a precise order, so that consultants do not have to complete one phase before attending to the next. At any point, consultants may be handling multiple activities or tasks despite their assigned stage.

Although the terms for specific consultation stages differ from writer to writer, each stage consists of a relatively standardized set of tasks and dynamics. By attending to these, consultants ensure a thorough approach to consultation that requires them to plan and organize their activities (Kurpius et al., 1993). In this chapter we discuss seven consultation stages:

1. Preliminary contact
2. Entry
3. Assessment and diagnosis
4. Goal setting
5. Intervention
6. Evaluation
7. Termination

Preliminary Contact

The preliminary contact stage most often begins when a consultee requests help from a consultant in relation to a work-related task or problem. At this preliminary stage, consultant-consultee explorations emerge from telephone calls, written correspondence, requests for proposals, face-to-face meetings, or even chance encounters. These contacts may be the first between a particular consultant and consultee or may be requests for re-peat or follow-up consultation (Cosier & Dalton, 1993). Though the preliminary contact stage is an introductory phase that precedes more formal actions, it represents a crucial part of the overall consultation process by establishing a basis for later actions.

Preliminary contact activities vary depending on whether the consultant is an inter-nal or an external consultant. **Internal consultants** are employed in the same organiza-tion as consultees; as insiders, they are often familiar with consultees and their needs. Thus, these consultants have the advantage of prior knowledge.

In contrast, **external consultants** come from outside the organization or setting. Although their outsider status may slow the consultation process because they must ori-ent themselves to the setting and consultation problem, they bring an unbiased or neu-tral perspective. Many consultation principles and practices are similar for both types of consultants, however (Kurpius & Fuqua, 1993).

Exploratory discussions emphasize many issues, including the **presenting con-sultation problem** (the work-related condition that prompts consultation). Indeed, an implicit assumption is that a work-related problem exists that the consultee has been unable to resolve. Initial discussions also provide an overview of the purpose and direction of consultation. Both parties should consider any constraints that could affect the consultation process, including logistical matters such as scheduling problems, travel demands, and so on.

At the preliminary contact stage, consultants should also attempt to assess an orga-nization's level of support for consultation and its potential for change. Consultants will usually want to find out how organizational members perceive outsiders. Consul-tants may also want to determine whether hidden motives or other barriers could inhibit the consultation process. Early meetings with consultees should focus on these kinds of issues.

Exploring the "Fit"

Exploratory discussions between the prospective consultant and consultee help to de-termine the **consultation fit**. Successful consultation obviously demands compatibility among the consultant, consultee, and consultation problem. One prerequisite is that consultants evaluate their own insights, skills, and knowledge as they relate to particu-lar consultation situations. Kurpius et al. (1993) advise consultants to continually en-gage in this process of self-assessment to "ensure that they are the right person for a particular situation" (p. 601). Kurpius and Fuqua (1993) list various questions consul-tants should ponder:

> As a consultant, how do you view humans? Are you more attracted to some than oth-ers? How do you listen and respond to leaders at the top of the organization as com-pared with workers at the bottom? What do you think and feel when consultees disagree with you and confront you or your ideas? What about your espoused theories versus your theories-in-use? (p. 601)

Consulting with individuals from diverse cultural and ethnic backgrounds imposes special requirements that should be considered in the preliminary contact period. Con-sultants working with consultees who have cultural characteristics different from their own will almost certainly need extra knowledge and sensitivity. Accepting consultation assignments for which one is uninformed or insensitive risks not only failed outcomes but ethical and legal complications as well (Gibbs, 1980).

Organizational Readiness

Organizational readiness is an issue that should concern the consultant throughout the preliminary contact period. Some experts believe the organization's readiness for change is as important to the success of consultation as the consultant's interventions themselves (Beer & Spector, 1993). Consulting with inflexible organizational leaders and members, for example, can be wasteful in terms of human and material resources. But organizational readiness is often difficult to assess; even the most detailed inspection can yield misleading conclusions.

Kurpius et al. (1993) present a straightforward model in which consultants evaluate readiness according to two critical variables: (1) the organization's openness to change (that is, its willingness to embark on a new course of action), and (2) the balance of forces—such as political elements, resources, or ideologies—inside the organization for and against change. To apply these criteria, consultants must understand the dynamics of the organizations in which they work. They should consider rejecting requests for help from closed or rigid systems that resist change. A situation where the internal forces appear equally balanced for and against a new course of action can be problematic. As Kurpius et al. (1993) point out, "Usually, this spells trouble with little or no opportunity for change to occur" (p. 602). The ideal consultation situation involves a system that is open and amenable to change. In this case, the forces for change will outweigh those against it.

Consultation Contracts

Consultants should recognize that each consultation request is unique with respect to the consultee's expectations, problems, and setting. Often, consultation proceeds despite the lack of clear, mutually respected agreements, with consultants and consultees clinging to different perceptions and goals. Without firm agreements, confusion and ambiguity, rather than fluid working conditions, are the potential by-products.

When the consultant and consultee are compatible and there is sufficient organizational readiness, both parties should draw up a contract. Brown, Pryzwansky, and Schulte (1991) point to the significance of such contracts: "A carefully drawn contract may be the most effective means of avoiding legal entanglements concerning contractual issues" (p. 369). **Contracting** requires the consultant and consultee to negotiate and agree on the relevant terms for working together. Contractual harmony among consultees and other **consultation constituents** (such as administrators, consultees, and policymakers) provides a sound foundation for the consultation process.

Consultation contracts take various forms. A formal written contract represents a legal agreement that identifies the responsibilities of all parties. Most agree that written contracts, especially those that spell out responsibilities in detail, are preferable. Another alternative is a brief letter of understanding that specifies the details of the consultation arrangement, including the relevant logistical matters. At times, especially for simple consultation assignments, oral agreements may be satisfactory. Even these agreements can be considered legally binding, however (see Chapter 11).

Guidelines for writing contracts vary somewhat for internal consultants. For the consultant who is an employee of the organization, many consultation tasks and expectations are addressed in job descriptions or employment contracts. Although the terms for providing consultation are often included in these documents, internal consultants should not casually assume that those involved with the consultation process always agree on or understand the terms of consultation. At a minimum, oral discussions and understanding should precede consultation.

Entry

The **entry stage** marks the consultant's formal entrance into the consultation process. At this time, both consultant and consultee will probably form impressions—often unspoken—about the process, including its likelihood of success. Although the entry stage is not a time for active problem solving, the way the consultant, consultee, and others manage the consultation tasks at this stage often determines the success of later phases of the process.

The consultant's entry into the consultation situation occurs on three levels—physical, psychological, and social. Each parallels the others, and all serve similar or overlapping functions. Success or failure at one level can affect outcomes at other levels. Together, the levels establish a sound infrastructure on which consultation proceeds.

Physical Entry

Physical entry refers to the consultant's initial visit to the organization as well as to any other physical movement required by the consultation process. Many practical issues arise; some are summarized below.

1. *Office or work station*   The consultant's work location can facilitate successful physical entry. Sufficient space and comfort not only add credibility to the consultation effort; these amenities indicate the organization's commitment to the process. The work location must be appropriate to the activities that take place there. For example, highly sensitive interviews or client assessments require more privacy than record reviews, short-term training programs, or informal dialogue.

2. *Consultant's movement*   Rarely are consultants permitted to visit all offices or units within an organization, nor should they conduct frivolous explorations or unwarranted interviews. A consultation assignment in which a psychologist must assist a case manager with complex cases, for example, does not require access to unrelated confidential records or unscheduled interviews with other staff. Thus, the consultant's physical movement should be consistent with the purposes, contractual expectations, and expected activities of consultation.

3. *Time considerations* Consultation can be disruptive to the organization. Thus, the timing of consultation visits and on-site activities deserves close scrutiny. The consultant should be sensitive to the consultee's normal flow of activities in arranging visits and should avoid surprise visits that intrude on the organization's work schedule.

Psychological Entry

A consultant—particularly one from outside the organization—is a stranger whose values and behaviors may differ from those that prevail in the organization. Even members of the organization strongly committed to the consultation process may find the consultant's personality, attitudes, and priorities uncongenial. Thus, psychological entry is most concerned with gaining acceptance and approval from consultees and other constituents (Dougherty, 1990).

Another objective of psychological entry is the creation of trust between the consultant and members of the organization. The consultant should demonstrate trustworthiness, since this quality cements the bond between the participants in the consultation process. As Gibb (1979) contends, "People accept help from those they trust. When the relationship is one of acceptance and trust, offers of help are appreciated, listened to, seen as potentially helpful, and often acted upon" (p. 109).

Egan (1986), who writes extensively about the qualities of skilled helpers, has prepared a list of recommendations that could help consultants develop trustworthiness. Although these guidelines were originally intended for therapists, they appear just as useful in a consultation framework. Consultants facilitate trustworthiness when they:

- Carry out the agreements cited in consultation contracts.
- Respect and adhere to the rules of confidentiality.
- Show respect for the needs and feelings of the consultee and other consultation participants.
- Are genuine, sincere, and open in addressing consultation tasks.
- Express realistic optimism about the consultee's ability to resolve the consultation problem.
- Give feedback to the consultee.
- Use all forms of social influence or authority in ways that reflect the best interests of the consultee.
- Invite feedback from the consultee.
- Avoid any behaviors or actions that imply ulterior motives.

Consultants must also recognize that each setting boasts a collection of beliefs, rules, and customs that form the **organizational culture.** Though the details of this culture may not be spelled out in policy manuals, it can be a powerful unifying force (Kilmann, Saxton, & Serpa, 1985). Thus, to win acceptance consultants must respect the organization's preferences in such matters as dress, conduct, language, attitudes, interests, and cultural harmony. Consultation success is often a product of "the degree to which the consultant's behaviors are congruent with those expected by and consistent with the staff" (Gallessich, 1982, p. 283).

Social Entry

Social entry refers to the personal or social dynamics surrounding the consultant's entry. In addition to the professional attributes consultants bring to the consultation role, they bring important social characteristics that potentially contribute to successful entry. While the activities connected with physical and psychological entry often occur exclusively within the consultee's work setting, social issues surround virtually all activities. Many consultees, for example, prefer special meetings or conferences that occur away from work, such as lunches, invitations for coffee, recreational activities, or social gatherings. Social meetings serve as opportunities to fashion the consultant-consultee relationship. Moreover, meetings at neutral sites allow person-to-person dialogue that is not overshadowed by normal work schedules or interruptions. Some consultants pursue their work in retreat-like settings that blend work and social engagements. To avoid questionable ethical practices in social settings, however, consultants should monitor all interactions to ensure that they support the purpose of consultation and are conducted in an atmosphere of professionalism.

Entry for internal consultants differs from that of external consultants. Because their primary job roles are internal to the organizational setting, internal consultants often have preexisting relationships with consultees. Indeed, their entry can be simpler and quicker when preestablished relations are effective and conducive to effective consultation. In contrast, negative or impaired relations should be a matter for concern when internal consultants are named. All consultants (whether internal or external) should consider methods to facilitate successful entry.

Relationship Building

Skillful assessment and specially tailored interventions alone do not ensure successful consultation outcomes. Although these measures add much to the consultation process, the relationship between consultant and consultee is paramount (Brown et al., 1991; Conoley & Conoley, 1982; Kurpius & Robinson, 1978; Pryzwansky & White, 1983). This relationship provides the vitality, encouragement, and trust necessary for positive consultation outcomes. With each new stage come new challenges for the relationship, but positive relations can insulate the consultation process against discord, conflict, or resistance. Bell and Nadler (1979) emphasize the importance of consultant-consultee relationships:

> Consultation is not simply the mechanical tossing of expertise toward a painful client; it is an experience in shared resources. There is an appropriate place for technique, tactic, and form. However, it is the substance and spirit in the helping process which gives consultation its unique humanness. (p. 1)

Positive consultant-consultee relationships are not automatic; they often require great effort. Establishing a collegial, collaborative atmosphere begins during the entry stage and continues throughout the consultation process. Although positive consultation relationships lead to a pleasant and harmonious working arrangement, the greatest advantage is the promotion of effective problem solving.

Rapport: Conditions and Strategies   As consultants encounter backgrounds, experiences, and perspectives different from their own, they observe the crucial importance of human relations skills. From the very beginning of the consultation process, they have to rely on these skills. One objective is the creation of **rapport** (a relationship characterized by agreement, cooperation, and harmony). McMaster (1986) points out that "rapport is generally defined by descriptions of the feelings which result from it, such as trust, comfort, openness" (p. 8).

In most consultation situations, rapport does not develop by chance; it is a relational ingredient that must be shaped and nurtured. To transform once-distant relations into synergistic problem-solving interactions, the consultant should:

1. *Promote acceptance.* Rapport in consultant-consultee relationships requires the same core conditions found in most therapist-client relationships. Although consultation relationships differ from therapeutic relationships in important respects, consultation relationships can benefit from the core helping conditions of warmth, acceptance, genuineness, and respect (Rogers, 1980, 1961).

2. *Establish common ground.* As consultants extend their services across diverse organizations or settings, they often collaborate with individuals representing different problem-solving methods, interpretations, and expectations. Consultants need to manage these differences effectively. Interactions that begin on common ground are desirable; that is, consultants should consider the fundamental characteristics, interests, goals, or concerns they share with consultees. When consultants and consultees emphasize commonalities rather than differences, the relationship is characterized by mutual respect and appreciation. Consultants should be committed to a framework that acknowledges interpersonal differences, but these differences should not divide participants in the process.

3. *Create a balance of power.* Although consultees are voluntary participants who have a certain degree of autonomy, they are often content to assume subservient or passive roles (Brown et al., 1991; Caplan, 1970). Though this effect occurs naturally, it is exaggerated when consultants abuse their power and create a relational imbalance. Rapport is best served when consultants behave, verbally and nonverbally, in ways that equalize the power in consulting relationships. Encouraging the consultee's participation and listening intently to and validating his or her ideas are helpful strategies that reduce a power imbalance.

4. *Demonstrate authenticity.* Effective consultation relationships cannot involve manipulation or deception. Consultants must be straightforward and truthful. Some writers emphasize the importance of authenticity in consultant-consultee relations (Block, 1981). Throughout the consultation process, the authentic consultant participates in dialogue marked by open and honest disclosures.

Collaboration and Empowerment   Though they often come from different backgrounds and professions, consultants and consultees must forge a relationship in which collegial interactions pave the way for constructive solutions. Most writers and practitioners stress the need for collaboration between constituents. Collaboration, as we noted in Chapter 1, refers to consultant-consultee relations that reflect a climate of shared responsibilities and commitments. Collaborative relationships are nonhierarchical and nonthreatening. Brown, Pryzwansky, and Schulte (1995) point out that the absence of collaborative exchanges during certain stages of consultation—assessment and goal setting, for example—dooms the overall process to failure.

One distinct advantage of collaboration is the sense of **empowerment** (increase in personal power) that the participants derive from the process. As equal partners, consultants and consultees engage in person-to-person interactions in which the contributions of each are integral to successful problem solving. Collaborative consultants value these principles as they emphasize and reinforce the consultee's contributions to problem solving. Not only are the consultee's suggestions, ideas, or hypotheses instrumental, their approval by the consultant serves a reinforcing and empowering purpose. A sense of empowerment often leads to optimal confidence, which, in turn, promotes positive outcomes and future problem solving. Parsons and Meyers (1984) offer these suggestions on how to facilitate collaboration and empowerment:

1. Allow the consultee freedom to accept or reject.
2. Encourage the consultee to contribute suggestions.
3. Encourage the consultee to make decisions.
4. Emphasize the consultee's contributions.
5. Encourage consultee responsibility.
6. Require effort from the consultee. (pp. 38–39)

Recognizing Tension, Resistance, and Conflict   In the earlier stages of the consultation process, consultants must anticipate the tensions often generated by consultation. Despite their recognition that problems exist and solutions are needed, many consultees are ambivalent as they enter the consultation relationship. Many possible sources of tension among consultees and other organizational members exist. To some people, for example, the consultant's presence implies disruptive changes that will undermine job assignments, status, and work methods. To others, proceeding with consultation is an indication that the organization and its members are incompetent or unwilling to resolve problems. Regardless of its source, consultants must prepare for **resistance**, an active or passive opposition to the real or anticipated changes accompanying consultation. Resistance is especially problematic when the consultant is unable to motivate the consultee to engage in problem-solving activities (Piersel & Gutkin, 1983).

Tensions may evolve into interpersonal conflicts. Some conflicts may already have been present in the organization or may arise after the consultant arrives. Some conflicts erupt without warning or have unpredictable causes. Organizational disagreement surrounding the decision to pursue consultation, for example, often leads to friction that is unrelated to the consultant's demeanor or relational skills. Some participants in the consultation process have negative attitudes toward consultation because of earlier experiences. Others may question the legitimacy of consultation as a helping process or feel that an existing organizational member should assume the consultant's role. Still others may view consultation as an unnecessary expense. Although most consultants recognize that tension, resistance, and conflict are common, their sources and influences should never be trivialized or ignored (see Chapter 5).

Assessment and Diagnosis

Assessment and diagnosis encompass the data gathering and analysis procedures that bring consultation problems into focus and point the way toward solutions. Although they are crucial at the beginning, these procedures play a role throughout the consultation process, as consultants reexamine findings and rethink problem-solving strategies. For assessment and diagnosis to be successful, collaboration between consultants and consultees is essential (Beer & Spector, 1993; Brown et al., 1995; Cooper & O'Connor, 1993; Furr, 1979; Kurpius et al., 1993). In particular, consultants and consultees need to agree on assessment methods, which should be the topic of contractual and other discussions. Privacy issues are also crucial. Consultants must protect the privacy of those participating in the process. The need to disclose information obtained through assessment and diagnostic practices can raise especially delicate issues that consultants should handle cautiously and sensitively.

Assessment

Assessment in consultation involves collecting, organizing, and interpreting information that can help consultants and consultees bring problems into focus and determine their causes. The importance of the assessment process cannot be overstated. Problem elements that are overlooked or misinterpreted during the assessment period are unlikely to be resolved later (Bergan & Tombari, 1976; Kratochwill & Bergan, 1990). Misdiagnosing causal elements produces similar undesirable consequences. To elicit helpful information, consultants often begin the assessment process with questions like these:

- What problems have prompted the request for consultation?
- What is the consultee's perception of these concerns?
- How do the problems affect the organization?
- Are the problems caused by human factors or structural deficiencies in the organization?
- What solutions has the consultee tried?
- Why are the problems still unresolved?

Scanning the Environment   As skilled observers and data analysts, consultants often begin their assessment by "scanning" the organizational environment (Gallessich, 1982, p. 315). **Scanning** requires the consultant to look beyond the scope of the consultation problems to observe a broad spectrum of conditions that may be relevant. The scanning process permits the consultant to verify or refine the consultee's interpretation of the problems, to correct biased or limited perceptions, and to recognize additional dynamics. Although the scanning process appears particularly relevant to consultation problems that have broad organizational implications, individual consultee- or client-related issues often have environmental dynamics that must be assessed as well.

Data Gathering Methods Information gathering is integral to the assessment process. Before discussing various data collection methods, however, we should call attention to two indispensable rules. First, as Kurpius et al. (1993) point out, "The traditional statement about good data is that they should be valid and reliable" (p. 603). Thus, consultants must ensure that their methods yield truthful and consistent data. Second, since assessment and data collection activities have strong ethical and legal implications, consultants must make sure that these activities are in compliance with ethical and legal guidelines (see Chapter 11).

As the need for data varies from setting to setting, so too, do the data collection methods consultants have at their disposal. Different methods are appropriate at different points in the consultation process. Data gathering methods also vary with respect to their obtrusive or unobtrusive nature (Dougherty, 1990). **Obtrusive** data collection procedures are highly visible and can cause disruptions in the consultation setting. In addition, obtrusive data gathering requires some response by consultees or others. Interviews, problem diagnosis sessions, surveys, and checklists are common examples of obtrusive methods. In contrast, data can be generated by **unobtrusive** methods that allow routine organizational activities to continue uninterrupted.

A common method of gathering information in consultation is the individual or group interview. The **interview** is a purposeful and directed meeting, usually conversational, with one person in the interview having the responsibility for its development (De Schweinitz & De Schweinitz, 1962). Because consultees often have opinions about the causes of problems and what to do about them, a sound beginning to the assessment stage is a formal interview with the consultee. Interviews are usually either standardized or nonstandardized (Molyneaux & Lane, 1982). *Standardized* interviews require the consultant to have a clear understanding of assessment needs; questions are prepared ahead of time. *Nonstandardized* interviews, which are often spontaneous, do not bind the consultant to any particular topic or format. Both types of interviews are normally conducted in a private setting and allow consultants to explore the attitudes and perceptions of consultees and others.

The purpose of a specific interview determines whether an individual or group format is most appropriate. Individual interviews are the method of choice when the consultant wishes to collect sensitive, private information, such as personal opinions or evaluations. Group interviews are often effective for collecting large amounts of information quickly. But like other types of public forums, they may limit disclosures to only the most vocal participants. Further, participants in group interviews may not express their true feelings or perceptions.

Consultants often explore problems together with consultees and other constituents in problem assessment groups. Group meetings can provide qualitative information about the consultation problem and have the added advantage of allowing for multiple vantage points. Brown et al. (1991), for example, endorse **problem diagnosis sessions** as forums in which various constituents can exchange information integral to client, program, or organizational problems. These groups encourage participants to apply their expertise to particular, rather than global, consultation problems. By pooling this expertise, the problem diagnosis sessions can yield productive strategies and solutions.

Surveys represent another alternative. As we are using the term here, **surveys** consist of questionnaires, completed anonymously, that elicit valuable information or perceptions about particular consultation issues or problems. This approach allows consultants to collect large amounts of information from many individuals in a short time. Gallessich (1982) points out that surveys are particularly useful in exploring personal attitudes, feelings, perceptions, and evaluations.

Surveys can be problematic, however. Two types of errors are common: sampling and nonsampling errors (Fienberg & Tanur, 1989). *Sampling errors* occur when consultants generalize the perceptions, ideas, or philosophies of respondents to the entire population being surveyed. Consultants should remember that the perceptions of respondents returning completed questionnaires may differ dramatically from the perceptions of others who failed to respond. Sampling errors can be reduced by distributing a larger number of questionnaires and by creating incentives that boost return rates. *Nonsampling errors* include the mistakes that respondents and consultants make in communicating ideas, interpreting the meaning of items, and collecting and analyzing data. Consultants usually find it helpful to test survey materials through pilot administrations with consultees, peers, or colleagues. Pilot distributions, where subjects provide feedback about survey items and questionnaire format, diminish nonsampling error by improving the survey's validity.

Like survey questionnaires, **checklists** are devised to include pertinent details about specific consultation issues. They are formal or informal lists of characteristics, conditions, or other items that consultees and other consultation constituents may mark as a way of providing relevant information. These lists vary in length and detail and have the benefit of expediency. They promote easy and timely feedback because consultees and other respondents simply check or mark preferences without having to elaborate.

To increase confidence in the data they obtain, consultants may want to use standardized checklists. These checklists are advantageous because they have built-in validity and reliability; they also simplify the assessment process. Less-standardized or "homemade" checklists offer consultants the convenience of custom design, though they risk less-valid data.

The data collection methods we have just reviewed are obtrusive. Unobtrusive methods are less visible. That is, they are designed to collect information without serious interference or interruption in the workplace. Ideally, such methods do not require an active response by others. Unobtrusive methods include making observations, reviewing records and documents, and exploring client history.

Observation, the consultant's intentional viewing of events (Dougherty, 1990), is a method of acquiring firsthand information about clients or programs. Consultant observations are particularly useful in formulating hypotheses about client characteristics or behaviors or about organizational processes that consultees do not recognize or acknowledge (Gallessich, 1982). Although observation cannot be described as purely unobtrusive, the process is less disruptive to the consultee's schedule than interviews, group meetings, surveys, and checklists.

Some situations demand that observational data be used cautiously. The presence of external observers in consultation settings can distort the natural environment and inadvertently influence the behavior of those observed (Dougherty, 1990). In these cases, client behaviors deviate from the norm. Thus, the most reliable observations are conducted by consultants who cannot be seen by clients. One-way mirrors and specially equipped observation rooms, for example, permit accurate observation while reducing the effects of observer influence.

The push for accountability in most human service organizations makes record-keeping and other documentation practices integral to organizational survival. Whether for individuals, programs, or systems, maintaining both temporary and permanent records is essential and in fact may be mandated by the organization. For our purposes, **records** are accounts, often chronologically arranged, of the actions or behavior of the consultee or organization in reference to the consultation problem. Relevant records may include formal client charts, progress notes, case files, and performance records, or informal, anecdotal accounts.

Records of organizational characteristics may be useful to consultants working with agencies or programs. Documents such as mission statements, organizational charts, correspondence, job descriptions, and reports resulting from accreditation or formal program reviews can provide valuable information. But consultants should not expect automatic access to these and other types of records, because access may be limited by ethical and legal restrictions.

Whether clients are individuals or systems, they have histories that have a bearing on the consultation problem. The **client history** is a collection of information, facts, and observations that provide a developmental account of the client's past. A review of historical information allows the consultant to clarify events, explore historical developments, and observe organizational trends. The client history answers important questions and crystallizes relevant information. Intake reports, usually integral to formal client records, provide a useful account of a client's past life. Testing and human appraisal information offer comparisons of present observations and past evaluations.

Programs and organizations also have identifiable histories. Consultants, for example, may review grant applications or program proposals that specify the basic needs or conditions giving rise to human service programs. Similarly, through their review of a program's annual reports, short- and long-term planning documents, and mission or philosophy statements, consultants formulate impressions of existing program or organizational characteristics.

Diagnostic Impression

Data collected during the assessment phase must be synthesized, categorized, and analyzed in order to formulate an accurate diagnostic impression. Without a complete and accurate understanding of assessment data, these data are of little use (Kurpius et al., 1993). **Diagnosis** as it relates to psychological consultation entails the identification or classification of consultation problems (client- or program-related) and their probable causes. Diagnostic impressions of specific problems, achieved through the collective actions of consultants and consultees, yield prescriptive ideas of the types of interventions needed to correct existing problems.

The consultation client, whether an individual, program, or system, influences the type of diagnosis. Brown et al. (1995) provide a useful model that categorizes consultation problems as occurring in three realms: consultee characteristics, client characteristics, and environmental characteristics. Each realm may collectively, interactively, or individually contribute to the consultation problems. Consultee characteristics include the weaknesses or deficiencies that have a bearing on client or organizational problems. Client characteristics may include problematic perceptions and behaviors. Environmental characteristics can be those of either the immediate or the larger environment; they are organizational features (for example, resources, policies, and constraints) that contribute to the need for consultation. To be thorough, consultants must examine each set of characteristics to determine its relevance to the consultation problems.

The primary objective of assessment and diagnostic activities is an accurate conceptualization of the consultation problem. These activities establish the purpose and direction of consultation.

Goal Setting

Assessment and diagnosis should lead to a succinct **problem statement** (a description of consultation issues, needs, or difficulties). Formulating a problem statement helps consultants and consultees identify substantive consultation goals. **Goal setting** in consultation is a broad term that refers to the processes in which consultants and consultees determine target objectives and anticipated outcomes. These processes are crucial and should not be rushed (Egan & Cowan, 1979). **Consultation goals** are the specific outcomes that will resolve or eliminate consultation problems. They provide a framework for the process by imposing a mission and channeling interventions in certain directions. Consultants and consultees can encounter difficulties if they "agree that there is a problem or that a change is desirable" (Lippitt & Lippitt, 1978, p. 15), then fail to address problems within the context of desirable outcomes. Consultation goals are often restorative or corrective. Thus, they are devised to reflect the need for change, the processes needed for change, and the end product of that change (Gutkin & Curtis, 1990).

Goal setting in consultation requires adherence to a standard set of principles, which we outline here.

1. *Consultants must recognize that goal setting is a collaborative process that involves consultees and other key participants.* Mutual commitment to specified goals establishes a blueprint that all parties can support. It also ensures that consultees will have adequate input and enhances everyone's understanding of the problem.

2. *The consultant and consultee should set realistic goals.* Lofty goals are potentially discouraging. Moreover, unrealistic goals create resistance or nonadherence to consultation interventions. In a collaborative format, consultation goals should be tailored to the consultee's or organization's resources (in terms of time, finances, and so on) and commitment.

3. *Goals must be specific.* Goals should be expressed in clear, precise terms. Vague or amorphous goal statements provide little direction to those involved in the consultation process. Dougherty (1990) describes goal setting as "a process of shaping, a movement toward concreteness and specificity from a broader, more general perspective" (p. 81).

4. *Complex or global goals are undesirable.* Some consultation problems are extremely complex and naturally require complex problem-solving methods (Egan, 1985). For such problems, the goal-setting process should focus on smaller, specific accomplishments that will move individuals or programs in the correct direction. Attaining these smaller goals can help keep the process on track and can provide useful information on the progress and direction of various interventions.

5. *The consultant and consultee should audit their progress.* Consultation goals are seldom accomplished without extensive planning and organizing. Well-conceived consultation goals specify time frames, deadlines, and related contingencies. Further, consultants and consultees must anticipate the obstacles or barriers that threaten goal accomplishment (Dougherty, 1990).

6. *Goals should be formulated in measurable terms.* Measurable goals make it easier to assess specific outcomes and ultimately to determine the overall success of the consultation process. Measurable goals also yield evidence that consultees can use in justifying the human and material resources needed for problem solving. Hutchins and Cole (1992) define such goals more precisely: "Normally, if goals are stated positively, have specified conditions for their achievement, and are broken down into achievable parts, goals will be measurable" (p. 141).

Intervention

Although the entire consultation process can be considered one large intervention (Brown, Kurpius, & Morris, 1988), a time-specific and action-oriented intervention stage represents the most visible problem-solving phase of the process. This stage is essentially a litmus test in which the success or failure of the process is evident. **Interventions** integrate the methods and strategies conceived by consultants and consultees to address problems. Carkhuff (1983) elaborates as follows:

> An intervention is both a response and an initiative. It is a response to a situation that defines a need. It is a response to a deficit or to what is not present. At the same time, it is an initiative to influence that situation—to fill in what is not present, to transform the deficits into assets. In short, an intervention is an attempt to make a difference. (p. 163)

Dougherty (1990) defines interventions with specific reference to consultation: "In consultation, interventions are the actions or activities that, when put together in a systematic manner, make up a plan to achieve a goal" (p. 84).

Strategy Selection

Substantive interventions should be tailored to the organization or setting and implemented according to available resources. Decisions at this point reflect intuitive planning that connects, both theoretically and practically, potential solutions with problems. Interventions are most successful when they are the products of collaboration and mutual endorsement. Kurpius et al. (1993) assert that "the best predictor of success for any intervention is to have an accurate problem definition that is owned by the consultee and the consultee's client" (p. 604). In addition, as Conoley, Conoley, Ivey, and Scheel (1991) note, consultees are more inclined to accept interventions matched to their own attitudes and choices.

The selection of interventions requires an atmosphere of openness in which a range of approaches are explored. For each proposed intervention, the consultant and consultee should investigate as many of the relevant issues as possible. For example, what is the best approach or model? What is the feasibility of the intervention? Does the intervention match identified needs? What about logistical and cost factors? Is the intervention complete? The answers to these questions provide important data that make selections less complicated.

Consultants should avoid interventions that involve convenience or favoritism or that reflect purely personal preferences. Basing interventions on expediency or convenience, for example, risks serious error (Kurpius et al., 1993). Thus, as a rule, consultants should gear interventions to the nature of the problem. They should also formulate interventions that reflect sound theoretical principles and conceptual models. Too often, consultants enter the intervention period with poor preparation. The probable result will be interventions whose usefulness is questionable.

Types of Interventions

Consultants and consultees can select from among various interventions. An important consideration is the target of the proposed interventions. That is, interventions can be delivered at multiple levels and, depending on assessment and diagnostic findings, they can be directed at individuals, groups, or organizations.

Individual Interventions   Much has been written about individual consultation interventions (Brown et al., 1988; Fuqua & Newman, 1985; Kurpius, 1985; Mathias, 1992). According to Fuqua and Newman (1985), individual interventions are most appropriate when:

1. the underlying problems are of an individual nature;
2. systems interventions are untimely or unlikely;
3. perceptions of problems are limited to individuals;
4. a system is highly resistant to change; and
5. individual behavioral change is grossly more efficient given the present condition of the system. (p. 391)

Individual interventions may target specific clients or consultees. Where problematic clients are at issue, case-oriented consultation is probably the most appropriate intervention. Like Caplan's (1970) client-centered case consultation, case interventions are directed at consultees who, although competent, are unable to resolve client problems. Case consultation methods often require face-to-face conferences that emphasize the consultee's client. Of necessity, case consultation methods take into account the client's psychological needs and novel strategies the consultee may use to address them.

When the consultee's behavior stems from a client's lack of progress, individual interventions focus more on the consultee's needs and less on the client's problems.

Caplan's (1970) consultee-centered case consultation model is perhaps the best-known individual model that targets the individual consultee's deficits (see the next chapter). Interventions in the form of face-to-face interviews, reviews or discussions of case strategies, and training are geared to remediating the consultee's deficits. In addition, coaching interventions are individually centered interventions that focus on consultees' level of awareness, behavior, and learning skills (French & Bell, 1978). Coaching methods require consultants to serve as tutors or mentors who encourage discipline, practice, and teamwork to help the consultee improve case-related weaknesses.

Group Interventions   In some work settings, consultation problems extend beyond the needs of individuals. Group interventions are appropriate when consultation problems stem from the performance deficits or needs of more than one person. Such interventions are based on the premise that particular elements of a group's functioning hamper the performance of the group as a whole (Kurpius, 1985). Examples of group interventions include training, conflict resolution, and team building. Because we give these interventions more detailed attention in Chapter 10, the discussions here are purposely brief and introductory.

1. *Training*   Training interventions are common in the consultation process. **Training** is the application of teaching or skill-building strategies that help consultees acquire information, learn new technologies, or build competencies. A training program is conventionally presented in a workshop atmosphere in which skill acquisition and rehearsal form indispensable activities. Further, training can serve a "retooling" purpose when participants need new technologies or existing skills need to be revitalized. **Seminars**—alternatives to the workshop format—focus less on skill building and more on the presentation of innovative information or practices to help participants stay abreast of developments in their field. Some seminars emphasize participants' enhancement and growth as individuals. Less-formal training can take the form of talks or other presentations.

2. *Conflict resolution*   Conflicts among individuals and groups are common and can represent extreme challenges to an organization. According to Johnson and Johnson (1975), conflicts generally result from differences in needs, values, and goals; scarcity of resources; or rivalry or competition among group members. Whether they emerge suddenly or evolve gradually, the range of factors contributing to conflicts can be perplexing and frightening. Although groups or individuals often dislike the conflicts that divide them, simply wanting to overcome these conflicts is usually not enough. Consultation can lead to interventions that resolve complex conflicts while preserving interpersonal relationships.

3. *Team building*   An increasingly popular strategy among efficiency-minded organizations is to create a "team" atmosphere where employees work together to accomplish their mission. Teams are effective when they are synergistic—that is, more than the sum of their parts (Dyer, 1987). Organizations of all kinds can be viewed as large teams or as consisting of multiple teams in separate programs and locations. Because of the push for quality programs, organizational leaders often look to team-building approaches to help employees work together. Psychological consultants, particularly those

skilled in group dynamics and processes, help groups to identify group obstacles, recognize group resources, and evolve into high-achieving teams.

Organizational Interventions   The push for top quality creates a need for consultants to assist in the planning and implementation of organizational interventions. Organizational interventions target the whole organization, whether a company, agency, or system, rather than separate individuals, clients, or employees. Although consultants may work predominantly with specific consultees (for example, managers, supervisors, or organizational leaders), the entire organization is actually the client and the direct beneficiary of any changes. There are numerous organizational interventions, and mentioning all of them is beyond the scope of this chapter. A few models include:

1. *Process consultation*   Process consultation is a style of consultation in which the consultant—a process-oriented organizational observer—provides expertise to the organization by observing and assessing processes related to organizational communication, meetings, decision making, and problem solving (Schein, 1987). Process consultants are invested in organizational processes and the empowering of consultees as active agents in organizational change.

2. *Organizational assessment and diagnosis*   The consultant serves a diagnostic role in consulting with organizational members to help them examine the organization's strengths, weaknesses, and overall health (Hanna, 1988; Morasky, 1982). Assessment and diagnostic activities target specific organizational units or subsystems or the organization as a whole.

3. *Strategic planning*   Strategic planning is a consultation function in which consultants help organizational leaders recognize the importance of setting their sights on the future, creating visions, and planning rather than speculating (Burack, 1972; Kaufman & Herman, 1991). Strategic planning, which can be either short- or long-range, reflects the belief that organizations should actively mold their own futures rather than passively allowing the future to unfold.

4. *Altering organizational paradigms*   Obsolete beliefs or values often become firm rules or paradigms that govern an organization's operations. When organizational leaders cling to these beliefs or values in making decisions, they risk stagnation and failure. Fuqua and Kurpius (1993) describe an innovative approach in which consultants help consultees recognize obsolete or inhibiting paradigms, accept the need for change, and implement paradigm shifts that move organizations to more adaptive and productive futures.

Implementing Interventions

Implementing interventions requires consultants and consultees to actualize planned interventions, initiate problem-solving behaviors, and resolve diagnosed problems. Since it requires action approaches, this phase of the consultation process is highly visible. Implementation considerations include logistical matters (for example, time, schedules, space, access, materials), the consultee's abilities and commitment to the intervention, and the reactions of consultees and other constituents.

Implementation activities yield important information about the accuracy of earlier consultation decisions. As intervention plans are transformed into action, consultants and consultees encounter the fallibility of their decisions, and despite their best efforts, mistakes or unanticipated obstacles often manifest themselves. According to Brown et al. (1991), "No matter how thorough strategy selection and planning have been, it is likely that the plan derived during consultation will be in need of adaptation and adjustment to meet unanticipated problems" (p. 161).

Implementing interventions puts the spotlight on the respective roles of consultant and consultee. In many forms of consultation, the responsibility for implementing planned interventions rests with the consultee, while the consultant remains a watchful, collaborative resource (Caplan, 1970; Dougherty, 1990). But interventions that involve specialized group approaches (such as training, conflict resolution, and team building) rely almost exclusively on the consultant as the chief agent in implementation.

Evaluation

Evaluation in a broad sense is a form of systematic inquiry about certain "activities, characteristics, and outcomes of programs" (Patton, 1987, p. 15). More specifically, **consultation evaluation** is the process of rendering judgment about the overall effectiveness of consultation interventions. Evaluation-minded consultants are usually interested in the extent to which interventions resolve consultation problems. Evaluation in consultation is often a multidimensional process that relies on various techniques to assess multiple variables. Though consultants are usually interested in the outcomes of the process, they should also examine the broad range of variables that influence the process. Evaluation measures, for example, may focus on the effects of decisions and procedures during any phase of consultation.

Regrettably, evaluating consultation processes often involves more rhetoric than action. That is, though most consultants would quickly agree that the evaluation of consultation is necessary to determine outcomes and credibility, many consultants plan haphazard evaluation strategies or resist evaluation practices altogether (Brown et al., 1988). Technical complexities, obsolete paradigms, and evaluation myths are a few of the numerous obstacles that exist. To overcome these and other barriers, consultants must first make evaluation a priority.

Although a broad range of questions arise in the course of evaluation, perhaps the most central is the following: "What about the consultation process should be evaluated or measured?" The response or responses to this question will determine the nature of the evaluation process, including the choice of techniques and methodologies. Although we do not present a standard formula or suggest that one is available for all consultation situations, some typical evaluation plans exist (see Chapter 4).

Although consultants may assume that evaluation occurs formally during the latter stages of consultation, evaluation processes, in actuality, should be continuous and "fully integrated" into each stage of consultation (Kurpius et al., 1993, p. 605). At distinct periods in the consultation process, consultants should take advantage of opportunities to attend to evaluation matters. Contractual agreements established during the entry stage of consultation, for example, should outline expectations about evaluation and authorization for data collection and dissemination. Goal-setting activities often include the formulation of measurable objectives that reflect the plan for evaluating goal attainment. Further, some evaluation designs require the collection of data before and after interventions, so that consultants must attend to evaluation at pre- and postintervention periods.

Evaluation takes many forms depending on the situation in which it is carried out. Evaluation also satisfies multiple purposes. Inquisitive consultants may feel overwhelmed by decisions about what to measure and what types of information to collect. Fortunately, Scriven (1967) offers a model that classifies evaluation into two broad types, formative and summative. Although originally devised for educational curriculum evaluators, Scriven's model can be applied to consultation decisions and actions. *Formative* strategies include evaluation tactics that target the full range of processes—including the consultant's decisions, actions, plans, and organizational strategies—as they unfold. Of necessity, the consultant carefully examines each stage of the consultation process, searching for a complete, valid assessment of the dynamics in progress. *Summative* evaluation focuses on consultation outcomes, including goal attainment and the effects of applied interventions.

Evaluation methods vary with respect to sophistication and formality (Schmidt & Medl, 1983) and must be tailored to the setting. Formal evaluation methods include standardized measures or carefully controlled evaluation designs. Applying the scientific method, controlling key variables, measuring changes from pre- to postconsultation periods, and using valid statistical procedures are examples of formal evaluation methods. Consultants should understand, though, that some evaluation techniques may require technical expertise beyond their knowledge and experience. When this is the case, they should seek supervision or assistance from more skilled evaluators.

Useful evaluation data can also be generated through informal methods that provide intuitive and practical impressions of consultation success. Informal methodologies can provide subjective or qualitative feedback on the consultant's performance, the quality of the consultation relationship, and subsequent outcomes. The consultee's degree of satisfaction and general impressions about the efficacy of consultation are examples of informal evaluative measures. Further, the consultant's qualitative observations on organizational variables can be useful. Interviews with consultees during or after the consultation process provide another informal source of information.

Admittedly, consultation evaluation deserves more attention than we provide in this general discussion. You are encouraged to review the more detailed information presented in Chapter 4.

Termination

The **termination stage** is the concluding phase of the consultation process. Kurpius et al. (1993) cite two reasons for termination: "First, it is the time when the consultant and consultee agree that the consultation should be terminated either because of successful completion of the project or because it is becoming more clear that success is unlikely" (p. 605).

If the sparse attention given termination in the consultation literature is any indication, the termination stage is the most devalued period of the entire process (Kurpius et al., 1993). But this stage has several important dimensions. Dustin and Ehly (1984) advise consultants to bring closure to the consultation arrangement with an **exit interview.** During the exit interview, consultants and consultees bring formal closure to the consultation process, identify residual issues or concerns, and discuss possible future actions. The interview provides indispensable feedback about the general effects of consultation and the consultee's feelings about these effects. The exit interview is also a forum that brings together all the consultation participants to exchange comments about the way the process met (or did not meet) the terms of the consultation contract.

Schein (1969) describes the importance of consultant-consultee discussions that clarify the possibility of future consultation. Since the consultation process is often the product of an intensive commitment and shared effort, and the familiarity of consultation relationships often makes consultees dependent on the consultant's help, consultees may sense a psychological tie to the consultant. This phenomenon appears significant when there is strong probability that existing problems will continue or new ones will arise. As Schein (1969) points out, the consultant's involvement in the organization may not be terminated in an absolute sense but may continue in some intermittent fashion.

The problems that result from inadequate termination can be substantial (Beisser & Green, 1972). Under certain circumstances, it is especially important that consultation not be brought to a close. Consultants, for example, should resist termination when consultees are confused about outcomes. The presence of unresolved problems means that the consultation process should probably be prolonged. Some consultees may be confused or uncertain about the future, and at the time of termination, they may ask, "What happens now that the consultant's role is substantially diminished?" Others may reflect on the work that remains and the problems that linger. The consultee's tentativeness regarding the future represents a readiness issue that consultants must assess in the termination period.

But termination should not be delayed unnecessarily (Hansen, Himes, & Meier, 1990). Although termination normally follows completed interventions and predetermined time frames, special circumstances may create the need for early termination. Political or budgetary concerns, a diagnosis revealing problems beyond the consultant's ability to resolve them, unsatisfactory relations between consultant and consultee, and distrust by either party are conditions that warrant early termination (Gallessich, 1982). For example, in settings other than mental health settings (such as schools, child development programs, industrial firms), unanticipated or acute mental health problems require consultants to disengage themselves and arrange for more direct psychological interventions (Caplan, 1970). In these cases, consultants provide immediate support for the distraught consultee or client and seek professional help through referrals and collaboration. Consultants also realize the need for early termination when they are unable to create effective interventions or when consultees become disenchanted with the consultation process.

A final termination action occurs following the exit period. Many consultants communicate with consultees through follow-up letters, telephone conversations, or fax correspondence. Follow-up correspondence can express appreciation and continued support. Further, follow-up efforts serve to check the durability of the consultation changes or the emergence of unexpected obstacles.

TABLE 2.1
Summary of consultation stages and activities

Stage	Focus	Consultant's Task	Philosophy
Preliminary Contact	Getting started Creating a basis for consultation Agreeing on working terms	Determining the "fit" Accepting the consultant role Contracting	To establish a solid foundation To explore applicable models
Entry	Entering the organization Establishing relationships	Accomplishing physical, psychological, and social entry Building solid working relations	To gain acceptance and trust To recognize and manage resistance
Assessment and Diagnosis	Identifying the consultation problem Creating a problem statement	Scanning Gathering data Forming a clear diagnosis Deciding on appropriate methods	To collect valid and reliable data To confirm presenting problems
Goal Setting	Establishing the direction of consultation	Setting measurable goals	To identify desired outcomes
Intervention	Applying strategies that address problems	Selecting and implementing change strategies	To resolve consultation problems
Evaluation	Determining the effectiveness of interventions	Measuring outcomes of interventions Evaluating the consultation	To determine the success of consultation
Termination	Ending the consultation process	Bringing closure to consultation Following up	To conclude consultation at an appropriate juncture

SUMMARY

Consultation consists of a series of interconnected processes that require careful planning and organization. Though there is a great diversity of models, settings, and consultees, consultation generally proceeds through a series of typical stages. This chapter has described seven consultation stages: preliminary contact, entry, assessment and diagnosis, goal setting, intervention, evaluation, and termination. Each stage consists of important dynamics and tasks that contribute to the overall process. By keeping the individual stages in mind, consultants are able to structure their work thoroughly and efficiently (see Table 2.1).

GLOSSARY

Assessment   In consultation, the multilevel process of collecting information specific to the consultation problem.

Checklists   Formal or informal lists of items on which consultees and other participants identify their perceptions or other items.

Client history   A collection of information, facts, and observations that provide a developmental account of the past.

Collaboration   Cooperation between consultant and consultee in working toward consultation goals.

Consultation constituents   Those who participate in the planning and implementation of consultation.

Consultation evaluation   Determination of the extent to which the consultation problems have been resolved or eliminated and of the usefulness of processes and decisions contributing to such outcomes.

Consultation fit   The degree to which a consultant is matched (in terms of competencies, interests, and values) to a consultation assignment.

Consultation goals   The specific outcomes that will resolve or eliminate the problems addressed in the consultation process.

Consultation stage   An identifiable interval—consisting of specific tasks and dynamics—in the consultation process. Consultation stages tend to be loosely structured and sequenced along a developmental continuum.

Contracting   The process through which a consultant and consultee negotiate and agree on terms for working together. The contract may be a formal document, an informal agreement, or a letter of understanding.

Diagnosis   In consultation, the act of identifying or classifying the consultation problem and its probable cause.

Empowerment   In consultation, increasing the client's or consultee's sense of personal power. Empowered consultees are able and motivated to resolve consultation problems.

Entry stage   The period during which a consultant comes into the consultation relationship and assumes a formal helping role. Consultants enter organizations physically, psychologically, and socially.

Evaluation   Systematic and coordinated inquiries and processes that attempt to determine the positive or negative worth of activities, variables, procedures, or changes.

Exit interview   A planned meeting, conducted during the termination stage of consultation, signaling the end of the consultation relationship.

External consultant   A consultant employed outside the general boundaries of the consultee's organization.

Goal setting   A stage of the consultation process during which realistic goals are devised. Goal setting presupposes the accurate assessment and diagnosis of consultation problems.

Internal consultant   A consultant employed within the same general setting or organization as the consultee.

Intervention   In consultation, a planned method or strategy of addressing consultation problems.

Interviews   Purposeful and directed meetings, usually conversational, with one person in the interview having the responsibility for their progress and development.

Observation   A popular method of gathering consultation information through the deliberate viewing of events.

Obtrusive data collection   Methods of gathering important consultation information that require some disruption of the consultee's schedule or flow of activities.

Organizational culture   The pattern of behaviors, norms, and values that prevails in an organization and shapes employee performance.

Presenting consultation problem   The problematic issue or need identified by the consultee during the preliminary contact stage of consultation.

Problem diagnosis sessions   Assessment meetings in which various constituents can exchange information integral to client, program, or organizational problems in a collaborative forum.

Problem statement   A succinct statement resulting from assessment and diagnosis of the consultation problem. Problem statements are an outgrowth of collaboration between the consultant and consultee.

Rapport   In consultation, agreement, cooperation, and harmony between constituents.

Records   Documented, chronological accounts of the actions or behavior of the consultee or organization in reference to the consultation client, program, or individual.

Resistance   Active or passive opposition to the real or anticipated changes accompanying consultation.

Scanning   Linked to assessment in consultation, scanning is the practice of observing or considering the various environments surrounding a consultation setting and problem.

Seminars   Workshops or classes that present current information, useful strategies, or innovative practices to help participants stay abreast of developments in their work.

Surveys   Written statements or questions designed to elicit valuable information or perceptions about particular consultation issues or problems.

Termination stage   The end of the consultation process.

Training   A structured, planned instructional process in which learners acquire information or skills intended to enhance their ability to perform their work. Inherent in these activities is an evaluation process assessing the learning accomplishments of students or trainees.

Unobtrusive data collection   Methods of gathering important consultation information without significantly disrupting the consultee's schedule or flow of activities.

ANNOTATED BIBLIOGRAPHY

For further information on the various consultation stages, June Gallessich's book *The Profession and Practice of Consultation: A Handbook for Consultants, Trainers of Consultants, and Consumers of Consultation Services* (1982) is must reading. In Chapters 11 to 15, Gallessich presents an in-depth discussion of consultation principles and practices. The practical examples she includes are especially useful.

Another key resource is *The Client-Consultant Handbook* (1979), edited by Chip Bell and Leonard Nadler. This is a collection of reprinted readings that focus on the stages of consultation in the business environment. Relational issues receive special attention.

In *Developing Consultation Skills* (1984), Parsons and Meyers offer both novice and professional consultants information on a wide range of consultation skills, strategies, and techniques. Chapter 11 provides valuable material for readers who wish to continue their study of consultation evaluation. The book also features many helpful exercises.

A more contemporary resource is A. Michael Dougherty's 1990 book *Consultation: Practice and Perspectives*. Four chapters provide detailed descriptions of the tasks and dynamics common to each consultation stage.

Finally, we should mention Duane Brown, Walter B. Pryzwansky, and Ann C. Schulte's *Psychological Consultation: Introduction to Theory and Practice* (3rd ed., 1995). Chapters 5 and 6 of this book explore the features of the various consultation stages.

REFERENCES AND SUGGESTED READINGS

Beer, M., & Spector, B. (1993). Organizational diagnosis: Its role in organizational learning. *Journal of Counseling and Development, 71*, 642–650.

Beisser, A., & Green, R. (1972). *Mental health consultation and education.* Palo Alto, CA: National Press Books.

Bell, C. R., & Nadler, L. (Eds.). (1979). *The client-consultant handbook.* Houston, TX: Gulf Publishing.

Bergan, J. R., & Tombari, M. (1976). Consultant skills and efficiency and the implementation and outcomes of consultation. *Journal of School Psychology, 14*(1), 3–14.

Block, P. (1981). *Flawless consulting.* San Diego, CA: University Associates.

Brown, D., Kurpius, D., & Morris, J. (1988). *Handbook of consultation with individuals and small groups.* Alexandria, VA: Association for Counselor Education and Supervision.

Brown, D., Pryzwansky, W. B., & Schulte, A. (1991). *Psychological consultation: Introduction to theory and practice* (2nd ed.). Boston: Allyn & Bacon.

Brown, D., Pryzwansky, W. B., & Schulte, A. (1995). *Psychological consultation: Introduction to theory and practice* (3rd ed.). Boston: Allyn & Bacon.

Burack, E. (1972). *Strategies for manpower planning and programming.* Morristown, NJ: General Learning Corporation.

Caplan, G. (1970). *The theory and practice of mental health consultation.* New York: Basic Books.

Carkhuff, R. (1983). *Sources of human productivity.* Amherst, MA: Human Resource Development.

Conoley, J., & Conoley, C. (1982). *School consultation.* New York: Pergamon Press.

Conoley, C., Conoley, J., Ivey, D., & Scheel, M. (1991). Enhancing consultation by matching the consultee's perspectives. *Journal of Counseling and Development, 69*, 546–549.

Cooper, S., & O'Connor, R., Jr. (1993). Standards for organizational consultation assessment and evaluation instruments. *Journal of Counseling and Development, 71*, 651–660.

Cosier, R., & Dalton, D. (1993). Management consulting: Planning, entry, performance. *Journal of Counseling and Development, 72*(2), 191–198.

De Schweinitz, E., & De Schweinitz, K. (1962). *Interviewing in the social services.* London: National Council of Social Service.

Dougherty, A. M. (1990). *Consultation: Practice and perspectives.* Pacific Grove, CA: Brooks/Cole.

Dustin, D., & Ehly, S. (1984). Skills for effective consultation. *School Counselor, 32,* 23–29.

Dyer, W. (1987). *Team building: Issues and alternatives* (2nd ed.). Reading, MA: Addison-Wesley.

Egan, G. (1985). *Change agent skills in helping and human service settings.* Pacific Grove, CA: Brooks/Cole.

Egan, G. (1986). *The skilled helper: A systematic approach to effective helping* (3rd ed.). Pacific Grove, CA: Brooks/Cole.

Egan, G., & Cowan, M. A. (1979). *People in systems: A model for development in the human-service professions and education.* Pacific Grove, CA: Brooks/Cole.

Fienberg, S., and Tanur, J. (1989). Combining cognitive and statistical approaches to survey data. *Science, 243,* 1017–1022.

French, W., & Bell, C. H., Jr. (1978). *Organization development: Behavioral interventions for organizational improvement.* (2nd ed.). Englewood Cliffs, NJ: Prentice-Hall.

Fuqua, D., & Kurpius, D. (1993). Conceptual models in organizational consultation. *Journal of Counseling and Development, 71,* 607–618.

Fuqua, D., & Newman, J. (1985). Individual consultation. *Counseling Psychologist, 13*(3), 390–395.

Furr, R. (1979). Surviving as a messenger: The client-consultant relationship during diagnosis. In C. Bell and L. Nadler (Eds.), *The client-consultant handbook* (pp. 119–128). Houston, TX: Gulf Publishing.

Gallessich, J. (1982). *The profession and practice of consultation: A handbook for consultants, trainers of consultants, and consumers of consultation services.* San Francisco: Jossey-Bass.

Gibb, J. R. (1979). Is help helpful? In C. Bell and L. Nadler (Eds.), *The client-consultant handbook* (pp. 108–118). Houston, TX: Gulf Publishing.

Gibbs, J. T. (1980). The interpersonal orientation in mental health consultation: Toward a model of ethnic variations in consultation. *Journal of Community Psychology, 8,* 195–207.

Gutkin, T. B., & Curtis, M. J. (1990). School-based consultation: Theory, techniques, and research. In T. B. Gutkin & C. R. Reynolds (Eds.), *The handbook of school psychology* (2nd ed., pp. 577–611). New York: Wiley.

Hanna, D. (1988). *Designing organizations for high performance.* Reading, MA: Addison-Wesley.

Hansen, J., Himes, B., & Meier, S. (1990). *Consultation: Concepts and practices.* Englewood Cliffs, NJ: Prentice-Hall.

Hutchins, D., & Cole, C. (1992). *Helping relationships and strategies* (2nd ed.). Pacific Grove, CA: Brooks/Cole.

Johnson, D., & Johnson, F. (1975). *Joining together: Group theory and group skills.* Englewood Cliffs, NJ: Prentice-Hall.

Kaufman, R., and Herman, J. (1991). *Strategic planning in education: Rethinking, restructuring, revitalizing.* Lancaster, PA: Technomic Publishing.

Kilmann, R., Saxton, S., & Serpa, R. (Eds.). (1985). *Gaining control of the corporate culture.* San Francisco: Jossey-Bass.

Kratochwill, T., & Bergan, J. (1990). *Behavioral consultation in applied settings: An individual guide.* New York: Plennum Press.

Kurpius, D. (1985). Consultation interventions: Successes, failures, and proposals. *Counseling Psychologist, 13*(3), 368–389.

Kurpius, D., & Fuqua, D. (1993). Fundamental issues in defining consultation. *Journal of Counseling and Development, 71*(6), 598–600.

Kurpius, D., Fuqua, D., & Rozecki, T. (1993). The consulting process: A multidimensional approach. *Journal of Counseling and Development, 71*(6), 601–606.

Kurpius, D., & Robinson, S. (1978). An overview of consultation. *Personnel and Guidance Journal, 56*, 321–323.

Lippitt, G., & Lippitt, R. (1978). *The consulting process in action.* La Jolla, CA: University Associates.

Mathias, C. (1992). Touching the lives of children: Consultative interventions that work. *Elementary School Guidance and Counseling, 26*, 190–201.

McMaster, M. (1986). *Performance management: Creating the conditions for results.* Portland, OR: Metamorphous Press.

Molyneaux, D., and Lane, V. (1982). *Effective interviewing: Techniques and analysis.* Boston: Allyn & Bacon.

Morasky, R. (1982). *Behavioral systems.* New York: Praeger.

Parsons, R., & Meyers, J. (1984). *Developing consultation skills.* San Francisco: Jossey-Bass.

Patton, M. Q. (1987). *Creative evaluation* (2nd ed). Newbury Park, CA: Sage.

Paul, S. C. (1979). Consultation evaluation: Turning a circus into a performance. In M. K. Hamilton & C. J. Meade (Eds.), *Consulting on campus (New Directions for Student Services)* (pp. 33–46). San Francisco: Jossey-Bass.

Piersel, W., & Gutkin, T. B. (1983). Resistance to school-based consultation: A behavioral analysis of the problem. *Psychology in the Schools, 20*, 311–318.

Pryzwansky, W., & White, G. (1983). The influence of consultee characteristics on preferences for consultation approaches. *Professional Psychology, 14*, 457–461.

Rogers, C. (1961). *On becoming a person.* Boston: Houghton Mifflin.

Rogers, C. (1980). *A way of being.* Boston: Houghton Mifflin.

Schein, E. (1969). *Process consultation: Its role in organizational development.* Reading, MA: Addison-Wesley.

Schein, E. (1987). *Process consultation: Lessons for managers and consultants* (Vol. 2). Reading, MA: Addison-Wesley.

Schmidt, J. J., & Medl, W. A. (1983). Six magic steps of consulting. *School Counselor, 30*(3), 212–216.

Scriven, M. (1967). The methodology of evaluation. In R. Tyler, R. Gagne, & M. Scriven (Eds.), *Perspectives of curriculum evaluation* (American Educational Research Association Monograph Series on Curriculum Evaluation) (pp. 39–83). Chicago: Rand McNally.

CHAPTER THREE

Consultation Models and Approaches

Summary

Glossary

Annotated Bibliography

References and Suggested Readings

Psychological practitioners in most specialty areas typically proceed by applying the knowledge and established rules of accepted, formal theories. Psychological consultants, however, are partial exceptions. Because psychological consultation is a somewhat amorphous and interdisciplinary field without strong unifying formulations, several authors have voiced major concerns about its theoretical imperfections (Bardon, 1985; Gallessich, 1985). This situation creates disenchantment for consultants who would prefer a unified model they can apply despite their discipline-driven orientations and regardless of particular consultation settings. But one should avoid generalizations that portray consultation as a practice without effective and reliable problem-solving methods. The opposite appears to be true, since the field has seen tremendous growth in the methods of conceptualizing and performing consultation tasks (Brack, Jones, Smith, White, & Brack, 1993; Dougherty, 1990; Gallessich, 1985).

Although the consultation field has yet to articulate formal, cross-disciplinary ideologies, consultants do have at their disposal several conceptual models or approaches (Hansen, Himes, & Meier, 1990). This chapter introduces three popular and enduring models: mental health consultation, organizational consultation, and behavioral consultation. We focus on these approaches because they appear most visible across the psychological specialties and, as modern consultants are aware, form the basis for other theoretical developments..Due to space limitations, however, the information we present is introductory, generalized, and condensed.

Mental Health Consultation

In **mental health consultation**, professional consultants address mental health issues through their work with providers of direct treatment services (Dougherty, 1990). This approach has been acclaimed for its efficacy in meeting both present and future needs. Consultation addresses current problems, for example, by attending to the dynamics of specific client or client program issues. Far-reaching, and hopefully preventive, purposes are served when consultees apply the skills gained from present consultation processes in intervening with future client or program matters. Thus, mental health consultation serves the explicit purpose of helping consultees help themselves.

Caplan's Mental Health Consultation Model

The mental health consultation model is closely tied to the work of Gerald Caplan. Caplan's contributions to the mental health field drew attention to the practice of consultation as a substantive alternative to traditional mental health treatment. His model, described in the now-classic book *The Theory and Practice of Mental Health Consultation* (1970), is grounded in the supposition that technical assistance, education, and emotional support are often insufficient to resolve complex consultation issues (Rogawski, 1978). Caplan hypothesizes that the client problems prompting the request for consultation are not the only important factor; consultees' performance deficiencies may also require much attention. Thus, he asserts, mental health consultation is often preoccupied with the work-related competencies of consultees as well as with the needs of clients.

Caplan's pervasive influence on the consultation field is evidenced by the many authors who describe his conceptual model in their publications. Caplan's (1970) definition of mental health consultation is quoted in most modern texts on the subject:

> A process of interaction between two professional persons—the consultant, who is a specialist, and the consultee, who invokes the consultant's help in regard to a current work problem with which he is having some difficulty and which he has decided is within the other's area of specialized competence. (p. 19)

As a prelude to this brief study of Caplan's model, we should note Caplan's background as a psychiatrist as well as the more specific impact of Sigmund Freud's theories on his thinking. Thus, Caplan's work should be interpreted with psychoanalytical principles in mind. Caplan contends, for example, that unconscious factors often create conditions within consultees that impede mental health treatment. He assumes, also, that disturbed consultee-client relationships frequently result from consultees' intrapsychic conflicts, biases, or excessive emotionality.

Distinguishing Features   Caplan's focus on strengthening consultees' work behavior in order to satisfy clients' needs distinguishes his approach. To meet this objective, consultants must integrate interpersonal and program skills that reflect complex role descriptions, responsibilities, and operating principles. We describe a few distinguishing features of Caplan's model below.

The Consultant's Role   As a skilled professional, the consultant has a challenging role. Consultation activities range from screening individual client characteristics and assessing organizational deficiencies to collaborating with consultees and providing recommendations for organizational leaders. Usually a member of a separate profession who is external to the consultee's organization, the consultant represents a trusted helper who offers informed and objective understanding of the problem or problems. As a general rule, the consultant brings no predetermined solutions or interpretations to the setting (Brown, Pryzwansky, & Schulte, 1995).

The Consultant-Consultee Relationship   According to Caplan, consultation occurs between professionals. The consultation relationship originates through the consultee's voluntary request for the consultant's specialized knowledge, skill, and experience. Caplan proclaims the consultant-consultee relationship "one of coordinate interdependence in which each side both gives to and takes from the other" (p. 81). This emphasis on reciprocal professional exchanges should lead to a collaborative format. Interactions must focus on work-related problems; personal or sensitive issues are excluded from overt discussions.

In mental health consultation, the consultant possesses no direct, supervisory authority in the relationship. Thus, the consultation relationship is marked by egalitarian principles. Consultants must rely on nonauthoritarian and inspirational incentives (such as the influence of useful ideas and insights) to encourage consultees' participation. In the relationship and throughout the entire consultation process, the consultee has substantial autonomy and authorizes all decisions and interventions.

The Consultation Problem   Mental health consultation problems are represented by a range of consultee, client, or program mental health issues that persist despite consultees' attempts to resolve them. Some consultation problems emerge from client or consultee disturbances that confuse treatment processes or lead to treatment impasses. Other problems stem from disturbed client or program functioning and consultees' inefficiency in resolving these problems. Thus, consultation problems are often obscure and indirect, and as assessment and diagnosis activities unfold, consultants must consider the influence of less-visible etiologies.

Processes, Interventions, and Outcomes   Mental health consultation can continue indefinitely if specific client or program problems persist (Caplan, 1970). Most often in situations involving client problems, consultation proceeds through a series of short interviews or meetings between consultants and consultees. When the focus of consultation is on program or administrative issues, the consultant should broaden the scope of the process to assess issues that are organization wide. Decisions on consultation interventions emerge from collaborative consultant-consultee dialogue guided by a mutual commitment to problem solving.

Consultation Types   Caplan delineates four types of consultation that are applied situationally depending on the focus and goals of the process: (1) client-centered case consultation, (2) consultee-centered case consultation, (3) program-centered administrative consultation, and (4) consultee-centered administrative consultation. Though the client-centered and consultee-centered approaches are appropriate for issues that reflect the interests of individual clients, the program-centered and consultee-centered administrative approaches address problems in administrative or planning functions.

Box 3.1
Case example: Client-centered case consultation

A psychologist (*consultant*) is employed by contract to provide mental health consultation to staff of a group home for delinquent youth. During a visit to the program, the psychologist was approached by a social worker (*consultee*) who is the supervisor of resident services. The social worker describes Resident X (*client*), who has become noticeably depressed following a recent visit to his mother's home. The social worker seeks consultation to evaluate the extent of Resident X's mood disturbance and its etiological factors. In addition, the social worker wishes to explore strategies for interacting with the resident during this period.

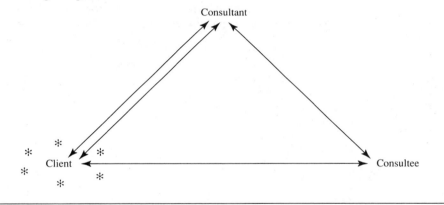

Client-Centered Case Consultation   Each client brings unique and often-perplexing issues to the mental health treatment setting. The difficulties associated with or stemming from such cases prompt the consultee's request for outside consultation. In **client-centered case consultation**, described by Caplan as the most "familiar" of the four types of consultation he proposes (p. 109), consultants rely on professional skills, insights, and experiences to help consultees with existing, possibly perplexing cases. While client-centered consultation requires a consultant to work predominantly with the consultee, direct client contact (for example, through observation, interviews, assessment) is often integral to the assessment process. A case example of client-centered case consultation is included in Box 3.1.

Consultee-Centered Case Consultation   Like the client-centered approach, **consultee-centered case consultation** addresses the needs of clients. This approach is distinguished, however, by its focus on the consultee's need for change rather than on the client's limitations. That is, as mental health consultants establish a relationship with mental health professionals, they often discover that the consultee's cognitive or emotional qualities impair, restrict, or bias the treatment process. Caplan recognized

---

Box 3.2
Case example: Consultee-centered case consultation

A counselor (*consultant*) is asked by a substance use counselor (*consultee*) to
provide consultation on her substance addiction cases. In the treatment program, the substance use counselor provides group and individual therapy for
alcohol addiction patients. The consultee is especially concerned about Patient
X (*client*), who has experienced little success since entering the program three
weeks earlier. The consultee describes Patient X's resistance, lack of progress,
and probable failure relative to the treatment goals of recovery. During the initial case conference, the consultee admitted that Patient X's case is remarkably
similar to that of her father, who was also alcohol-dependent. The consultee
described her father as a "hopeless case" who never wanted to overcome his
addiction. Most of the case session entailed the consultee's recollections of her
father's failures.

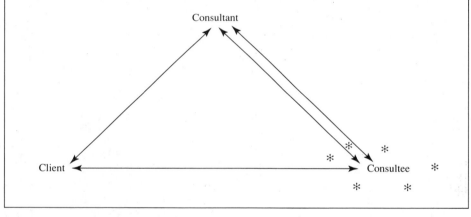

---

that distorted expectations, for example, can infiltrate the consultee-client relationship,
creating disturbed or biased treatment dynamics. Consultee-centered case consultation
is illustrated in Box 3.2.

Caplan identifies four deficit areas that may give rise to consultee-centered case consultation. When consultees have *knowledge deficits,* they lack the formal training or
theoretical or practical understanding to resolve clients' psychosocial problems. *Skill
deficits* occur when consultees possess adequate information to recognize and understand
client problems but lack the necessary skills to devise or implement successful treatment
strategies. *Deficits in self-confidence* exist when consultees view themselves as inadequate because of personal or professional characteristics (for example, inexperience, age,
gender, poor health). *Deficits in objectivity* result when consultees exhibit "defective
judgment" that results in the lack of professional objectivity (Caplan, 1970, p. 131).

Caplan emphasizes the intrapsychic and relationship issues that impair consultees'
objectivity. He categorizes these deficits according to five potential sources: (1) **direct**

personal involvement—consultees often misperceive the therapist-client relationship as a personal relationship rather than a professional exchange; (2) **simple identification**—this bias occurs when consultees identify with clients or other constituents to the extent that they lose perspective; (3) **transference**—consultees allow feelings or fantasies from former relationships to invade a current therapist-client relationship; (4) **characterological distortions**—consultees experience serious psychiatric disturbances that interfere with the treatment processes; and (5) **theme interference**—consultees inadvertently restrict clients' success because of beliefs or frustrations that emerge from past personal experiences (p. 132).

Regardless of the source and nature of the consultee's objectivity disturbances, Caplan advises consultants to avoid confrontive actions that undermine the consultee's confidence. Consultants must resist insinuations or accusations that consultees are inadequate or incompetent. Further, consultants should never misconstrue a consultant-consultee relationship as a therapy relationship. Rather, as Caplan suggests, consultants should initiate a series of nonthreatening case consultation meetings that include **displaced discussions**. These indirect, but relevant, discussions target problem areas through circuitous methods. Such discussions are grounded in the hypothesis that consultees will connect indirect information to unconscious, intrapsychic sources, correct biases, and subsequently reflect correct thinking in their conscious actions.

Caplan emphasizes consultee-client problems that emerge when a consultee allows personal biases to interfere with objective and impartial treatment. According to him, a consultee develops **themes** (narrowed or disturbed thinking) that result from personal experiences, failures, or frustrations. Unresolved emotional conflicts persist in the unconscious or preconscious until they emerge as repetitious, stereotypical thinking. When the treatment dynamics of an existing client trigger the consultee's unresolved conflict or thinking biases, theme interference is the potential consequence. Until corrected through the help of a knowledgeable mental health consultant, disturbing themes can interfere with the client's progress in treatment.

Caplan advises that biases can manifest themselves in the form of a **syllogism** (if A exists, then B must be true) in which the consultee assumes an inevitable link between two statements or conditions (p. 145). For example, following years of counseling relationships with female victims of domestic violence, a consultee has adopted the exaggerated belief that battered wives always return home regardless of their expressed desire to leave abusive relationships. The consultee forms the syllogism in which statement A— "since all female victims of domestic violence return home"—is true, then statement B—"my current client will return home despite her intent to leave the relationship"— must also be valid. The therapist forms a theme that asserts that "all women victims of domestic violence eventually return to their abusive relationship despite their plans to terminate the relationship." Although this conviction contains elements of truth, the theme is distorted and overgeneralized to the extent that it leads to superficial support and effort with respect to abused women who truly wish to end abusive relationships.

Themes consist of the *Initial Category,* the condition or situation included in statement A, and the *Inevitable Outcome,* the disturbed belief or bias included in statement B (Caplan, 1970, p. 158). Although addressing theme interference is often a sensitive and intricate process, the central tasks are to: (1) identify the initial category through observations of the consultee's emotional or cognitive responses to specific questions, and (2) "weaken the obligatory link between the initial category and its inevitable outcome" (Mendoza, 1993, p. 632). The expectation is that the consultee will link case conference information and material with unconscious variables. Caplan (1970) describes four indirect or displaced strategies that can reduce theme interference. First, by *verbally focusing on the client,* the consultant makes the true and factual details of the case the overt focus of the consultation process. This approach helps to undercut the consultee's unfounded assumptions. Mental health consultants may also rely on *parables or stories* to address the consultee's unconscious beliefs or conflicts. Creative parables, though seemingly distanced from the current case, allow the consultant to communicate with the consultee's unconscious rather than through accusations or blame. A third strategy endorses the consultant's *nonverbal focus on the client.* The consultant addresses inappropriate themes through a confident and poised demeanor. By appearing relaxed, the consultant gives the impression that the outcome the consultee anticipates is remote. Caplan recommends a fourth strategy in which the consultant *focuses nonverbally on the consultant-consultee relationship.* When the consultee transfers a disturbing or inhibiting theme into the relationship, the consultant accepts the truth of the theme's Initial Category. Then, through nonverbal behavior inconsistent with the theme's Inevitable Outcome, the consultant provides observable evidence of the theme's false nature.

Program-Centered Administrative Consultation   The **program-centered administrative consultation** approach extends consultation efforts to program, rather than human, deficits. This approach is similar to client-centered case consultation, with the exception that, in the latter situation, the client is a program or organization. The types of organizational issues consultants encounter in program-centered consultation are multifaceted, requiring competencies in organizational theory and practice (see Box 3.3).

Assignments involving programs and organizations require mental health consultants to broaden consultation boundaries. Consultants must view the client as a program rather than as an individual. In this type of consultation, the consultant is responsible for providing a comprehensive assessment of organizational efficiency as well as feedback and recommendations on program problems. Caplan urges consultants, following their assessment of organizational imperfections, to prepare a report detailing the need for and dynamics of program changes. Such changes often demand organizational changes, altered job descriptions, or the disclosure of sensitive information. Caplan cautions, however, that consultants must formulate recommendations that are considerate, timely, and realistic. Idealistic or global suggestions that have little relevance to the organizational setting result in only superficial or inappropriate solutions.

Consultee-Centered Administrative Consultation   The **consultee-centered administrative consultation** approach is similar to the consultee-centered case approach except that the consultee's request for help is related to deficient administrative, rather than treatment, skills. Although consultees often perceive this type of consultation as focusing on existing administrative problems, the underlying purpose is to strengthen the consultee's problem-solving and management skills so as to be able to cope with future administrative problems (see Box 3.4).

Box 3.3
Case example: Program-centered administrative consultation

A community psychologist (*consultant*) is asked by the director (*consultee*) of a community mental health center to help establish a staff development and training program. State regulations require mental health agencies to offer such programs so that all employees have access to a system of ongoing education and skill-building opportunities. The program (*client*) should be based on state guidelines and conform to licensure and certification laws. The consultant is asked to help with program development.

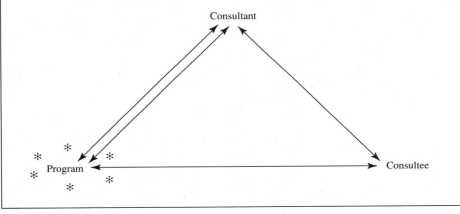

According to Caplan, consultee-centered administrative consultation often presents substantial challenges for the mental health consultant. Consultation focusing on consultees' skills, knowledge, and performance requires the consultant to exercise skill in individual and group processes, be knowledgeable about the dynamics of social systems, be prepared to address the needs of multiple consultees, and be able to manage potential conflicts.

In consultee-centered administrative consultation, consultants must be able to overcome many obstacles. Negotiating firm agreements about what makes up the consultant's role is an immediate task. In addition, consultants must garner support from all levels of the organization, particularly consultees. Because consultants often cross intraorganizational boundaries, access information from multiple levels, and disrupt normal organizational activities, they must be able to recognize and manage tension and resistance. Consultants must also be skilled at addressing the divided loyalties that emerge when consultees and subordinates have contrasting attitudes or goals. Overcoming these hurdles is necessary if trusting relationships and collaborative problem solving are to be maintained.

Consultee-centered administrative consultation interventions target organizational practices that contribute to program problems. Caplan identifies seven possible outcomes of consultee-centered administrative consultation. First, the consultant, through

Box 3.4
Case example: Consultee-centered administrative consultation

A counseling psychologist (*consultant*) enters into a consulting agreement with the supervisor (*consultee*) in a hospital's employee assistance program (*client*). The program is in its first year of operation. In addition, the program has employed all new staff. The supervisor describes his frustration with the resistance he senses from hospital staff. Referrals have been sparse, and few have even inquired about the program. Despite accreditation standards that require such programs, staff appear frustrated with the cost of the program and with hiring practices that bring "outsiders" to the hospital. The supervisor admits he has never encountered such resistance and fears serious conflict will emerge.

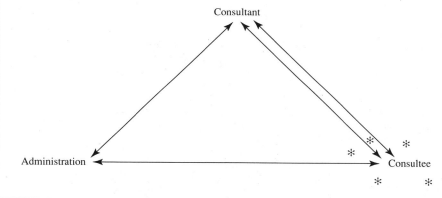

collaborative interactions, hopes to enhance the consultee's understanding of particular problems, and as a future concern, to increase the consultee's awareness of systematic methods of problem solving in general. Second, consultees often encounter organizational or client situations that result in uncomfortable emotional consequences (such as frustration, anger, fear, depression). The consultant should recognize these negative emotions, should help the consultee accept the normalcy of emotional discomfort, and when necessary, should prescribe appropriate action. Third, as they cross organizational boundaries to observe work processes or interact with members at different levels, consultants often recognize deficient communication practices. One focus of consultation, then, is to address organizational communication deficits, particularly those that result from the consultee's actions.

Fourth, since distorted or prejudicial thinking can interfere with work relationships or undermine the consultee's problem-solving efforts, consultants must often implement interventions that foster objectivity and perceptual awareness. Fifth, because leaders often have few opportunities to share their concerns with trusted associates, mental health consultants provide an objective, supportive atmosphere in which confidential

Box 3.5
Comparison of Caplan's types of mental health consultation

Consultation Type	Consultee's Identity	Focus of Consultation	Goal of Consultation
Client-centered case consultation	Direct-service deliverer	Client	Improvement in the client's problem
Consultee-centered case consultation	Direct-service deliverer	Consultee	Improvement in the consultee's treatment skills
Program-centered administrative consultation	Manager, supervisor, administrator	Program or organization	Improvement in program functions
Consultee-centered administrative consultation	Manager, supervisor, administrator	Consultee	Improvement in consultee's management skills

exchanges free leaders of the anxieties and pressures of their positions. Sixth, consultants remain alert to, and communicate to the consultee, the importance of balancing work and human contentment. Throughout the consultation process, consultants remind consultees and other organizational members of the human needs that influence work performance and policy implementation. A final potential outcome emerges when mental health consultants deliver information about the complex interpersonal factors that affect organizational functions. The consultant fulfills an educational role in helping consultees meet the psychological needs of organizational members and groups.

Mental health consultation places a high priority on accurate assessment and diagnosis. Consultants, for example, must assess consultees' characteristics and organizational problems to discern which type of consultation is most appropriate. Failing to distinguish properly among the consultation types risks ill-informed decisions and actions—conditions that may ultimately lead to failed outcomes. The four types of consultation are summarized in Box 3.5.

To reiterate, Caplan's (1970) mental health consultation model offers a sound approach to client or organizational change. A philosophy that encourages consultees to learn to help themselves has many advantages. Through the mental health consultation relationship, the consultee strengthens professional competencies, works through treatment impasses, and implements strategies to resolve present and future organizational and client problems. The goal of consultation is achieved when consultees (and their organizations) accept responsibility for their own work problems, and through a sense of self-empowerment, for their own futures.

Organizational Consultation

From large corporate entities and small businesses to human service and family systems, **organizations** consist of people working together to achieve a common purpose (Hanna, 1988). Specified or implied goals shape the mission of the individuals and groups making up an organization. Most organizations institute regulatory policies and procedures to govern their practices. A characteristic feature of larger organizations is the presence of multiple layers of leadership and supervision denoting lines of authority.

Organizations are affected by both internal and external forces promoting growth or other forms of change. Most modern organizations are immersed in an endless cycle of adaptation, problem solving, and planning, leading to an increasingly visible role for organizational consultants. These consultants are professionals from diverse backgrounds (for example, psychologists, organizational development specialists, counselors, counseling psychologists, industrial or occupational psychologists) who espouse multidisciplinary approaches and methods (Pugh & Hickson, 1989). Dougherty (1990) views organizational consultation as a comprehensive process:

> *Organizational consultation* is the process in which a professional, functioning either internally or externally to an organization, provides assistance of a technical, diagnostic/prescriptive, or facilitative nature to an individual or group from that organization in order to enhance the organization's ability to deal with change and maintain or enhance its effectiveness in some designated way. (p. 187)

Systems Theory: A Lasting Framework

Organizations have often relied on piecemeal approaches to solve problems or adapt to the future. This tendency can be seen in their somewhat compulsive integration, in various historical periods, of machine theories, group dynamics, human relations, and leadership theories into their philosophies (Gordon, 1991). In their preoccupation with singular or fragmented success formulas, organizational leaders have often overlooked the fact that organizations must incorporate multiple components and processes to achieve success (Hanna, 1988). This principle teaches that a combination of many interdependent processes determines the success of the whole organization. **Systems theory**, rooted in the field of biology (Hanna, 1988), is a widely held organizational philosophy that depicts the whole organization as one large entity or system composed of smaller, interconnected divisions. Because systems theory principles appear generalizable across organizational settings (Kurpius, 1985), organizational consultants should consider the systems implications of consultation problems.

Open Systems   According to systems theory, organizations are open, dynamic, and adaptive entities responsive to external influences (Hanna, 1988). Open systems are, as Katz, Kahn, and Adams (1980) observe, dependent on regular transactions with their surroundings: "We cannot develop an internal system of mechanics to describe organization functioning without reference to its ongoing commerce with its surroundings" (p. 5). **Open systems**, much like living organisms that breathe fresh air, contain

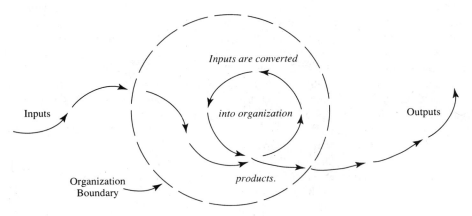

FIGURE 3.1
Open-system inputs and outputs

porous boundaries allowing a stream of organization-sustaining inputs to enter and flow throughout the organization. Once inside, inputs are converted into viable products that ultimately leave the organization as products or other outputs (Figure 3.1). Since open systems engage in continual transactions with changing, often-volatile surroundings, they must constantly import new information and adapt internal processes accordingly. Organizations that fail to adapt to fluctuating demands risk gradual decline or exhaustion (Katz, Kahn, & Adams, 1980).

Human service organizations that depend on an assortment of external inputs (community needs, trends, financial support, volunteerism, demographic data, and feedback, for example) are considered open systems.

Structural Characteristics   When consultants view organizations through a systems framework, they discover that organizations possess a relatively standard set of characteristics regardless of their setting. Most organizations have a structure consisting of a whole system and smaller divisions or other units that Brown, Pryzwansky, and Schulte (1995) describe as **subsystems**. Together, subsystems form part of an **organizational structure** (a strategic configuration of organizational functions, jobs, and policies in a pattern that best serves organizational goals).

In systems organizations, subsystems are inevitably dependent on the whole system of which they are important components. This relationship entails a supportive reciprocity in which the needs of both entities are system priorities (Kurpius, 1985). Moreover, subsystems exist in interdependent relationships in which the deficiencies in one subsystem can spread throughout the entire system. When the staff of a drug treatment program experiences morale problems, for example, surrounding subsystems (such as subsystems responsible for treatment, productivity, employee relations, and leadership) feel the effects. Ultimately, the entire drug treatment program must resolve the multiple consequences of low staff morale.

Each subsystem is systematically tied to other subsystems. Interventions that target the deficiencies in one subsystem should propose collateral or complementary changes within surrounding subsystems (Chin & Benne, 1976). Solutions to systems problems, therefore, must be multifaceted and comprehensive. Katz and Kahn (1966) define the principle of **equifinality**, which emphasizes that there are no single solutions to systems problems and that organization revitalization can occur through many alternative actions. Returning to the example of the drug treatment program with staff morale problems, organizational leaders who adhered to the principle of equifinality could choose from a range of potential solutions (for example, salary adjustments, workload reduction, stress management training, management-staff dialogue).

Organizations naturally vary in size; the larger the organization, the greater the need for specialization and differentiation (Brown et al., 1995). Each organization, therefore, must devise its subsystem structure and composition according to the available human and material resources. The professional literature describes a number of structural models and approaches that illustrate subsystem composition and interrelatedness (Brown et al., 1995; Fuqua & Kurpius, 1993; Hanna, 1988; Katz et al., 1980; Beer, 1980; Kurpius, 1985). Figure 3.2 depicts a generic structural model highlighting the relational quality of organizational subsystems.

Each subsystem is composed of interactive elements, processes, and responsibilities that serve the whole organization. While the specific configuration and description of subsystems in particular organizations depend on the organization's size, values, resources, and need for specialization, a number of general structural descriptions dominate the organizational literature (Fuqua & Kurpius, 1993). For purposes of discussion, we present a somewhat generic model:

1. *Administration subsystem* Organizations require a broad framework that dictates operating principles, actions, and priorities. Personnel policies, job descriptions, performance and program evaluations, and employee incentives are examples of administration subsystem priorities. Further, the administrative subsystem provides order to the organization by defining lateral and hierarchical work relationships.

2. *Planning subsystem* The planning subsystem prepares the organization to meet existing and future demands. Planning enables the organization to respond to internal and external inputs (including emerging trends, fiscal constraints and opportunities, and human or material resources) to set the organization's course. Strategic planning, visioning, and environmental scanning are examples of planning subsystem activities.

3. *Authority subsystem* The organization's governance authorizes decisions, prescribes and enforces rules, and directs work behavior. The organization's leadership, from the board of directors to middle managers and field supervisors, represents a legitimate, respected form of authority. The authority subsystem defines the organization's structure and the composition of subsystems.

4. *Production subsystem* The production subsystem specifies how internal operations manufacture and deliver products to the external environment. Products can consist of services (for example, teaching, advocacy, and networking), ma-

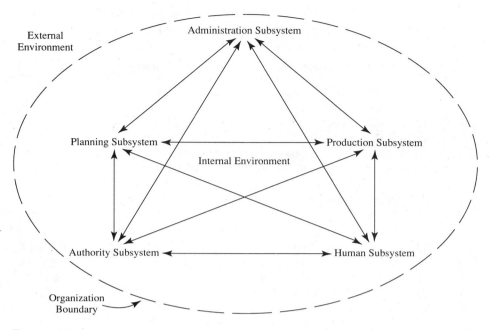

FIGURE 3.2
Subsystem interrelatedness and structure

terials (including goods and marketable products), or intangible human conditions (such as psychological well-being and adjustment). Further, technological specialization and the application of work efficiency principles represent production subsystem responsibilities.

5. *Human subsystem*　Organizations are made up of people with diverse characteristics who are engaging in complex social relations. Human behaviors, norms, and values contribute to the culture of the organization. Moreover, such human factors as motivation, morale, teamwork, and commitment are often integral to organizational productivity and longevity.

Organizational Variables and Consultation

Considerable variability exists from organization to organization, and consulting rarely proceeds according to standardized formulas or processes. Despite the variation, consultants can expect certain organizational variables to influence the consultation process. Among the more prominent variables are the organization's leadership, readiness for consultation and change, and culture.

1. *Organizational leadership* The leadership within most organizations is the medium through which organizational problems are identified, consultation processes are initiated, and organizational change is articulated. Much has been written about the influence of organizational leaders on the consultation process and related problem-solving efforts (Beer, 1980; Brown et al., 1995). Although consultants may deal directly with leaders at multiple organizational levels, their work usually occurs under the auspices of top leadership. Regardless of the source and nature of the organizational difficulties and the focus of interventions, consultants can expect the authority structure to exert powerful influences on the consultation process. Leaders typically authorize consultation, approve the direction it takes, and oversee the associated processes. Moreover, when organizational changes emerge from consultation, the attitude of leadership toward the planned changes is critical. Consultants must recognize the influence of organizational leaders, value their support, and provide incentives that reinforce their participation.

2. *Organizational readiness* The organization's acknowledgment of problems and decision to pursue consultation do not guarantee that needed organizational changes actually occur. Change requires organizational members to be open to transitions and solutions. Indeed, the organization's readiness is perhaps more important to successful consultation outcomes than the consultant's methods and interventions (Beer & Spector, 1993). A positive state of readiness requires organizational members and consultants to address a range of potentially inhibiting factors. Gordon (1991) summarizes the conditions that often impede an organization's readiness and hence the consultant's success:

> Specific forces against change include employees' distrust of a change event, fear of change, desire to maintain power, and complacency; lack of resources to support the change; conflicts between individual and organizational goals; and organizational inertia against changing the status quo. (p. 700)

3. *Organizational culture* The **organizational culture** represents the unique pattern of acceptable rules, beliefs, rituals, and behaviors that define organizational processes and responsibilities. The organization's culture evolves from organizational members' need to adapt to their surroundings and represents a powerful influence on the consultation process. Fuqua and Kurpius (1993) provide three explanations that clarify the importance of cultural variants. First, the organization's culture is the medium through which organizational members greet outside constituents and adapt to the unfamiliar conditions connected with consultation. Next, the organizational culture is often integral to the organization's recognition of problems. How problems are conceptualized and interpreted, for example, often depends on cultural norms and values. Further, the culture of the organization has often preserved core values and beliefs over a long period. Because it is enduring and resilient, the culture often resists necessary change. This can become a significant part of the consultation problem. How the consultant addresses organizational culture issues can be critical in determining the outcome of the process. Consultation interventions and subsequent organizational changes must be developed and articulated with a clear vision of how the organization's culture will be affected (Gordon, 1991).

Organizational Consultation Processes

Organizational consultation lacks a standardized, theoretical formula to define its processes and methods across organizational settings. Ultimately, consultants' roles and techniques are delineated within the context of the organizations they serve, the problems they address, and the theoretical orientation to which they subscribe. Despite the absence of a generalizable model, however, the primary objectives of organizational consultation processes are to help organizations overcome deficiencies, restore momentum or equilibrium, and provide interventions that move the organization toward its goals. These goals require several core consultation activities.

Diagnosing Organizational Problems   **Organizational diagnosis** is the process through which consultants and consultees attempt to understand the dynamics of organizational problems. Further, diagnostic processes apply "concepts and methods from the behavioral sciences to assess an organization's current state and find ways to increase its effectiveness" (Harrison, 1987, p. 1). The accuracy of diagnostic processes is considered the best predictor of successful organizational interventions (Kurpius, Fuqua, & Rozecki, 1993).

Although consultants utilize diverse diagnostic frameworks and associated techniques, a set of activities appear relatively standard. The following list of steps, based on an earlier proposal by Beer and Spector (1993), provides general guidelines for diagnosing organizational problems.

1. *Problem recognition*   The organization's leadership recognizes that a problem exists and must be addressed. Organizational problems may be complex, poorly understood, and require specialized interventions.
2. *Selecting consultants*   The organization searches for internal or external consultants to identify, assess, and conceptualize organizational problems.
3. *Data gathering*   The consultant must initiate a data gathering process that targets organizational problems and isolates causal factors.
4. *Analyzing valid information*   Consultants and consultees explore valid data sources that can yield information about organizational problems. They synthesize and analyze assessment data to determine the relationship between problems and diagnostic discoveries.
5. *Diagnostic feedback*   To complete the diagnostic process, consultants must analyze and synthesize their findings into meaningful diagnostic formulations. Feedback to consultees allows consultants and consultees to develop a conceptual framework through which corrective actions are planned and implemented.

Consultants select from a range of assessment methods to complete the diagnostic process. The most common data gathering methods include individual and group interviews, observation, questionnaires, reviews of organizational documents, surveys, and standardized organizational assessment instruments. Assessment data can be quantitative (objective and measurable) or qualitative (subjective and intuitive). The consultant's primary concern is that diagnostic data are reliable (consistent) and valid (truthful).

Organizational consultants should adhere to several technical principles in the diagnostic process. First, because each organizational problem occurs within a unique organizational environment, *diagnostic processes must be tailored to the organization's characteristics and consultation goals.* The nature of the consultation problem and the purpose of consultation provide early direction for the consultant's diagnostic efforts.

Second, because organizational problems differ with respect to the organizational territory they afflict, *organizational assessment practices often target multiple organizational levels.* Cooper and O'Connor (1993) describe assessment strategies suited to specific processes at individual, group, and organizational levels. Problems at individual levels include process issues involving individuals (such as job satisfaction, skill deficits, and role clarification). Problems at group levels are those pertaining to groups (for example, teamwork and interface conflict). Problems at organizational levels encompass systemwide issues (such as organizational policies, culture, and structure).

Third, because of the broad scope of many organizational problems, *assessment processes should integrate multiple methods* (Brown et al., 1995). Cooper and O'Connor (1993) contend that consultants should implement a "triangulation of psychometrically sound quantitative instruments, process-oriented 'soft' surveys, and qualitative methods" (p. 658). These tactics are especially suited to multifaceted organizational problems. They enable consultants, for example, to extend organizational assessment activities beyond singular assessment approaches that limit insight, suggest one dimensional interventions, and produce inadequate outcomes.

Fourth, *organizational diagnosis methods should acknowledge that organizations are made up of human behavioral (attitudes, values, knowledge) and organizational structural (organization policies, rewards, resource alignment) processes.* Deficiencies within either realm may contribute to organizational problems. Morale and stress problems among employees, for instance, represent complex human issues that suggest behaviorally oriented interventions. Conversely, unclear job descriptions or policy guidelines represent organizational structural deficits. On most occasions, consultants must acknowledge that behavioral and structural elements are rarely mutually exclusive (Aplin, 1978). This appears particularly valid for systems organizations where human problems (such as low morale) and structural solutions (for example, improvement in work incentives) are inevitably interwoven. Thus, organizational consultants must always be cognizant of both approaches to problem solving (Kurpius et al., 1993); otherwise they may propose inappropriate interventions (Aplin, 1978).

A final principle stresses that *the assessment process should be conceived and implemented through collaborative efforts.* Though consultants can facilitate the process, the involvement of key organizational members is usually necessary for a favorable outcome. For example, when consultees help to generate key organizational information, they express greater acceptance of and commitment to the problem-solving process (Beer & Spector, 1993; Harrison, 1987). Moreover, a strong partnership between consultants and organizational members adds to consultees' understanding of organizational problems and patterns of defensiveness (Cooper & O'Connor, 1993). Further, Harrison (1987) points out that "participation . . . enhances the possibility that members will develop the capacity to assess their own operations" (p. 9).

Organizational Intervention Models   Consultants and consultees have a choice of several organizational intervention models. Which they select depends on their personal and professional competencies and experience and on the unique needs of each organization. A detailed discussion of every approach is beyond the scope of this chapter, but we highlight a few representative models.

Content and Process Consultation   Although consultants generally agree that consultation is meant to be a purposeful helping process, many disagree about what constitutes effective helping (Schein, 1978). To some, consultation implies a supervising, directing, or technical assistance role in which the consultant adopts responsibility for the organization's problems. Others view consultation as a collaborative, empowering process in which consultees are active, integral participants. To distinguish between content and process strategies, Schein (1978) advises that "content refers to the actual task to be performed or problem to be solved, while process refers to the *way* in which the problem is attacked" (p. 340). In content-oriented consultation, consultants presume that consultees lack understanding or awareness. Thus, providing specialized information or expertise is essential to successful problem solving. Content-oriented consultation would be required, for example, by the director of a mental health center who is confused about the implementation of a computer-based client tracking system. In this example, the consultant's role primarily involves the sharing of expertise and information.

Schein (1987) suggests two types of content-oriented helping models: (1) the *purchase-of-expertise* model (p. 340), in which the consultee understands that deficiencies exist and wants the consultant to correct them, and (2) the *doctor-patient* model (p. 341), in which the consultee has neither a clear idea of what the problem is nor an idea of how to resolve it. In both, the expert-based consultant's role is active and influential, while the consultee's participation is passive and minimal.

According to Schein (1987): "Process consultation is a set of activities on the part of the consultant that help the client [consultee] to perceive, understand, and act upon the process events that occur in the client's [consultee's] environment" (p. 34). Content and process models are compared in Box 3.6.

The decision to engage in process-oriented consultation must take several factors into account. Schein (1987) outlines some of these conditions. Consultees, for example, must own the consultation problem and commit to active participation with respect to problem solving. If they are active participants in the process, all decisions and solutions must reflect their insight and judgment. This, Schein believes, leads to a positive disposition in which consultees accept and commit to consultation processes. Next, he contends that consultees, to perform consultation tasks and propose appropriate solutions, must possess the necessary cognitive and behavioral competencies. Through the collective experiences brought by their participation, consultees learn how to solve future organization problems.

Schein (1987) emphasizes that consultants must identify and suggest improvements to inefficient organizational processes, including those that entail "problem solving, decision making, and organizational effectiveness in general" (p. 39). The process consultant must, therefore, be adept in understanding the fundamental task and interpersonal

Box 3.6
A comparison of content and process consultation models

Style of Helping	Focus of Consultation	Consultant's Role	Consultee's Role
Content-oriented consultation	Provide knowledge that facilitates organizational solutions	Expert-based; to assume responsibility for solutions	Passive and compliant; responsive to consultant's solutions
Process-oriented consultation	Identifiy the processes that contribute to organizational problems	Process-based; to work jointly with consultees to solve problems	Active and participatory; owns the consultation problem

processes that enable individuals, groups, and organizations to function smoothly. Although Schein (1969) initially introduced content and process consultation approaches as separate, exclusive models, he later proposed a revised model that reflects the interconnecting and overlapping qualities of content and process consultation (Rockwood, 1993).

Altering Organizational Paradigms An organization's structure, operating regularities, and production methods are often dictated by generational and deeply entrenched values that govern key organizational elements. As organizational beliefs are passed on, especially when they lead to success, they evolve into invariable and often unchallenged rules, or **paradigms**. According to Barker (1992): "A paradigm is a set of rules and regulations (written or unwritten) that does two things: (1) it establishes or defines boundaries; and (2) it tells you how to behave inside the boundaries in order to be successful" (p. 32). Paradigms are powerful and resilient. They are more implacable than many of the rules and biases that come and go with organizational trends. Indeed, many organizational leaders adhere so firmly to paradigms that they fail to recognize the need to challenge those that are no longer in the organization's best interests. Beer and Spector (1993) could be writing about organizational paradigms in a description of the blindness that besets many executives:

> Organizational members become committed to a pattern of behavior. They escalate their commitment to that pattern out of a sense of self-justification. In a desire to avoid embarrassment and threat, few if any challenges are made to the wisdom and viability of these behaviors. (p. 642)

Early writings about the influence of paradigms suggest that change and discovery are often linked more to established paradigms and their associated rules than to truth, reality, and the need for change (Kuhn, 1962). Although the notion of paradigms was advanced by Kuhn (1962) to explain the nature of scientific change, they hold useful explanations for organizational decision making. As Barker (1992) puts it: "The points Kuhn makes about scientific paradigm shifts are true for any situation where strongly held rules and regulations exist" (p. 40). As they relate to organizations, paradigms are firmly grounded rules that have proven successful in the past. Dilts, Epstein, and Dilts (1991) explain that "we often limit our creativity because it's so easy to go back to what we've always done" (p. 44).

As long as organizational paradigms and the associated rules match environmental trends, demands, and technologies, they serve organizations faithfully—even to the point that organizations become totally reliant on them. Organizations decline or even fail, however, when their leaders are unwaveringly committed to paradigms that operate in contradiction to the organization's needs. Since organizations cannot survive when their products are no longer valued by their environments, organizations must occasionally alter or shift their paradigms. A **paradigm shift** represents an alteration in the conceptual thinking that people use to interpret their circumstances (Fuqua & Kurpius, 1993).

Paradigm shifts are often the products of slow and arduous change, and for many organizations, such change occurs only after their "typical problem-solving strategies have failed" (Fuqua & Kurpius, 1993, p. 615). Fuqua and Kurpius (1993) have proposed a novel approach in which consultants help organizational leaders accelerate the paradigm shift process. Helping organizations identify obsolete paradigms and replace them with organization-sustaining practices is not easy, however. The work of consultants attempting to facilitate paradigm shifts is eased somewhat when they observe these guidelines:

1. Organizational members must recognize obsolete beliefs and be open to the paradigm shift (Fuqua & Kurpius, 1993). Without recognizing the need for change, leaders can drive organizations into chaos and decline.
2. Consultants should involve the organization's leaders and members in the analysis of repetitive patterns of behavior that do not match environmental demands (Beer & Spector, 1993). Acceptance of paradigm shifts is fueled by collaborative and empowering strategies.
3. Because paradigm shifts are often responsive to anticipated events, trends, and conditions, consultants must anticipate the organization's future (Barker, 1992).
4. Consultants must anticipate and address strong resistance to the paradigm shift. Many organizational constituents will remain committed to old standards despite the apparent futility of these standards.
5. Consultants must dispel unrealistic or fearful thinking that paradigm shifts are "risk-everything" change strategies (Dilts et al., 1991; Fuqua & Kurpius, 1993). Consultants can help organizations address the most pressing needs and, as a matter of caution, change gradually.
6. Consultants must help organizational members cope effectively with the changes that emerge when new beliefs and practices are integrated into the organization's infrastructure. The transition period often represents a period of crisis.

Strategic Short- and Long-Range Planning   Even well-established organizations risk failure when they do not plan for changing and often volatile circumstances.

Strategic planning, whether short- or long-range, is a broad process through which organizational leaders scan existing realities and envision trends to help the organization prepare for and achieve its future. In contrast to stagnant, nonplanning organizations that react passively or impulsively to whatever the future brings, strategic planning organizations create and guide their own futures. Consider, for example, a child development program that anticipates major program expansion, higher enrollments, and broader service demands. The program recognizes that strategic planning is necessary to arrange staffing patterns and construct physical facilities to meet the challenges of the future. Through strategic planning, the program eases into the future by actualizing preplanned program alternatives.

Strategic planning processes encompass sequential and developmental activities that help organizations prepare for expected realities. Scanning potential environmental trends and pressures, both current and future, represents strategic planning's most unique feature (Fuqua & Kurpius, 1993). Strategic planning consultants help organizational members learn strategic planning processes, promote a framework to conduct planning, and facilitate the organization's efforts to develop a specific plan. Although the literature offers a number of strategic planning models and approaches (Barry, 1986; Bryson, 1988; Fuqua & Kurpius, 1993; Goodstein, Nolan, & Pfeiffer, 1992), a relatively standard set of activities makes up an effective planning process. They are presented here in condensed and simplified form:

1. *Operationalize the planning process.* Organizations must prepare to plan by arranging for organizational resources and personnel.
2. *Prioritize organizational values.* Organizations must identify their products and ensure the planning process begins with conceptual understanding of the most important needs.
3. *Envision the future.* Anticipating future trends and developments is a prerequisite to present planning.
4. *Ascertain the organization's mission.* The organization's mission is the overarching goal that defines the organization's reason for existence.
5. *Generate strategic options.* Taking various courses of action into account will add substance to the plan.
6. *Plan for obstacles and contingencies.* Planning must prepare for the resistance and other barriers imposed by organizational constituents.
7. *Translate plans into visible organizational practices.* Without concrete actions, planning remains a wasteful and superficial organizational endeavor.
8. *Continue planning.* Planning is never complete. Even the most effective strategic plan must be evaluated, modified, or updated to reflect new trends and environmental demands.

The list of possible organizational interventions far exceeds those described in this chapter. As consultants and organizational leaders search for the best solutions to problems, they will find many other useful approaches. A few other alternatives deserve mention in this section, although again the list is far from complete:

- Organizational effectiveness (Ridley & Mendoza, 1993)
- Organizational culture (Fuqua & Kurpius, 1993; Schein, 1985)
- Organizational development (Huse, 1978)

- High-performance organizations (Hanna, 1988; Nelson & Burns, 1984)
- Data-based consultation (Newman & Fuqua, 1984)
- Cyclical organizations (Blake & Mouton, 1976)

In summary, given the complexities of organizations and the environments in which they operate, the consultant must be able to participate in diverse activities and formulate a broad range of conceptual interventions. Recognizing that organizations are dynamic, adaptive systems is also critical. Organizational consultation encompasses multiple, often overlapping processes that require the consultant to enter complex systems, diagnose organizational deficiencies, and apply conceptual interventions tailored to specific organizational problems.

Behavioral Consultation

In **behavioral consultation**, the principles of behavioral psychology are integrated into the framework of consultation. As consultants who help consultees solve client or work-related issues through a triadic, problem-solving approach, behavioral specialists apply the processes of mediation, collaboration, and instruction. Behavioral consultation has evolved to the point where consultants can choose from among a wide range of applications and ideologies to address behavioral changes in client populations.

Behavioral consultants utilize philosophies rooted in the larger domain of behavioral or learning theory. The ideologies, methods, and applications selected vary with the consultant's preferences. Some writers, for example, describe consultation approaches that apply behavioral principles only to clients' overt behaviors (Bergan, 1977; Dougherty, 1990; Gallessich, 1982). Others outline a social learning approach to the consultation process in which cognitive factors and observational learning are major determinants of one's behavior (Brown et al., 1995). Still others describe behavioral consultation within a cognitive-behavior framework that blends overt (that is, observable behaviors) and covert (for example, cognitions, thoughts) processes to define and resolve consultation problems (Brack et al., 1993). Regardless of the approach selected, however, all are founded on theoretical learning principles that "share the scientific heritage of behavioral psychology and are therefore similar in a number of ways" (Brown, Pryzwansky, & Schulte, 1991, p. 68).

Behavioral consultants must have a knowledge base that reflects the views of behavioral psychologists and theorists and that reflects the following premises about human behavior:

1. Human behavior, whether adaptive or maladaptive, is the product of learning (Gallessich, 1982).
2. Behavior occurs according to distinct, lawful, and systematic principles (Corey, 1986; Dougherty, 1990).
3. Human behavior is measurable and can be empirically validated (Russell, 1978).
4. Human behavior is the product of the interaction between behavior and environmental influences (Bandura, 1969).
5. Human behavior consists of overt and covert processes (Brack et al., 1993).

Behavioral consultation is most often a client-oriented approach in which consultants and consultees prepare behavioral plans to correct a client's maladaptive behavior (Bergan, 1977). Consultants are attracted to behavioral consultation approaches because they offer well-defined methods of problem solving and are relatively standardized with respect to theories of human behavior and behavioral change technologies.

Bergan's Behavioral Consultation Model

J. R. Bergan (1977) is credited with extending behavioral principles to the psychological consultation field. Because he has formulated a cogent model, the present discussion draws heavily on his work. Bergan views consultation as an indirect, problem-solving process in which an expert consultant utilizes psychological data in interpreting consultation problems and designing behavioral interventions.

According to Bergan, three constituents interact in behavioral consultation: the behavioral consultant, the consultee, and the client. Each has distinct behaviors and role responsibilities that contribute to the consultation process. Since consultation problems are conceptualized within a behavioral framework, consultation activities must conform to behavioral principles.

The Consultant's Role   The behavioral consultant's role is that of a behavioral expert who assesses the client's maladaptive behavior and its effects. The consultant follows a systematic approach to helping and strives to "establish the stages in the consultation process and to guide the consultee through them" (Bergan, 1977, p. 11). Consultants help devise the intervention plan and monitor its implementation. Because the consultant's specialized skills and knowledge are integral to behavioral consultation, he or she has a degree of authority that encourages the consultee to comply with consultation goals. The consultant, though having a general responsibility for the consultee's client, has no formal, direct relationship with the client (Bergan, 1977).

The Consultee's Role   The consultee's role is integral to the consultation process. Consultees must work directly with clients, put behavioral plans into action, and evaluate the success of behavioral change strategies. Bergan describes four prominent functions that make the consultee's role critical to the success of consultation: (1) specification or description—the consultee must describe the client's problem or behavior that prompts the consultation request; (2) evaluation or decision making—the consultee must judge the validity of suggested behavioral plans and evaluate their efficacy; (3) working with the client—the consultee must assess the client's behavior or performance and implement behavioral strategies designed to alter such behavior in desirable directions; and (4) supervision or monitoring—the consultee is responsible for supervising the client's behavioral changes relative to consultation interventions.

The Client's Role   Depending on clients' maturity and sense of responsibility, their participation in consultation planning can be highly beneficial in terms of their cooperation and commitment to consultation goals. Bergan and Kratochwill (1990) observe that a client's participation in behavioral consultation may result in more self-directed behavior and less reliance on temporary incentives. Often, however, clients are intellectually, developmentally, or behaviorally unable to conceptualize consultation problems and proposed changes. On these occasions, clients are recipients of and re-spondents to the behavioral conditions established through the consultation process.

Problem-Solving Processes   Behavioral consultation is most often initiated by a consultee who requests help with the management of a client (for example, child, student, employee, or other individual). Should consultation proceed through a case-oriented approach, the consultant and consultee address the behavior of a specific individual with whom the consultee has engaged in some type of formal care. Throughout, behavioral principles guide a consulting process that has the explicit goal of helping the consultee assess problem behaviors and identify conditions that encourage such behaviors. Bergan's (1977) advice for consultants can be summarized with a few general guidelines:

1. Consultees must be active participants throughout the behavioral consultation process. They have specific responsibilities for identifying behavioral problems and implementing interventions.
2. An integral function of the behavioral problem-solving process is the development of problem-solving skills in clients.
3. Problem solving encompasses a range of strategies for the design and implementation of systematic psychological principles.
4. Problem-solving decisions are grounded in convincing research evidence about human learning.
5. Consultation problem solvers view a client's problems as extraindividual and accept responsibility for implementing conditions that promote behavioral change.
6. Problem-solving endeavors recognize the contributions of environmental factors to human behavior.
7. Problem solving emphasizes evaluative and goal attainment processes rather than the client's individual characteristics.

Problem-Solving Stages   Case-oriented behavioral consultation requires a collaborative relationship in which consultants and consultees address the maladaptive or problematic behaviors of individual clients or groups. The consultant brings substantial expertise to bear on a process that identifies problems, analyzes information, implements a change-oriented behavioral plan, and evaluates consultation success. The behavioral consultation model that Bergan (1977) espouses proceeds through a series of four stages that, cumulatively, afford structure and direction to the consultation process. Bergan's stages, each having specific objectives and tasks, include the problem identification stage, the problem analysis stage, the plan implementation stage, and the problem evaluation stage.

1. *The problem identification stage*   Behavioral consultants as a group contend that the collection of precise, discerning information leads to accurate recognition of

behavioral problems (Bergan & Tombari, 1976). Thus, the importance of correctly identifying and assessing problems cannot be overstated. Identifying problem behaviors requires the consultant and consultee to form a problem-solving relationship in which the specification and synthesis of case-related information is paramount. Through data collection processes and a "problem-identification interview" (Bergan, 1977, p. 89), consultants and consultees orient themselves with respect to the client's target behaviors. During this phase, the consultant relies on specialized expertise to define the client's behavior within the context of behavioral principles. Formulated in succinct behavioral terms rather than in terms of ambiguous psychological or mental states, the consultation problem represents the discrepancy between a client's actual behavior and the behavior desired by the consultee (Kaufman, 1971). The ultimate consultation objective, according to Kaufman (1971), is to eliminate this discrepancy.

2. *The problem analysis stage*   The behavioral approach to consultation is predicated on a thorough study of the client's behavior and the creation of a framework in which behavioral interventions can be applied. The problem analysis stage represents a critical period in which consultation focuses on the variables that influence problem behaviors and their resolution. One objective at this point is the isolation of the environmental conditions that exert important influences on a client's behavior. Bergan (1977), in keeping with his emphasis on operant principles, advises consultants to identify **antecedents** (conditions that occur immediately before the behavior), **consequences** (conditions that occur immediately following the behavior), and **sequential conditions** (pattern of times or days in which the behavior occurs) that characterize the client's behavior. Although the consultant-consultee relationship is generally described as collaborative, the consultant exerts a leading role in the interpretation of information within a behavioral framework. Ultimately, the problem analysis stage results in a **behavioral plan** that prescribes the conditions necessary to correct or eliminate the client's maladaptive behavior.

3. *The plan implementation stage*   Because they interact in important ways with the client, consultees must implement behavioral plans and monitor clients' behavior in response to them. Translating a substantive behavioral plan into action, however, is a difficult process in which the consultee must apply appropriate behavioral techniques (a few representative methods are illustrated in Table 3.1). Successful consultation at this juncture depends on the precision and consistency with which behavioral plans are enacted. At this point, consultants also monitor plan implementation, work to repair consultee skill deficits, and propose revisions when unexpected outcomes emerge.

4. *The problem evaluation stage*   Consultants and consultees must integrate evaluation procedures into the consultation process to determine to what extent a client's behavior has changed. Evaluation of the overall success of consultation is achieved through measuring the client's behavior relative to consultation objectives. Evaluation data emerge from observations, documented rating forms and checklists, and comparisons between pre- and postintervention behavior. Depending on the degree to which consultation objectives are met, the consultant and consultee determine whether consultation should terminate, the behavioral plan must continue, or plan revisions must be implemented.

An example of case-oriented behavioral consultation is presented in Box 3.7.

TABLE 3.1
Common behavioral methods

Method	Process
Positive reinforcement	To increase the occurrence of desirable behavior, the application of positive conditions (praise, attention, privilege, tokens) if the subject's performance warrants it
Negative reinforcement	The removal of an aversive condition if the subject engages in desirable behavior
Punishment	To decrease the occurrence of undesirable behavior, the application of aversive conditions depending on the subject's performance
Extinction	Eliminating an undesirable behavior by terminating the conditions that reinforce the subject's performance
Ignoring	Eliminating the subject's undesirable behavior through inattention to it
Shaping	Changing the subject's undesirable behavior through the positive reinforcement of successive approximations of the desirable behavior
Differential reinforcement	Increasing the subject's performance of desirable behaviors through the selective reinforcement of desirable behaviors and ignoring the undesirable behaviors
Environmental cues	Environmental stimuli that prompt the subject's behavior
Inadvertent reinforcement	Inadvertently or unintentionally reinforcing the subject's behavior by creating conditions that have an effect opposite of that anticipated
Contingency contracting	The process of formalizing an agreement that specifies the behavioral conditions or plans associated with behavioral change
Behavioral rehearsal	An educational learning process in which subjects practice new, adaptive behavior in a controlled setting

Verbal Processes Problem solving requires the acquisition of information and the subsequent translation of client-related information into a behavioral framework (Bergan, 1977). For these reasons, Bergan (1977) and Bergan and Kratochwill (1990) contend that the verbal exchanges between consultants and consultees are at the heart of the entire consultation process. Brown et al. (1995) allude to Bergan and Kratochwill's comprehensive model of verbal interaction:

> Although the importance of the verbal interchange in consultation is recognized by all consultants, they place more emphasis upon this area because they view the consultant's utterances as the key not only to eliciting the information required to assess the problem but to influencing consultee behavior as well. (p. 54)

Box 3.7
Case example: Case-oriented behavioral consultation

A counseling psychologist is asked to help the teacher in a child development program reduce the "wandering" behaviors of a four-year-old boy. The child is compliant most of the time with the exception of story time, in which all the children are asked to sit in a circle, listen quietly, and participate in interactive story-telling activities. The boy rarely joins the group; he prefers wandering around the classroom, randomly playing with toys or puzzles. The behavioral consultant arranges a case oriented discussion with the teacher, collects data through a brief interview and child observation, and reviews the associated records and documents. The child observation reveals that the boy resists group activities until the teacher admonishes him several times and eventually takes him by the hand and requires him to sit beside her in the group circle. The consultant realizes that this action reinforces his wandering behavior. Together, the consultant and teacher agree to a behavioral plan in which the teacher ignores the boy's wandering behavior, offers positive attention only when he joins the group, and focuses on positively reinforcing social peers who join the group cooperatively. The teacher agrees to try the plan for three weeks, until the next consultation meeting.

The consultant's delivery of behaviorally oriented statements and questions influences, even directs, the consultee's responses. The purpose, according to Dougherty (1995), is not to "control the specific content of the consultee's verbalizations" (p. 289), but to solicit the types of responses needed to solve consultation problems. For the benefit of consultants, Bergan (1977) devised a classification system that categorizes verbal interactions according to their content, process, and method of control. This model incorporates seven content subcategories that form the data gathering content of consultant-consultee verbalizations:

1. *Background-environment*   This subcategory includes discussions that focus on the client's background and environmental conditions. The consultant's verbalizations elicit information that, although remote in time and location, could have a delayed or prolonged effect on the client's current behavior.
2. *Behavior setting*   Verbalizations in this subcategory elicit information about the client's immediate environment and its influence on the problematic behavior. The conditions that occur immediately before and after the behavior and the pattern (the specific times or days in which the behavior occurs) are the subject of verbalizations in this subcategory.
3. *Behavior*   Behavior subcategory verbalizations elicit information that leads to a precise understanding of the client's behavior. Consultants want to know the frequency, strength, and duration of the behavior—characteristics that will affect behavioral intervention plans.

4. *Individual characteristics*   These verbalizations identify individual client characteristics that may influence the problem behavior. Personality attributes, physical build, and intelligence are among relevant client characteristics.
5. *Observation*   Verbalizations that elicit information about data gathering and behavior assessment are integral to the observation subcategory.
6. *Plan.* Verbalizations that refer to the approaches or plans aimed at behavioral change are included in this subcategory. Plan verbalizations may be specific or general.
7. *Other*   This content subcategory represents a residual category for verbalizations that cannot be categorized elsewhere.

Bergan (1977) advises consultants to use an assortment of "message processes" to derive information from consultees (p. 37). While content subcategories reflect the nature of information about client behavior, message processes refer to the dynamics of how information is presented and discussed (Dougherty, 1990). Five types of message processes can assist the behavioral consultant in securing information on client behavior: (1) specification—verbalizations designed to elicit precise information; (2) evaluation—verbal processes that indicate how the consultee feels about or reacts to the client's behavior; (3) inference—verbalizations that rely on judgment rather than fact; (4) summarization—verbal processes that review earlier information or findings; and (5) validation—verbal processes that seek agreement or disagreement.

Message processes serve planned or purposeful strategies in consultant-consultee interactions. Consultants, for example, can direct dialogue by posing the types of questions or statements presented to consultees. Bergan presents two types of "message control" verbalizations that, when expressed by the consultant, direct consultee verbalizations into specific content and process subcategories (p. 43). According to him, **elicitors** are verbal behaviors that call for a response to content and process questions. For instance, when a behavioral consultant asks a fourth-grade teacher, "What happens when Tommy kicks Lenny?," the verbalization guides the consultee's response. With this verbal elicitor, the consultant targets the behavior-setting content subcategory and the specification message process subcategory. Bergan describes **emitters** as verbal responses that react to the verbalization of the speaker. Emitters include content and process categories without calling for a specific response. For example, when a behavioral consultant responds to a parent, "I can see that Timmy has behaved this way for quite a while" (background-environment content subcategory and inference emitter), the parent's response is spontaneous, open, and flexible, governed only by personal or intuitive reasoning.

Other Behavioral Consultation Approaches

Bergan's behavioral consultation model emphasizes an operant approach (the use of reinforcement, punishment, and shaping) to learning (Brown et al., 1991). Though it is a now-classic approach that warrants the attention of students and beginning consultants, dramatic shifts have taken place in the learning field, giving rise to new methodologies (Brack et al., 1993). **Social learning theory,** for example, is based on the principle that, while all human behavior is learned, complex human learning cannot be explained adequately by classical or operant mechanisms alone (Wallace, 1986). Bandura (1969) contends that people are able to observe, construe, and evaluate their environment, and indeed that human learning must entail distinct cognitive factors. The role of **self-efficacy** (the belief in one's ability to succeed or accomplish something) can be a critical determinant in behavioral learning (Bandura, 1989). Social learning theory (SLT) emphasizes the dynamic interactions among a client's behavior, interpersonal elements (for example, cognitions and perceptions of self-efficacy), and environmental factors (Brack et al., 1993). Human behavior involves a process of **reciprocal determinism**, in which behavioral factors interact and influence each other (Wallace, 1986). Brown et al. (1991), known for their advancement of social learning principles as a consultation model, suggest two assumptions that must guide the application of these principles to consultation. First, consultants must examine the consultee's and client's behavior within a social learning framework, and, more specifically, with reference to the principle of reciprocal determinism. Second, the consultant's task is to facilitate change in the existing relationship among the consultee's behavior, intrapsychic elements, and environmental forces that inhibits successful client treatment. The consultee learns, in turn, to apply these two principles to client relationships.

The prominent role of cognitive factors in learning fuels the emergence of cognitive-behavior approaches that emphasize the role of covert thinking processes (Adler, 1969; Beck, 1976; Ellis, 1962, 1973; Meichenbaum, 1977). **Cognitive-behavior theory** is rooted in the belief that human thoughts and images are integral to behavior and emotions. Disturbances within cognitive processes, therefore, contribute to the client's maladaptive state. Within a consultation framework, the cognitions, behaviors, and life experiences of consultants, consultees, and clients often contribute to problems (Brack et al., 1993). Cognitive-behavior consultation, for example, may be extended to the consultee who demonstrates distorted, irrational demands in the area of personal performance. The cognitive-behavior consultant, like the operant or case-oriented behavioral consultant, follows a systematic process of assessment, goal setting, and evaluation, except that each is conducted within a cognitive-behavior framework.

To reiterate, behavioral consultation offers specialized, scientifically formulated models emphasizing the potential for patterned, problem-focused consulting. Based on the principles of behavioral theory and advanced through scores of research inquiries and hypotheses about human behavior, behavioral consultation practices emphasize the relationship between clients and their environments and maladaptive learning. Bergan's (1977) behavioral consultation model, Bandura's (1978) social learning model, cognitive-behavior perspectives, and behavioral training provide a foundation for effective behavioral consultation.

SUMMARY

Consultation is a complex and diverse professional activity that lacks strong unifying theories and ideologies. Consultants across the psychological disciplines rely on selected models or approaches to supply the structure and methodologies needed to perform consultation tasks. The chapter highlighted three approaches. In the first approach—the mental health consultation model—consultants collaborate with the deliverers of direct mental health services to meet the needs of clients and consumers. A second approach, organizational consultation, emphasizes the application of consultants' expertise to organizational or systems problems. The third model, behavioral consultation, integrates behavioral psychology and the data generated by behavioral research into the framework of consultation. The chapter defined each approach, explored process issues, and offered representative case examples.

GLOSSARY

Antecedents   In behavioral theory, a term describing the conditions that occur immediately before a specific behavior.

Behavioral consultation   An approach to consultation that integrates behavioral psychology and research into consultation practices.

Behavioral plan   In behavioral consultation, a framework through which consultees implement changes within the client's environment that eliminate problem behaviors.

Characterological distortions   In Caplan's (1970) mental health consultation model, a source of consultee-client impasse in which the consultee's psychiatric disturbances distort perceptions of the client's behavior.

Client-centered case consultation   A type of mental health consultation in which a professional consultant extends specialized knowledge to help a consultee with an existing client-related issue.

Cognitive-behavior theory   A learning theory that posits that human learning integrates cognitive (thoughts, interpretations, images) and behavioral (emotions, actions) factors.

Consequences: In behavioral theory, a term that describes the conditions that occur immediately following a specific behavior.

Consultee-centered administrative consultation   A type of mental health consultation in which a professional consultant extends specialized knowledge to address a consultee's deficient administrative or program skills.

Consultee-centered case consultation   A type of mental health consultation in which a professional consultant extends specialized knowledge to address consultee characteristics that inhibit a client's treatment.

Direct personal involvement   In Caplan's (1970) mental health consultation model, a source of consultee-client impasse where the consultee replaces the professional relationship with a personal relationship.

Displaced discussions   Consultant-consultee interactions that avoid confrontation. A consultee's biases or stereotypes are displaced onto or approached through parables, anecdotes, or dramatic portrayals.

Elicitor   A term proposed by Bergan (1977) to describe the direct and information-specific questions used by behavioral consultants to control the consultees' responses. Elicitor questions direct the content of consultant-consultee interaction.

Emitter   A term proposed by Bergan (1977) to describe open-ended, noncontrolling questions or statements used by behavioral consultants to acquire information from consultees about a client's behavior. Emitter statements encourage consultees to respond with autonomy and spontaneity.

Equifinality   A principle that emphasizes that there are no single solutions to organization systems problems and that organizational revitalization can occur through many alternative actions. The principle was defined by Katz and Kahn (1966).

Mental health consultation   A model of consultation in which professional consultants work directly with consultees to address the mental health needs of clients and consumers.

Open system   An organization dependent on its external environment for survival. Such systems are open to the influences of the external world.

Organization   A group of people working together to achieve some goal or purpose; an organization requires cooperation among people to perform work activities prescribed by established policies and procedures.

Organizational culture   The pattern of behaviors, norms, and values that prevails in an organization and shapes employee performance.

Organizational diagnosis   The process through which consultants and consultees assess organizational problem areas, isolate causal elements, and conceptualize organizational needs.

Organizational structure   The arrangement of individuals, groups, and programs (subsystems) that make up the whole organization. The primary purpose of an organization's structure is to arrange work processes and jobs to accomplish organizational goals.

Paradigm   Within an organizational context, a pattern of thinking that defines the practices, principles, and rules leading to success.

Paradigm shift   An alteration in the fundamental, conceptual thinking that organizations apply to explain their work and their future.

Program-centered administrative consultation   A type of mental health consultation in which a professional consultant addresses program, rather than human, deficits.

Reciprocal determinism   Bandura's (1978) term that describes the dynamic and reciprocal interactions among an individual's behavior, interpersonal processes, and environment.

Self-efficacy   In a social learning context, the belief in one's ability to succeed or accomplish something.

Sequential conditions   In the behavioral consultation model, a term that describes the pattern of times or days in which a specific behavior occurs.

Simple identification   In Caplan's (1970) mental health consultation model, a source of consultee-client impasse where the consultee identifies rather than empathizes with the client.

Social learning theory   The process of learning in which people learn by observing, construing, and evaluating the behaviors of others.

Strategic planning   The process through which organizational leaders scan existing realities and envision impending trends to help the organization plan for and achieve its future.

Subsystem   In systems organizations, a term that describes the smaller divisions or elements making up the total system.

Syllogism   In Caplan's (1970) mental health consultation model, the form that themes assume when consultees believe that if a specific condition exists, then an inevitable result is linked to the condition (if A exists, B must be true).

Systems theory   A widely held philosophy that depicts the organization as a whole as consisting of smaller, interactive subsystems.

Theme   In Caplan's (1970) mental health consultation model, a term that describes an unrealistic, emotionally laden belief or perception that potentially impairs therapy and other relationships.

Theme interference   In Caplan's (1970) mental health consultation model, a source of consultee-client impasse where the consultee anticipates unsuccessful client outcomes.

Transference   A source of consultee-client impasse where consultees project feelings (of past relationships or fantasies) onto the client.

ANNOTATED BIBLIOGRAPHY

Those interested in a more detailed account of mental health consultation should read Gerald Caplan's classic book, *The Theory and Practice of Mental Health Consultation* (1970). This work provides an extensive account of the experiences, views, and processes that make up Caplan's mental health consultation model. Excellent summaries of Caplan's approach can be found in Danielle Mendoza's 1993 article "A Review of Gerald Caplan's *Theory and Practice of Mental Health Consultation*" as well as in Alexander Rogawski's 1978 article "The Caplanian Model." An updated account, presented by Caplan and Caplan in their book *Mental Health Consultation and Collaboration* (1993), discusses the modifications consultants often make in modern mental health consultation practices.

For students who desire more in-depth reading in organizational consultation, we suggest several sources. *The Study of Organizations*—edited by Daniel Katz, Robert Kahn, and J. Stacy Adams (1980)—is a book of readings that examines various organizational issues. The first volume of a more recent book, *Organizational Consultation: A Casebook,* edited by Robert Conyne and James O'Neil (1992), presents a series of brief narratives that focus on critical organizational consultation issues. This book is written especially for counseling psychologists. In addition, a special 1993 issue of the *Journal of Counseling and Development,* volume 71, includes several excellent articles on organizational consultation issues. Of particular note is the article by Dale Fuqua and DeWayne Kurpius titled "Conceptual Models in Organizational Consultation."

Readers interested in behavioral consultation philosophies and methods should consider J. R. Bergan's *Behavioral Consultation* (1977). This book is a classic that outlines, in a detailed, elaborate discussion, the process of behavioral consultation. Michael Russell's article "Behavioral Consultation" (1978) offers a thorough account of the behavioral consultation process, while G. Roy Mayer's article "Behavioral Consulting: Using Behavior Modification Procedures in the Consulting Relationship" (1973) provides a practical discussion of the behavioral principles influencing consultant-consultee relationships. Chapter 11 of A. Michael Dougherty's 1995 book, *Consultation: Practice and Perspectives in School and Community Settings* (2nd ed.), is another source that addresses alternative behavioral consultation approaches.

REFERENCES AND SUGGESTED READINGS

Adler, A. (1969). *The practice and theory of individual psychology*. Paterson, NJ: Littlefield, Adams.

Aplin, J. (1978). Structural change vs. behavioral change. *Personnel and Guidance Journal, 56*(7), 407–411.

Bandura, A. (1969). *Principles of behavioral modification*. New York: Holt, Rinehart & Winston.

Bandura, A. (1978). The self system in reciprocal determinism. *American Psychologist, 33*, 344–358.

Bandura, A. (1989). Human agency in social cognitive theory. *American Psychologist, 44*(9), 1175–1184.

Bardon, J. (1985). On the verge of a breakthrough. *Counseling Psychologist, 13*(3), 355–362.

Barker, J. (1992). *Paradigms: The business of discovering the future*. New York: HarperCollins.

Barry, B. (1986). *Strategic planning workbook for nonprofit organizations*. New York: Amherst H. Wilder Foundation.

Beck, A. T. (1976). *Cognitive therapy and the emotional disorders*. New York: International Universities Press.

Beer, M. (1980). *Organizational change and development: A systems view*. Santa Monica, CA: Goodyear.

Beer, M., & Spector, B. (1993). Organizational diagnosis: Its role in organizational learning. *Journal of Counseling and Development, 71*, 642–650.

Bergan, J. R. (1977). *Behavioral consultation*. Columbus, OH: Merrill.

Bergan, J. R., & Kratochwill, T. R. (1990). *Behavioral consultation and therapy*. New York: Plenum Press.

Bergan, J. R., & Tombari, M. (1976). Consultant skill and efficiency and the implementation and outcomes of consultation. *Journal of School Psychology, 14*(1), 3–14.

Blake, R., & Mouton, J. (1976). *Consultation*. Reading, MA: Addison-Wesley.

Brack, G., Jones, E., Smith, R., White, J., & Brack, C. (1993). A primer on consultation theory: Building a flexible worldview. *Journal of Counseling and Development, 71*, 619–628.

Brown, D., Pryzwansky, W., & Schulte, A. (1991). *Psychological consultation: Introduction to theory and practice* (2nd ed.). Boston: Allyn & Bacon.

Brown, D., Pryzwansky, W., & Schulte, A. (1995). *Psychological consultation: Introduction to theory and practice* (3rd ed.). Boston: Allyn & Bacon.

Bryson, J. (1988). *Strategic planning for public nonprofit agencies*. San Francisco: Jossey-Bass.

Caplan, G. (1970). *The theory and practice of mental health consultation*. New York: Basic Books.

Caplan, G., & Caplan, R. B. (1993). *Mental health consultation and collaboration*. San Francisco: Jossey-Bass.

Chin, R., & Benne, K. (1976). General strategies for effecting changes in human systems. In W. G. Bennis, K. D. Benne, R. Chin, & K. D. Corey (Eds.), *The planning of change* (3rd ed., pp. 45–63). New York: Holt, Rinehart & Winston.

Conyne, R., & O'Neil, J. (1992). *Organizational consultation: A casebook*. Newbury Park, CA: Sage.

Cooper, S., & O'Connor, R., Jr. (1993). Standards for organizational consultation assessment and evaluation instruments. *Journal of Counseling and Development, 71*, 651–660.

Corey, G. (1986). *Theory and practice of counseling and psychotherapy* (3rd ed.). Pacific Grove, CA: Brooks/Cole.

Dilts, R., Epstein, T., & Dilts, R. (1991). *Tools for dreamers: Strategies for creativity and the structure of innovation.* Cupertino, CA: Meta Publications.

Dougherty, A. M. (1990). *Consultation: Practice and perspectives.* Pacific Grove, CA: Brooks/Cole.

Dougherty, A. M. (1995). *Consultation: Practice and perspectives in school and community settings* (2nd ed.). Pacific Grove, CA: Brooks/Cole.

Ellis, A. (1962). *Reason and emotion in psychotherapy.* Secaucus, NJ: Lyle Stuart.

Ellis, A. (1973). *Humanistic psychotherapy: The rational-emotive approach.* New York: McGraw-Hill.

Fuqua, D., & Kurpius, D. (1993). Conceptual models in organizational consultation. *Journal of Counseling and Development, 71*, 607–618.

Gallessich, J. (1982). *The profession and practice of consultation: A handbook for consultants, trainers of consultants, and consumers of consultation services.* San Francisco: Jossey-Bass.

Gallessich, J. (1985). Toward a meta-theory of consultation. *Counseling Psychologist, 13*, 336–351.

Goodstein, L., Nolan, T., & Pfeiffer, J. (1992). *Applied strategic planning: A comprehensive guide.* San Diego, CA: University Associates.

Gordon, J. (1991). *A diagnostic approach to organizational behavior* (3rd ed.). Boston: Allyn & Bacon.

Hanna, D. (1988). *Designing organizations for high performance.* Reading, MA: Addison-Wesley.

Hansen, J., Himes, B., & Meier, S. (1990). *Consultation: Concepts and practices.* Englewood Cliffs, NJ: Prentice-Hall.

Harrison, M. (1987). *Diagnosing organizations: Methods, models, and processes.* Newbury Park, CA: Sage.

Huse, E. (1978). Organization development. *Personnel and Guidance Journal, 56*, 403–406.

Katz, D., & Kahn, R. (1966). *The social psychology of organizations.* New York: Wiley.

Katz, D., Kahn, R., & Adams, J. (1980). *The study of organizations.* San Francisco: Jossey-Bass.

Kaufman, R. (1971). A possible integrative model for the systematic and measurable improvement of education. *American Psychologist, 26*, 250–256.

Kuhn, T. (1962). *The structure of scientific revolutions.* Chicago: University of Chicago Press.

Kurpius, D. (1985). Consultation interventions: Successes, failures, and proposals. *Counseling Psychologist, 13*(3), 368–389.

Kurpius, D., Fuqua, D., & Rozecki, T. (1993). The consulting process: A multidimensional approach. *Journal of Counseling and Development, 71*, 601–606.

Mayer, G. (1973). Behavioral consulting: Using behavior modification procedures in the consulting relationship. *Elementary School Guidance and Counseling, 7*(2), 114–119.

Meichenbaum, D. (1977). *Cognitive-behavior modification: An integrative approach.* New York: Plenum.

Mendoza, D. (1993). A review of Gerald Caplan's *Theory and practice of mental health consultation. Journal of Counseling and Development, 71*, 629–635.

Nelson, L., & Burns, F. (1984). High performance programming: A framework for transforming organizations. In J. Adams (Ed.), *Transforming work* (pp. 226–242). Alexandria, VA: Miles River Press.

Newman, J., & Fuqua, D. (1984). Data-based consultation in student affairs. *Journal of College Student Affairs*, *30*, 206–212.

Pugh, D., & Hickson, D. (1989). *Writers on organizations*. Newbury Park, CA: Sage.

Ridley, C., & Mendoza, D. (1993). Putting organizational effectiveness into practice: The preeminent consultation task. *Journal of Counseling and Development*, *72*, 168–177.

Rockwood, G. (1993). Edgar Schein's process versus content consultation models. *Journal of Counseling and Development*, *71*, 636–638.

Rogawski, A. (1978). The Caplanian model. *Personnel and Guidance Journal*, *56*(6), 324–327.

Russell, M. L. (1978). Behavioral consultation: Theory and process. *Personnel and Guidance Journal*, *56*(6), 346–350.

Schein, E. (1969). *Process consultation*. Reading, MA: Addison-Wesley.

Schein, E. (1978). The role of the consultant: Content expert or process facilitator? *Personnel and Guidance Journal*, *56*(6), 339–345.

Schein, E. (1985). *Organizational culture and leadership*. San Francisco: Jossey-Bass.

Schein, E. (1987). *Process consultation: Lessons for managers and consultants* (Vol. 2). Reading, MA: Addison-Wesley.

Wallace, W. (1986). *Theories of counseling and psychotherapy: A basic issues approach*. Boston: Allyn & Bacon.

◆ CHAPTER FOUR

Measuring Consultation Efficacy

Annotated Bibliography
References and Suggested Readings

Despite increased attention in the professional literature, courses in academic programs, and numerous practice opportunities, the field of psychological consultation has yet to evolve into a formal profession. As we hinted earlier in this book, consultation suffers from conceptual growing pains and has yet to achieve the status predicted (Bardon, 1985; Gallessich, 1985). One deficiency—discussed in the present chapter—is the inconsistent evidence for the effectiveness of consultation (Dustin, 1985; Froehle & Rominger, 1993; Heller, 1984). Not surprisingly, some authors have expressed concern that the field has grown so quickly despite the lack of validating evidence (Dustin, 1985).

We can only speculate, at least for now, about how long the field can continue to thrive without convincing empirical backing. What can be said with confidence is that consultation must eventually confront the same challenges facing other human service professions. One challenge is the call for accountability on the part of human service professionals and programs (Bloom & Fischer, 1982; Sze & Hopps, 1978). Sze and Hopps (1978), writing about the growing emphasis on performance accountability in human service programs, could be addressing an audience of consultants: "In the past it was assumed that any program with the stated purpose of helping people and solving human problems necessarily had great social value and therefore would be supported without question. This assumption is no longer accepted" (p. 1).

Accountability in consultation refers to the obligation of consultants to be answerable and responsible with respect to professional commitments. To be accountable, consultants must reflect the standards of their field as they approach major consultation assignments, especially those that are arranged by legal contracts, are fee-based, and involve significant problem-solving actions. Consultation accountability is advanced, also, when consultants demonstrate that their performance is effective. Thus, if the consultation field is to realize the bright future once forecast, consultants must attend to the need for evaluation.

This chapter elaborates on the concept of **consultation evaluation**, including the practical and theoretical issues that influence evaluation decisions and methodologies. In a broad sense, **evaluation** refers to "a systematic collection of information about the activities, characteristics, and outcomes of programs for use by specific people to reduce uncertainties, improve effectiveness, and make decisions with regard to what those programs are doing and affecting" (Patton, 1987a, p. 15).

As Gallessich (1982) observes, "Consultants are finding that a careful evaluation is an increasingly important aspect of their work" (p. 337). Evaluation assesses the efficacy of consultation in a given setting and situation. Although evaluation serves the immediate purpose of determining the extent to which interventions reduce consultation problems, it can examine a broader range of variables. An assumption implicit in consultation evaluation is that, in addition to measuring the impact of consultation (effects or changes), consultants should give equal attention to the viability of the "processes" that contribute to outcomes. The consultant's decisions, attitudes, and relationships, for example, are known to exert substantial influence on the overall success of interventions (Dougherty, 1990).

Evaluation Barriers and Myths

Evaluation-minded consultants often encounter obstacles that impede the evaluation process. Evaluation practices are seldom implemented without attention to the diverse barriers, theoretical and practical, affecting consultation. One barrier stems from the paradox in which, despite its potential to affirm consultation's credibility as a professional endeavor, evaluation appears to offer relatively weak support at present. Indeed, concerned consultants and investigators lament the growing tendency to overlook the usefulness of evaluation (Brown, Kurpius, & Morris, 1988; Parsons & Meyers, 1984).

Many of the difficulties that impede evaluation originate inside the consultation setting, and at first glance, appear beyond the consultant's control. Some obstacles stem from consultees' preferences for certain types of interventions. For example, consultees often appear most interested in "quick-and-early" measures that alleviate work-related problems (Kurpius, Fuqua, & Rozecki, 1993, p. 604). Parsons and Meyers (1984) express a more fundamental concern: "Evaluation of the consultation process and its impact is very often viewed by consultants and consultees as superfluous or as only tangential to the primary function of consultation" (p. 207).

Evaluation can be plagued by the "organizational and political context in which it must be performed" (Sze & Hopps, 1978, p. 206). Although consultants may be professionally committed to evaluation, they often serve organizations where uninformed or self-serving opinions, rather than substantive data, mold perceptions of the effectiveness of consultation. Moreover, some organizational members are blinded by long-standing, antiquated paradigms that lead to dogmatic and uncreative evaluation measures (Patton, 1987a). Another obstacle results when consultees obstruct evaluation practices out of an obsessive or unreasonable determination to protect organizational data from external visitors.

Evaluation plans are thwarted, also, by the technical processes required by measurement and evaluation activities. Some evaluation designs entail intricate and elaborate operations, and as a result, exceed the consultant's experience and knowledge. With these technical issues in mind, several consultation writers advise both beginning and experienced consultants to become familiar with professional evaluation techniques before engaging in evaluation and to seek the input of evaluation experts if necessary (Dougherty, 1990; Gallessich, 1982; Kurpius et al., 1993).

Despite the presence of political dynamics, biases, obsolete paradigms, and technical barriers, consultants should not abandon their commitment to the evaluation imperative. They must accept responsibility for evaluation problems in many cases, since these problems often stem from the haphazard methods they have employed or from their tendency to deny the relevance of evaluation to their work (Brown et al., 1988). Part of the difficulty appears related to consultants' adherence to a number of misconceptions or myths, a few of which are described here:

Myth 1: Evaluation and research are identical endeavors with identical purposes. A common misconception is that evaluation is synonymous with research. For some consultants, thoughts about evaluation summon images of complex research designs, scientific methods, or intricate statistical analyses. Although similar in their mission to uncover information, the two endeavors have separate and distinct purposes (Weiss, 1972). Consultation **research** entails tightly controlled investigations that attempt to explain theoretical hypotheses or stimulate knowledge of consultation as a field of study (Hansen, Himes, & Meier, 1990). While research objectives focus more on comparing consultation interventions or theoretical applications, evaluation is more concerned with consultees' immediate problems or situations. That is, consultation evaluation strives to answer specific questions about a single consultation situation as it exists in a distinct setting (Gallessich, 1982; Kurpius et al., 1993; Parsons & Meyers, 1984).

Myth 2: Evaluation is the least important consultation activity. Insufficient time, inadequate resources, a lack of skills, and other factors are cited as reasons consultants place evaluation at the bottom of their list of priorities. Regrettably, the devaluation of consultation evaluation often reflects an underlying belief that "evaluation is not important and not worth the investment." To the contrary, consultants must recognize the potential advantages of evaluation. With outcome data in mind, consultants provide information "that can then be applied to program management, accountability, and planning decisions" (Paul, 1979, p. 34). Evaluation data help confirm that consultation interventions are devised and implemented correctly. Further, because evaluation provides useful data on the status of problems following interventions, it may indicate whether residual needs exist. Other advantages have to do with the potential of evaluation to enhance the credibility of consultation. In view of Heller's (1984) concern that "the field is long on theory and short on empirical confirmation" (p. 267), the empirical data provided by evaluation are welcome (Parsons & Meyers, 1984).

Myth 3: Evaluation processes occur exclusively near the end of the consultation process. A common misconception is that evaluation must occur late in the consultation process (Dougherty, 1990; Parsons & Meyers, 1984). Consultants who subscribe to this view tend to carry out evaluation only when earlier consultation stages and processes have been completed. But many experts advise that evaluation should be an ongoing process permeating every phase of consultation (Brown et al., 1988; Hansen et al., 1991; Kurpius et al., 1993; Parsons & Meyers, 1984).

Myth 4: Evaluation is only concerned with measuring specific consultation outcomes. Consultants who believe that evaluation is concerned exclusively with end products risk overlooking less obvious but equally important criteria. Paul (1979) points out, for example, that "we often worry about our outcomes without checking our inputs" (p. 35). In practice, evaluation plans must consider the multidimensional nature of consultation, where success is a function of numerous variables. As an example, many authors emphasize that the consultant-consultee relationship is indispensable (Bell & Nadler, 1979; Brown, Pryzwansky, & Schulte, 1991; Caplan, 1970; Gallessich, 1982). Bell and Nadler (1979) point to dynamics of consultation that empower consultees to learn important skills through experience. Others emphasize the importance of evaluating decisions and processes while also examining the consultees' response to consultation (Brown et al., 1991).

Myth 5: Consultees do not require evaluation, so why should consultants? Consultants and consultees often enter the consultation relationship with different expectations. Consultees who express great interest in resolving work-related problems may perceive evaluation as superfluous. This attitude can be contagious; consultants can also become complacent, particularly if they are not knowledgeable about evaluation concepts and techniques. Conscientious consultants must commit to the full range of stages and processes without allowing negative or biased influences to undermine successful consulting.

Myth 6: Evaluation practices are the same for all consultation situations. Some consultants, for convenience or because of insufficient knowledge, proceed as if evaluation practices can be standardized across all consultation settings. In reality, they may be applying formulas that have little relevance or validity. Though evaluation practices are and should be governed by rules and technical guidelines, consultation issues and settings vary, and as a result, evaluation can take many different forms (Brown et al., 1991). Each consultant should adopt an evaluation plan tailored to the specific needs of a specific setting.

Myth 7: Consultants do not need to justify their performance. Some consultants neglect evaluation tasks because they believe that, since they are experts, their work should be accepted without verifying performance data. Other consultants may hold that consultees are directly liable for consultation outcomes and any failures belong to them. Whatever their suppositions, consultants who fail to justify their performance risk short consulting careers. Several powerful arguments support this claim. For example, increased professional competition, the costs of consultation (in terms of time, resources, and money), and the push for accountability all exert pressure on consultants to excel. Further, since consultants often perform their work on a contractual basis, they cannot afford to be complacent with respect to consultation outcomes. Poor consulting can also have traumatic consequences, including organizational or human turmoil. Perhaps the most succinct argument is offered by Phillips (1991), who states that "consultants are expensive and their costs must be justified" (p. 288).

Myth 8: Evaluation is the exclusive job of the consultant. Some consultants adopt the position that evaluating the effects of consultation is their responsibility and consultees should not be expected to invest time and effort in these tasks. Others may be concerned that consultees lack the technical skills or insights necessary to participate in evaluation procedures. While both arguments appear plausible, several authors write about the advantages of consultees' active participation (Beer & Spector, 1993; Brown et al., 1988; Harrison, 1987; Cooper & O'Connor, 1993). Brown et al. (1988) explain that "the central point here is to involve the consultee in as many aspects of the evaluation process as possible so that the intent and utility of the effort is understood and supported" (p. 45).

Characteristics of Evaluation Data

Consultation evaluation entails the collection and analysis of information. Implicit in these functions is the assumption that, to be credible and meaningful, information should be verifiable. Without confidence in the data they collect, consultants are unable to render sound decisions or judgments about consultation's effects. Consultants should ensure that their methods satisfy the requirements detailed in the following checklist:

1. *Validity*   **Validity**—arguably the most important feature of evaluation information—refers to its truthfulness. Evaluation information is valid "to the extent that it measures what one wants it to measure and not something else" (Katzer, Cook, & Crouch, 1982, p. 93). In consultation, data from a consultee satisfaction scale may not be a valid measure should the consultant wish to evaluate the overall effectiveness of consultation or the actual reduction of consultation problems.

2. *Reliability*   **Reliability** refers to the degree of dependability of information. Data are reliable when they are consistent, stable, and trustworthy through time. A measure approaches reliability to the extent that it "gives the same or very similar results each time it is used" (Katzer et al., 1982, p. 91). A consultant, for example, observes high scores on a test following an assertiveness training seminar. Test reliability is confirmed when similar results occur on retesting.

3. *Usability*   Evaluation data have good **usability** when they are articulated or synthesized in helpful forms. For consultation evaluation processes to translate into viable decisions or judgments, data must be presented in comprehensible ways. As Bloom and Fischer (1982) point out, "There is little advantage in selecting a measurement system that won't be used" (p. 45). Consider the team-building consultant who evaluates the results of consultation by administering a team-effectiveness scale. The results, though valid and reliable, are not very useful when articulated in terms of complex psychological concepts or diagnoses that participants cannot understand. Usefulness is restricted, also, when information is presented in meticulously detailed reports without practical application to the problems in question.

4. *Feasibility*   **Feasibility** is a feature of data that assesses its suitability for the situation and setting. Data feasibility is enhanced by the extent to which information gathering processes are workable and practical. Feasible measures are matched to the resources in the setting. For example, measures that violate the consultees' policies due to high costs and excessive effort score poorly in feasibility. Consider the consultant who conducts an empathy training program that teaches innovative psychological interviewing. Following the training, the consultant evaluates the effects of the program by observing each trainee during on-the-job intake interviews. Though such data are potentially useful, the method of data collection is time consuming, disruptive to trainees' schedules, and potentially invasive to clients' privacy.

Consultants must also consider the various forms in which data are presented. A standard division that holds true for consultation evaluation data is the classification of information into quantitative and qualitative forms. **Quantitative data** include evaluation information that documents the effects of consultation according to observable, objective, and measurable criteria. Consultants may search for process or outcome data that can be synthesized and expressed numerically. Examples of quantitative evaluation information include frequency data, cost-savings comparisons, and numerical scores on standardized tests.

Qualitative data include information that can be expressed in nonnumerical, subjective form. Consultants often derive information through interpretation and intuition. Van Maanin (1979) explains that *qualitative* is:

> At best an umbrella term covering an array of interpretative techniques which seek to describe, encode, translate, and otherwise come to terms with the meaning, not the frequency of certain more or less naturally occurring phenomena in the social world. (p. 520)

As it relates to consultation evaluation, qualitative information includes perceptual information, the results of interviews, satisfaction feedback, intuitive feelings, or opinions that can be judged or analyzed rather than counted.

A perpetual debate in the human service fields concerns the respective merits of quantitative versus qualitative methods. Some believe that a need exists to "expand assessment and evaluation approaches beyond those evolved from traditional deductive, positivistic, experimental methods" (Cooper & O'Connor, 1993, p. 651). Others cling to a purist perspective that espouses objectivity rather than subjectivity. Cooper and O'Connor (1993) suggest that the trend toward implementing measures that blend both types of data is welcome, since it may provide more complete data. They point out that each method has merit: "Many researchers believe that qualitative approaches have strength in answering discovery questions and in uncovering the meanings that individuals attach to their perceptions, whereas quantitative approaches are better for validation and theory" (p. 651).

Types and Levels of Evaluation Information

In Chapter 2, we described consultation as a process made up of an array of mutually interdependent processes (for example, relationship building, assessment, goal setting, and intervention implementation). An assumption that appears generalizable across settings is that these processes interconnect to produce the effects of consultation. Thus, evaluation methodologies, to be thorough, must assess the respective merits of a range of activities that contribute to end products. To observe the many variables that contribute to consultation one needs to consider only a few simple questions:

1. What is the effect of consultation on consultation problems?
2. What interventions appear to have the greatest positive effect?
3. Are the decisions about assessment, diagnosis, and goal setting appropriate and accurate?
4. What is the consultee's perception of the value of consultation?
5. How did the consultee change as a result of the consultation experience?
6. What were the effects of consultation on the consultee's client or clients?
7. How did the consultant perform?
8. Are program or organizational changes necessary?
9. What are the needs for additional interventions?
10. Which qualities of the consultant-consultee relationship contributed to the success of consultation?

Against the background that the success of consultation is often a function of multiple, interacting processes, the consultation literature has classified evaluation processes into two broad types. The first emphasizes "formative" evaluation methodologies that investigate the effects of ongoing consultation activities. The second is "summative" evaluation, in which consultants evaluate consultation through careful examination of the specific end products of the process (Scriven, 1967, p. 43). When Michael Scriven (1967) advanced these concepts, he detailed their advantages for interested educators with respect to curriculum evaluation. Since that time, several authors have applied Scriven's concepts to the field of consultation (Brown et al., 1991; Dougherty, 1990; Parsons & Meyers, 1984).

Formative Evaluation in Consultation

Formative evaluation examines the effectiveness or usefulness of an activity, program, or exercise as it is happening (Scriven, 1967). In Scriven's (1967) words:

> Unless entirely ignorant of one's shortcomings as a judge of one's own work, [the evaluator] . . . is also presumably engaged in field-testing the work while it is being developed, and in so doing he gets feedback on the basis of which he again produces revisions; this is of course, formative evaluation. (p. 43)

Consultants who follow Scriven's approach apply formative evaluation techniques during each stage of the consultation process. Their primary aim is to examine ongoing stage-related dynamics in order to "form" effective decisions and sound practices while they are occurring (Parsons & Meyers, 1984, p. 209). Formative data supply consultants with information needed to either validate or modify consultation processes (Dougherty, 1990). Ultimately, formative methodologies establish the course of consultation, and they subsequently evaluate that course as it unfolds.

Formative evaluation can be accomplished through a combination of informal techniques (for example, dialogue, processing, and progress checks) and formal methods (including systematic data gathering, surveys, and rating forms) applied situationally at each stage of consultation (Parsons & Meyers, 1984). Exhibit 4.1 provides an example of a formative evaluation checklist.

Informal dialogue and questions can lead to considerable insight. Consultants, for example, are often interested in the questions proposed by Swartz and Lippitt (1979), who refer to the consultee as a client:

1. Does the consultant form sound interpersonal relations with the client?
2. Does the consultant build dependence on his resources with the client?
3. Does the consultant focus upon the problem?
4. Does the consultant respect the confidences of the client?
5. Does the consultant achieve influence appropriately in the organization?
6. Does the consultant indicate the skills he possesses relative to the client's problem?
7. Does the consultant clearly inform the client as to his role and contributions?
8. Does the consultant express willingness to have his services evaluated? (pp. 218–219)

As a rule, consultants should be conscious of the need for formative data throughout the entire consultation process. Through formal and informal instruments, introspection, dialogue, and intuitive observation, they maintain an opinion of consultation that is frequently updated.

Formative Evaluation Checklist for Consultants

Directions: For each stage of the consultation process, feedback and request for corrective feedback from institutional representatives and consultees are both appropriate and desirable. The checklist provides a broad framework from which to conceptualize the specific formative function to be used within your particular consultation relationship.

Name of Institution _____   Name of Consultee _____   Date of Initial Contact _____

Formative Issue	Consultation Stage				
	Entry	Goal Identification	Goal Definition	Intervention	Assessment
1. Record of contacts (record dates, length of sessions)					
2. Special focus of contacts—concerns emerging for later consideration					
3. Provide feedback to highest relevant administrator (acceptable direction, time line, cost tone)					
4. Request feedback from consultee: Expectations met? Specific concerns? New needs? Suggestions for modification of program? Consultant style? Or administrative details (meeting times, rooms, and so on)					
5. Stage-specific concerns	All relevant personnel contacted? Collaborative atmosphere? Relationship skills?	Agreement on level of entry? Optimal entry point? Possible recontact?	Consultee's skill; cooperation; Facility in data gathering/ reporting? Data complete?	Feedback to consultee on joint ownership? Consultee accept? Agree? Understand? Modifications? Joint agreement?	Outcome/Inputs? Process? Design? Decision options? Assessment as collaborative effort?
6. Consultant's perception of process to date—new paths tried					

From *Developing Consultation Skills: A Guide to Training, Development, and Assessment for Human Services Professionals*, p. 210. Copyright © 1984 by Jossey-Bass Inc., Publishers. By permission of the publisher.

EXHIBIT 4.1
Formative evaluation checklist for consultants

Summative Evaluation in Consultation

Summative evaluation refers to evaluation methodologies that address the extent to which specific outcomes are achieved (Scriven, 1967). Applied in a consultation framework, this type of evaluation has the primary aim of determining the success of interventions in resolving consultation problems. Thus, summative techniques, in contrast to formative strategies, are aimed at the end products of consultation (changes, effects, and results). Although the advantages of ongoing dynamic evaluation are numerous, the ultimate benefits of the overall consultation process can only be determined by assessing the reduction of problems and other changes brought about by the consultation interventions. Parsons and Meyers (1984) emphasize that the examination of outcomes is the heart of consultation evaluation:

> Although it is valuable for a consultant and consultee to periodically share their perceptions of the quality or efficacy of the relationship, the bottom line to be assessed is whether the goal has been achieved—sales increased, achievement improved, absenteeism reduced. (p. 212)

Since the intent of summative evaluation is to demonstrate the efficacy of consultation in achieving desirable outcomes, such techniques emphasize a "results-oriented" philosophy. That is, consultants have the potential to fine-tune their evaluation expectations in order to examine desirable and recognizable outcomes (Robinson & Robinson, 1989). A number of results-oriented variables can be investigated. Although a complete discussion is beyond the scope of this chapter, we cover a few representative outcomes.

Goal Attainment   In Chapter 2, we discussed the dynamics of goal setting in consultation and the formation of viable and measurable goals. When measurable goals are established for interventions, they offer concrete indications of whether consultation has accomplished its mission.

An example of evaluation within the context of consultation goals is provided by the **goal attainment scaling** (GAS) model. Developed by Kiresuk and Sherman (1968) and discussed within a consultation framework by Brown et al. (1991), GAS involves a standardized process consisting of weighted measures and estimates of the degree of accomplishment for each goal. GAS is unique in focusing on the degree of goal accomplishment rather than employing global or "all-or-nothing" measures. Consultants have at their disposal quantitative scores that provide sound estimates of goal accomplishment at the end of the GAS process.

Reactions   One broad set of criteria, incorporating a diverse collection of variables, includes the range of **reactions** on the part of consultation participants and observers. These measures, according to Swartz and Lippitt (1979), "report feelings, attitudes, points of view, as these change over time" (p. 217).

One specific reaction that has received attention in the consultation literature is the degree of satisfaction consultees and others experience with the consultation process and final outcomes. **Satisfaction measures** represent the contentment or comfort consultees and other participants express relative to consultation outcomes (Brown et al., 1991; Parsons & Meyers, 1984). Satisfaction data can be derived from informal tactics (such as open dialogue and interviews) or through formal instruments (for example, consultee satisfaction surveys and checklists). An example of a standardized instrument is the *Consultee Satisfaction Form*, developed by Parsons and Meyers (1984).

Cost Justification   Consultation is costly, and the ultimate impact of consultation cannot be determined solely within the context of human behavioral or organizational changes. Levine (1981) summarizes the rationale for considering cost justification as an evaluation criterion: "What is required is a systematic procedure for comparing the cost of producing outcomes to the value of a 'stream of services' that these outcomes yield over time" (p. 21).

Levine describes **cost-benefit evaluation** as a method that measures the value of outcomes against the costs required to produce those outcomes. Consultants can compare the benefits of consultation outcomes to the expenses incurred by the purchase, design, and implementation of interventions (that is, investments of fiscal resources, time, materials, and effort). For example, when a psychologist is asked to design and implement a new client tracking system for a community mental health center, the outcome is a system that supplies data pertaining to the diagnosis and disposition of present and former clients. Projecting the cost-benefit ratio of this outcome requires the consultant to compare the cost of consultation (including fees, training time, and technical or computer software costs) to the potential advantages of the new system.

Human Behavioral Change   One variable that evaluation methodologies are often concerned with is human behavior: "Most evaluation research projects attempt to assess the impact of some type of intervention or treatment program upon individuals" (Cline & Sinnott, 1981, p. 1). Whether consultants take a strict behavioral position or adopt any of the change-oriented approaches, evaluation frequently measures the effects of interventions on the behavior of individuals, including consultees, clients, and possibly other organizational members. Although evaluating behavioral change is a complex process, the early formulation of measurable and achievable goals, written in specific behavioral terms, facilitates the consultant's actions.

Organizational Change   The consultation field's perpetual attention to the health of organizations demands that consultants evaluate the multitude of **organizational changes** (the redesign or reconstruction of any of the various organizational conditions and processes) that emerge from consultation. Though the prospects of change often bring anticipation and excitement, "planned interventions always produce unanticipated consequences" (Cline & Sinnott, 1981, p. 18). Thus, in addition to targeted change, evaluation must consider the peripheral or inadvertent effects on neighboring programs or subsystems. While the range of measurable organizational factors appears vast and fragmented, a few common organizational variables include program efficiency, cost savings, productivity, communication patterns, human relations, and organizational health.

Evaluation at Multiple Levels

As we have seen, the consultation framework usually consists of an assortment of human and organizational factors. The triadic structure of consultation, along with the reality that most consultation occurs in some type of organizational setting, suggests that the process should be evaluated at multiple levels. Implicit is the assumption that each level may respond differently to the various consultation activities. Though soliciting feedback from multiple levels may complicate the evaluation process, the potential for obtaining comprehensive and credible information is enhanced.

Each level has an investment in the success of consultation, and presumably, constituents at each level offer a unique vantage point on the process. Conventional levels include those of the consultee, consultant, and client.

1. *Consultee level* The consultee is the representative of the organization or setting who has a strong commitment to the consultation process and its outcomes. Consultees can be valuable sources of evaluation data since they are integrally involved in arranging for consultation, observing its progress, and appreciating consultation solutions. The consultee's firsthand observation of the effects of consultation often yields well-founded, intuitive impressions that add to the information secured through more formal and substantive means. According to Lockwood and Luthans (1980), the range of consultee reactions includes attitudes, emotions, insights, and behavioral changes.

2. *Consultant level* Consultants represent helping agents, often external to the consultation setting, who Paul (1979) claims are in "the unique position of being responsible to two possibly independent systems—the consultee system and their own" (p. 40). They are heavily invested in evaluation outcomes that both meet the needs of the consultee or organization and reflect well on their own professional performance. Feedback at this level often targets consultants' skills, knowledge, and related attributes, qualities that contribute heavily to overall performance.

3. *Client level* Clients, whether people, organizations, or programs, are the conventional beneficiaries of interventions, so that changes at this level represent a central measure of the effectiveness of consultation. Although human clients are usually inactive during evaluation in the sense that they rarely have overt or direct responsibilities, their reduction of problems, psychological growth, therapeutic gains, and mental health are common targets of evaluation measures. When clients are programs or organizations, changes in structural systems in response to interventions also represent measurement criteria.

Designs, Data Collection Methods, and Process Steps

Earlier in this chapter, we saw that evaluation actions should not be the products of sudden afterthoughts. Instead, careful, organized planning is preferred. Consultants' proactive thoughts about evaluation bring clarity and coherence to evaluation plans. Unless evaluation goals are consolidated into a cogent plan, consultants risk evaluation strategies that are fragmented, chaotic, or wasteful. To avoid these problems, consultants should begin the evaluation process with collaborative dialogue and exploration (Brown et al., 1988). Consultants may seek answers to a range of questions that illuminate the potential direction of consultation. Professional exchanges, though often informal and somewhat intuitive, include many fundamental questions that guide early decisions about evaluation. For example:

1. What is the purpose of consultation?
2. What should be evaluated?
3. What is the purpose of evaluation and how will information be used?
4. Which constituents (consultant, consultee, or other participants) are responsible for which aspects of the evaluation process?
5. What resources and logistical features (such as time, materials, people, instruments) are available?
6. Which data collection methods are necessary?
7. How will evaluation results be disseminated?
8. Is the evaluation process worth the investment?

Evaluation Designs

Evaluation decisions result from proactive planning in which consultants prepare a workable design that indicates how and when data are collected. The **evaluation design** refers to the architecture of the entire evaluation process, including the timing, methodologies, and control of conditions that surround data collection. Although the following definition offered by Verhonick and Seaman (1978) is aimed at researchers, their appraisal appears generalizable to consultant-evaluators:

> The design is the plan for the study [evaluation], providing the overall framework for collecting data. Once the problem has been concretely formulated, a design is developed in order to provide a format for the detailed steps in the study. The design is relatively specific, consisting of a series of guidelines for systematic data gathering. (p. 30)

The evaluation design also provides a blueprint indicating how, when, and under what conditions the consultant should measure or collect information. Sound evaluation designs should be tailored to the consultation situation and the organization's available resources (in terms of costs, time, effort, materials, and personnel). Well-matched designs enhance the probability that valid information can be generated (Kerlinger, 1973).

Consultants are sometimes hesitant to implement research designs. Many fear that they cannot control the "threats to internal and external validity" (Parsons & Meyers, 1984, p. 225) or that they lack the time or resources to implement the type of investigation common to scientific practices. Others must contend with the reality that evaluation designs in consultation cannot always meet strict standards of soundness and purity. Further, many of the conditions suggested by research purists to control for extraneous variables, for example, do not exist in the consultation setting. Thus, consultants must plan their designs by anticipating that some scientific practices (for example, randomization, tight controls, and control groups) are not available or convenient. In view of these limitations, consultants should adhere to the advice of evaluation experts as they explore several conventional designs (Brown et al., 1988; Gallessich, 1982). Campbell and Stanley (1963), mindful of the deficiencies presented by unpure or tainted research conditions, propose a series of "quasi-experimental" designs that appear adaptable to the consultation evaluation framework (p. 2). Since a complete discussion of all relevant designs is beyond the scope of this chapter, we briefly introduce a few of the most common. Our discussion is intended to provide a general overview of the various diagrams that seem applicable to consultation evaluation rather than to present a theoretical discourse on experimental designs.

One-Group Postintervention Design   Despite the threats to validity and the concerns of evaluation purists, the one-group postintervention design provides a structure that appears common in many evaluation situations. According to Campbell and Stanley (1963), this format generally furnishes a one-time measure that "conforms to a design in which a single group is studied only once, subsequent to some agent or treatment presumed to cause change" (p. 6). The one-time evaluation design requires consultants to measure consultation effects once the impact of interventions is felt and without reference or comparison to other groups. With X denoting the consultation intervention and O denoting the evaluation measure, we can represent the postintervention design by the symbols below (Campbell & Stanley, p. 6):

$$X \quad O$$

Since consultation often occurs in settings that restrict the application of elaborate evaluation schemes, the one-group postintervention design is sought for its practical, rather than scientific, merits. Despite its ideological shortcomings, this design is arguably "better than nothing." A case example illustrates the use of a one-group postintervention design in Box 4.1.

One-Group Pre- and Postintervention Design   A basic design that appears adaptable to some consultation settings is the pre- and postintervention design. This design requires data collection at two intervals. First, consultants gather problem data in the early stages of consultation (during assessment and diagnosis); second, an intervention is implemented; and third, consultants gather data on a second occasion to determine the differences between the two measurements. Campbell and Stanley (1963, p. 7) symbolize this design with the following diagram:

$$O_1 \quad X \quad O_2$$

The evaluator assumes that observed differences between the pre- and postintervention measures should be attributed to the effects of consultation decisions and solutions. Box 4.2 contains a case example of this design.

Box 4.1
Case example: One-group postintervention design

A licensed professional counselor is asked by the clinical director at a mental health center to provide a staff development training program for paraprofessionals employed in the transition/aftercare program. The clinical director designates "The Techniques of Case Management" as the workshop theme. The clinical director adds that because of the employees' caseloads and schedules, time for the training is restricted and there are no opportunities to meet with them before the training program. In addition, the clinical director wishes to have all center case managers participate. The consultant-trainer accepts the consultation assignment and begins to plan the training design that includes the workshop objectives, learning strategies, and methods of evaluating the workshop's success. Recognizing the limited time schedule, full agenda, and absence of a comparison group, the trainer plans an evaluation process that examines the knowledge and satisfaction of participants following the workshop. Thus, the trainer prepares a test assessing how well trainees have learned the concepts addressed in the workshop. Also, the trainer prepares several items that ask participants to rate on a Likert scale how well the program met their needs, increased their knowledge, and prepared them for existing work assignments.

Postintervention with Comparison-Group Design   A potential problem with one-group designs is the influence of nonconsultation factors that affect, often significantly, evaluation outcomes. According to Campbell and Stanley (1963), a range of "extraneous variables," including subjects' maturation, history, and the effects of testing, confound final measures and distort the opinions that result from such measures (p. 5). Should consultants desire to control for these influences, the addition of a closely matched comparison group isolated from consultation processes and interventions can be useful (Gallessich, 1982). In ideal circumstances and, indeed, to generate the most valid data, consultants should use randomization when comparison groups are involved in the evaluation process (though in many settings this process is not feasible). The postintervention with comparison-group design mandates the presence of two groups measured during the postintervention phase only. One group receives the consultation intervention and a second group does not. Campbell and Stanley (1963, p. 12) refer to this arrangement as the *static-group comparison* design; it is symbolized by the following:

$$(\text{group 1}) \quad X \quad O_1$$
$$(\text{group 2}) \quad \quad O_2$$

We include a case example of this design in Box 4.3.

Box 4.2
Case example: One-group pre- and postintervention design

A licensed social worker, specializing in team-building consultation, is asked by the social services director at a large nursing home to address the poor teamwork exhibited by her staff. The staff work on a social services unit that employs ten social service aides who visit patients, assess home and community needs, and consult with visiting family members to resolve issues related to patient care. Recently, the aides have become isolated in their work, have few opportunities for meetings, and exhibit poor communication. The consultee reports that the unfortunate results are low morale, duplication of medical treatments, and significant increases in the number of complaints by patients. Also, these deficiencies have created lower scores on program performance measures. The consultant accepts the request and decides to visit the home to observe the aides during their rounds and general duties. The consultant determines that assessing the group's teamwork skills is necessary, and asks all aides to complete a standardized team-effectiveness scale that examines their perceptions of group dynamics and processes. A compilation of scale results reveals that the unit appears to suffer from various team deficiencies, including poor communication, lack of trust, and an absence of commitment to the unit's goals. The consultant designs and implements a series of team-building sessions that include skill-building and rehearsal exercises. Following these interventions, the team consultant repeats the assessment tactics used prior to the intervention. The consultant next compares the pre- and postintervention scores to determine whether the aides perceive changes in team functioning.

Pre- and Postintervention with Comparison-Group Design   Though consultants may be satisfied with designs that compare groups or outcomes at postintervention periods only, they increase the soundness of their measures when they integrate preintervention comparisons into their evaluation plan. The collection of data from a consultation group and comparison group during pre- and postintervention periods allows comparisons of the groups' characteristics before the intervention and then following the intervention. Thus, the consultant can have increased confidence in consultation outcomes. In practice, this design requires consultants to measure variables for two matched groups before interventions take place. One group then receives the planned intervention while the comparison group remains separate. During the postintervention period, the measurements made in the preintervention phase are repeated for both groups to derive comparison data. This design is symbolized by the following structure:

$$\text{(group 1)} \quad O_1 \quad X \quad O_2$$
$$\text{(group 2)} \quad O_3 \qquad \quad O_4$$

Box 4.3
Case example: Postintervention with comparison-group design

A counseling psychologist consultant is contracted by a child development program to help classroom teachers implement child behavioral management tactics to reduce the number of discipline problems across the program. Several classroom teachers have reported significant discipline issues that distract from educational goals and create a modeling effect in which once-obedient children are becoming defiant and aggressive. The consultant, based on these reports and expressed needs, designs a training program emphasizing an experiential approach. The program allows teachers to apply the principles of learning to simulated cases as the consultant observes and provides feedback. Following three workshop sessions, the consultant wishes to evaluate the effects of training by comparing the number of reported discipline problems by teachers who attended the training sessions to the number of reports filed by teachers who did not attend. The consultant relies on this comparison with confidence because the different classrooms are similar in location, teaching methods, and child composition.

While this design is advantageous in the sense that extraneous variables (for example, maturation and history) can be controlled, it raises feasibility and usability questions. Consultants will also discover that many consultation settings do not afford the practical resources needed to implement this design (that is, control groups, time, commitment, or technical skills). A case example highlights this design in Box 4.4.

Single-Subject Design   Psychological consultants often respond to consultation requests in which the predominant concern is the behavior of an individual. Consultation interventions must address the needs of specific individuals without reference or comparison to others (Caplan, 1970; Fuqua & Newman, 1985). The evaluation of a single client, rather than groups or programs, assumes a single-subject format (Brown et al., 1991). The utility of single-subject evaluation should not be underestimated. While other designs attempt to discover knowledge and make broad contributions to a field of study, one should not devalue the importance of "specificity" (Lazarus & Davison, 1971, p. 209). That is, though data from larger groups promote inference and generalizability, one distinct advantage of single-subject designs is their capacity to resolve consultation questions within a specific setting, with a specific individual, and under specific conditions. Some researchers endorse the single-subject evaluation model because it allows a laboratory-type approach in which the subject is the only control and can be observed at different intervals during the research (Lazarus & Davison, 1971). Single-subject designs usually require "a series of observations over some period of time in order to determine both the degree and direction of change" (Anton, 1978, p. 122).

Box 4.4
Case example: Pre- and postintervention with comparison-group design

---

An internal organizational consultant is asked by the head of a consumer complaint division in a corporate setting to help complaint telephone operators handle more calls. Division statistics indicate that the average call is quite lengthy, and as a result, the phone lines are jammed with waiting calls. The division head wants the consultant to design and implement a communications program that trains the operators to shorten the time required by each call without jeopardizing consumer satisfaction. In an extensive assessment period, the consultant determines that the operators greet consumer complaints with insensitive responses that reflect little concern or empathy with the caller's frustration. As a result, consumers often become agitated or argumentative, thus lengthening the time needed for each call. The consultant's hypothesis is supported by the complaint division head, and the two agree that a comprehensive sensitivity training program should be considered. The consultant, recognizing the need to substantiate the effects of the program, randomly selects 20 of the 40 complaint operators to participate in the training program. The consultant begins the evaluation plan by creating a pre- and postintervention design that allows training- and nontraining-group comparisons at intervals before and after the training program. From division records, the consultant compares the total number of calls taken on a typical day by both groups. Pretraining comparisons suggest the two groups complete approximately the same number of calls. Next, only the training group receives an intensive one-week course in sensitivity training. The program emphasizes empathic interviewing that addresses active listening, voice tone, and pacing. In addition, the training program allows much time for practice, videotaped role playing, and feedback. Following the training program, the consultant repeats the group comparisons used during the pretraining period to determine whether the program helped operators handle more consumer calls than the nontraining group. Through this design, the consultant is confident that any differences in the posttraining period reflect the effects of sensitivity training.

One consultation model that often demands the implementation of single-subject designs is the behavioral model. A case example with a graphic representation of a single-subject evaluation is displayed in Figure 4.1.

Evaluation Data Collection Methods

Despite their purpose, utility, and idiosyncratic nature, evaluation designs require the collection, synthesis, and analysis of data. A sound evaluation design integrates the structure of evaluation with the actions needed to collect information in a particular

Case description: A psychological consultant is asked by a teacher in a child development program to help design a behavioral management program to reduce aggression by a four-year-old child in the classroom. Examples of aggressive behaviors include hitting, kicking, throwing objects, and biting. Following a data collection baseline phase (days 1–7) in which the teacher manages the behavior as usual, the consultant proposes a behavioral intervention that includes the use of logical consequences and separation. On subsequent days, the teacher applies the behavioral management program during a trial phase (days 8–16).

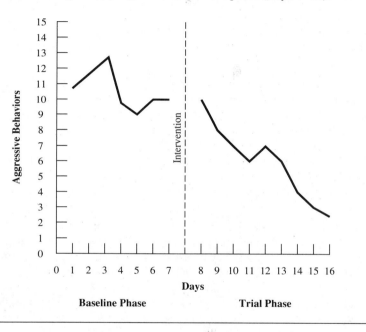

FIGURE 4.1
Single-subject evaluation using a behavioral framework

setting and with reference to a specific consultation problem. Although detailed descriptions of the immense assortment of the data collection methods are beyond the scope of this book, we provide an introduction to a few select methods. To begin, however, we caution readers that "evaluation can take many forms depending on the purpose(s), methodology, and resources available to conduct it" (Brown et al., 1991, p. 309). Decisions about data collection must consider the source of information and the desired form of the data (for example, qualitative versus quantitative data). Although data collection methods are generic in the sense that they serve multiple purposes in consultation (including evaluation, assessment, and diagnosis), their exact use is determined by the requirements of the situation. The methods we describe below are discussed in an evaluation framework rather than in the context of information gathering for the purpose of diagnosing consultation problems. We discuss the material in general terms, with the caveat that each method can satisfy formative or summative evaluation goals.

Observation   Observation is an evaluation tool that requires the systematic and intentional viewing of events (Dougherty, 1990). The detailed analysis of firsthand observations can provide credible and often decisive sources of evaluation data. Observation and documentation of human behavior or organizational processes, for example, allow the consultant to analyze evaluation data with the aid of other documentation or more technical evaluation methods. Conventional observational approaches have several distinct advantages. According to Patton (1987b), observation allows program evaluators to:

1. Understand the *context* within which program activities occur.
2. Directly experience the program as an experience unto itself, thereby making the most of an inductive, discovery-oriented approach.
3. See things that may routinely escape conscious awareness among participants in the program.
4. Learn about things that program participants may be unwilling to talk about in an interview.
5. Move beyond the selective perceptions of others. (p. 73)

Evaluation Interviews   Interviews are multipurpose tools in consultation; they can play a key role in evaluation (Gallessich, 1982). They help consultants determine the perceptions or values of key participants in consultation. Spitzer (1986) describes evaluation interviews as "powerful information gathering techniques, since they allow highly personal and focused discussions" related to a specific intervention (p. 133). Further, interviews have the potential to reinforce the accomplishments created by interventions (Spitzer, 1986). Patton (1987b) points out that:

> The primary data of in-depth, open-ended interviews are quotations. What people say, what they think, how they feel, what they have done, and what they know—these are the things one can learn from talking to people, from interviewing them. (p. 136)

Instrumentation   The use of psychometric instruments in consultation evaluation has received considerable attention (Cooper & O'Connor, 1993). Instruments include "specifically designed data collection devices whose purpose is to stimulate individual feedback about a situation" (Swartz & Lippitt, 1979, p. 218). Dougherty (1990) calls attention to an assortment of prospective evaluation instruments, including "rating scales, surveys, checklists, or questionnaires, which can be developed by the consultant and consultee or can be available in some standardized form" (p. 128).

Some authors lament the absence of a detailed and comprehensive taxonomy of standardized tools for evaluating consultation (Perloff & Perloff, 1977). This situation does, however, encourage practitioners and authors to develop their own user-friendly scales and survey reports. Several instruments can provide feedback on the consultant's performance. The *Consultant On-Site Evaluation Form*, developed by the Head Start Resource and Training Center of Region III (1994), is a practical example. Completed by consultees or other participants to evaluate the consultant's technical performance in Head Start settings, this instrument incorporates a relatively standardized checklist of consultant characteristics (see Exhibit 4.2).

Another instrument that provides detailed evaluation of consultants is Gallessich's (1982) *Consultation Evaluation Survey*. This instrument contains 34 items that require consultees or other participants to rate consultants' helping attributes. Such scales appear useful as outcome measures, or if consultees prefer, as formative measures used at any stage of the consultation process. An example of a more formalized and standardized evaluation instrument is the *Job Descriptive Index* (JDI), developed by Smith, Kendall, and Hulin (1969). Instruments like this may be useful for organizational consultants who want to evaluate the effects of consultation on workers' job satisfaction. Since organizational interventions often create changes in the roles and responsibilities of employees, their satisfaction is an important measure of the impact of consultation.

Case Studies   Perhaps readers will equate case studies with analytic reports that serve evaluation purposes in clinical or therapy settings (Barlow, Haynes, & Nelson, 1984). The need for clinical case studies is explained by Goldman (1978): "Usually when a case is considered in depth it will be discovered that data not supplied through the usual agency activities are necessary to a further understanding of the individual" (p. 229). In consultation evaluation, case studies use descriptive techniques to evaluate the specific effects of consultation on consultees and clients (Dougherty, 1990). They allow the assessment of consultation effects that more global evaluation methods are unable to detect. Used to trace the behavior and reactions of an individual to an intervention, case studies are chronologies of the specific dynamics, processes, and outcomes of consultation.

Case studies offer several advantages. Lazarus and Davison (1971) provide a cogent discussion of the potential benefits of case study methodologies. Though their principles were formulated with clinical research and evaluation goals in mind, we have adapted them to a consultation evaluation framework:

1. Evaluation data uncovered by a consultation case study may call into question the findings of global consultation evaluation approaches or methodologies.
2. The case study often elicits evaluation data that contribute substantively to more formal, traditional, and better-controlled evaluation data.
3. The case study approach allows consultants to evaluate atypical consultation situations not amenable to traditional evaluation methods.
4. The case study method permits consultants to apply traditional evaluation methodologies in innovative ways.
5. The case study, through the consultant's attention to tight control and scientific principles, has the potential to contribute valid evaluation data.
6. The case study allows consultants to add substance and depth to theoretical evaluation data.

Consultant Name:

Date(s) of Visit:

Name of Person Completing This Form:

Position:

Grantee Name:

Case Manager:

Number of On-Site Hours:

PLEASE RATE THE CONSULTANT ON THE FOLLOWING JOB PERFORMANCE ITEMS:

Timeliness and Preparation:	**High**	**Average**	**Low***	**N/A**
Punctuality				
Making and keeping appointments				
Preparation for purpose of on-site visit				
Presenting a schedule for the day				
Allocation of adequate time for tasks				
Use of appropriate materials for tasks				
Communication:				
Meeting with all appropriate staff members				
Respect for others				
Supportive and encouraging of staff				
Clear communication with staff				
Good listening skills				
Clear and concise written materials				
Review of planned objectives for the visit				
Clear instructions				
Clear and appropriate feedback				
Review of planned objectives for the NEXT visit				
Consultant Knowledge:				
Knowledge of Head Start				
Technical knowledge in area of expertise (management, health, etc.)				
Knowledge of resources (agencies, materials, A-V)				
Consultant Skills:				
Encouragement of problem solving process				
Solicitation of active participation from staff				
Focus on task identified by objectives				
Support for program's self-development				
Logical and clear planning process				
Identification of training or Technical Assistance needs				
Creating a productive environment				
Facilitating communication				
Meeting objectives of visit				

*Please comment on items marked in this column

Comments:

Signature _____   Date _____

EXHIBIT 4.2

Consultant on-site evaluation form

Reprinted by permission of Region III Head Start Resource and Training Center, University of Maryland.

Process Steps

The evaluation of consultation, whether through formative or summative strategies, varies with the consultant and setting (Paul, 1979), and as a result, the standardization or generalization of evaluation processes across consultation situations must be done on a case-by-case basis. Several authors have proposed models that systematically guide evaluation processes (Brown et al., 1991; Paul, 1979; Parsons & Meyers, 1984). The framework we have selected for inclusion here draws heavily on the model developed by Parsons and Meyers (1984).

Step 1: Specify consultation outcomes and relevant measures. Consultation evaluation must begin with decisions about the purposes of interventions. Consultants determine important consultation outcomes through the processes of "identification" and "specification" (Parsons & Meyers, 1984, p. 214). *Identification* refers to the examination of a broad array of possible consultation outcomes, and *specification* moves to more tangible and concrete descriptions of outcomes.

The selection of measurement techniques follows the identification and specification processes. In this period, consultants decide which techniques have the greatest potential for validity and reliability and are the most feasible and useful. Contributing to such decisions are estimates of the organizational resources, both material and human. Moreover, how measures are collected, synthesized, and interpreted within the context of consultation are important questions as well.

Step 2: Specify and evaluate program inputs. At this point, consultants look beyond potential outcomes to assess the program's inputs that can facilitate interventions. Parsons and Meyers (1984) point out that "modifications in consultee style, materials, techniques, or work-space environment may all be active inputs in the intervention plan" (p. 221). Inputs can also include the consultee's characteristics, facilities, problem intensity, and problem duration.

Step 3: Identify a substantive design. To create a blueprint that guides the evaluation process, consultants must devise an evaluation design consistent with the purpose of evaluation. The evaluation design adds structure to evaluation activities so that, at any stage of the evaluation process, consultants can easily discern what they must do next. Although several evaluation designs are potentially useful, decisions about their implementation should be shaped by the realities of the setting with respect to consultees' interests, time schedules, resources, and general planning needs.

Step 4: Implement the evaluation plan. Presumably, at this point all important decisions about evaluation measures and designs have been made. The next step involves putting plans into action. Parsons and Meyers (1984) emphasize the importance of collaborative decisions that resolve such questions as "who does what and when?" Important, also, are practical considerations having to do with the time and effort required by the evaluation processes along with anticipatory planning that prepares evaluators for unexpected obstacles or delays. Parsons and Meyers point out that mutual commitment to implementation decisions and responsibilities is critical at this juncture.

Step 5: Make decisions and disseminate results. Once data have been gathered, consultants should analyze them to assess the intervention's effects. Indeed, before they draw specific inferences, consultants must, as an evaluation imperative, ensure that the data are credible. Substantial errors in the measurement process may lead to superficial

Box 4.5
Case example: Step-by-step evaluation process

A professional counselor, with specialized training and experience helping organizations with stress, is asked by the vice president of a large urban bank to help alleviate the apparent stress in the organization. During the past year, the bank has realized considerable financial loss due to clerical errors. Also, medical leave requests have doubled, and resignations have increased dramatically. The consultant accepts the assignment and determines that bank officials wish to implement a comprehensive stress management program that includes wellness seminars, stress therapy, job enrichment opportunities, and employee support groups. The consultant plans the intervention and gives considerable thought to methods of evaluating the new program's success. The consultant decides that evaluation should have two purposes: (1) to determine the extent to which the organizational symptoms of stress have been alleviated, and (2) to determine the efficacy of the stress management program. Desirable outcomes are represented by significant reductions in the dollars lost through accounting errors, number of medical leave requests, and turnover rate. The consultant decides to measure these criteria because they seem to represent indirect consequences of stress, and alleviating these problems indicates that the stress program is effective. The consultant seeks permission to review organizational records to measure accounting error losses, sick days, and resignations. The consultant selects a one-group pre- and postintervention design that allows comparisons of categorical measures for the year preceding the stress management intervention to the same measures during the year following program implementation. Of concern, also, are the bank's commitment to the program, the intensity of stress problems, employee attitudes, and general factors that facilitate stress reduction. At the end of the program's initial year, the consultant collects comparison information and reports relevant data in written form during an exit conference. Also, understanding the bank's interest in finances, the consultant converts frequency data (accounting errors, sick leave days, and resignations) into estimates of cost savings.

or meaningless interpretations. Parsons and Meyers (1984) suggest that a final review of the technical merits of the evaluation process can prevent false or misleading reports. In addition, plans must be made to provide feedback to consultees with respect to the purposes of evaluation. Oral or written reports, presentations before select members of the consultee's organization, and exit interviews are common. Final outcome reports allow consultees to anticipate how the results of consultation fit into future decisions about interventions or programs.

The case example in Box 4.5 illustrates how these action steps are implemented.

SUMMARY

This chapter has explored consultation evaluation. Key themes have included the increasing need for accountability in human service settings and the potential benefits of evaluation in specific situations. We have noted that the consultation field has flourished despite its broad and somewhat amorphous nature and despite a lack of supporting empirical data. To give the field a more solid foundation and to justify their professional status, consultants must commit to a framework that includes documentation of the value of their work.

In this chapter, we have also discussed several barriers to successful evaluation, including the common myths that distort understanding of evaluation principles. In addition, we have reviewed the characteristics of evaluation data that add credibility and usability, presented an overview of evaluation designs, described evaluation data collection methods, and concluded with a condensed discussion of a step-by-step process model.

GLOSSARY

Accountability In the consultation field, the obligation of consultants to be answerable and responsible with respect to professional commitments.

Consultation evaluation Determination of the extent to which the consultation problems have been resolved or eliminated and of the usefulness of processes and decisions contributing to such outcomes.

Cost-benefit evaluation Within the framework of consultation, comparing the value of outcomes with consultation costs (for example, fiscal, time, materials, and effort).

Evaluation Systematic and coordinated inquiries and processes that attempt to determine the positive or negative worth of activities, variables, procedures, or changes.

Evaluation design The nature or structure of the plan for collecting data about the consultation process. The design reflects critical decisions and establishes practices relative to data collection.

Feasibility Suitability and practicality of data for a particular situation and setting.

Formative evaluation In consultation, a form of evaluation that examines the ongoing decisions, actions, and processes of consultation while they are occurring.

Goal attainment scaling A process of evaluating goal accomplishment in consultation in which each objective is measured with respect to the degree of accomplishment rather than in an all-or-nothing manner.

Organizational changes Alterations in any of the various organizational conditions and processes that emerge from consultation.

Qualitative data A type of subjective data that provides important generalizations or estimates of quality. Qualitative data are often informal estimates expressed in nonnumerical form.

Quantitative data Observable, objective, and measurable information that can be synthesized and expressed numerically. Quantitative results often yield important factual information about a hypothesis or variable.

Reactions   Consultees' and other participants' thoughts, feelings, attitudes, and opinions about the consultation process.

Reliability   The dependability of information over time. Data are reliable when they are consistent, stable, and trustworthy.

Research   Investigation or experimentation that attempts to explain particular phenomena or issues. Research contributes to the knowledge in a particular field.

Satisfaction measures   Indications of the contentment consultees and other participants experience with the consultation process and its outcomes.

Summative evaluation   In consultation, a form of evaluation that focuses on consultation outcomes and goal attainment.

Usability   The degree of helpfulness and practicality of evaluation data. Data are useful when they are presented in ways that translate into viable decisions or judgments.

Validity   With respect to evaluation, the degree to which data measure what they are intended to measure.

ANNOTATED BIBLIOGRAPHY

Before engaging in substantive evaluation activities, both beginning and experienced consultants should expand their knowledge of evaluation. An important first step in building competencies is examining evaluation from a conceptual perspective to gain insight into fundamental principles. Such knowledge forms a foundation on which consultants can construct and implement evaluation plans.

Fortunately an extensive literature on evaluation is available. A basic source is *Evaluation and Accountability in Human Service Programs,* edited by William Sze and June Hopps (1978). This book discusses key conceptual and methodological issues. A second source for beginning evaluators is Martin Bloom and Joel Fischer's *Evaluating Practice: Guidelines for the Accountable Professional* (1982). Also useful are Michael Patton's *How to Use Qualitative Methods in Evaluation* (1987b) and a book edited by Leo Goldman, *Research Methods for Counselors: Practical Approaches in Field Settings* (1978). In another evaluation book, *Creative Evaluation* (1987a), Patton provides a meticulous discussion of unique and practical evaluation techniques. This book will prove invaluable for consultants who must often handle assignments not conducive to traditional evaluation procedures. Included in Part II are numerous examples of evaluation methodologies readers will not find in many other sources.

For basic and reader-friendly information about research designs, Donald Campbell and Julian Stanley's classic work, *Experimental and Quasi-Experimental Designs for Research* (1963), is must reading. These authors address the typical sources of extraneous influence that jeopardize the validity of research conclusions. Also, they describe several "quasi-experimental" designs that, though not purely scientific, are almost so (p. 2). A source that discusses evaluation designs within the more specific context of consultation evaluation is Duane Brown, DeWayne J. Kurpius, and Joseph R. Morris's *Handbook of Consultation with Individuals and Small Groups* (1988). In Chapter 5, the authors present general information and illustrations of numerous designs.

A number of authors include book chapters that discuss evaluation as an element of the consultation process. Suggested readings include Chapter 11 of *Psychological Con-*

sultation: Introduction to Theory and Practice, by Duane Brown, Walter Pryzwansky, and Ann Schulte (1995). This chapter provides a thorough overview that can guide the consultant-evaluator's work. It includes illustrations of instruments or scales used by consultants. Another source is Chapter 15 of June Gallessich's *The Profession and Practice of Consultation: A Handbook for Consultants, Trainers of Consultants, and Consumers of Consultation Services* (1982). Gallessich provides a detailed and practical discussion to help prospective evaluators formulate sound evaluation plans. A thorough analysis of evaluation measures integrated into each consultation stage is included in Chapter 6 of Michael Dougherty's 1990 book, *Consultation: Practice and Perspectives*. Dougherty also cites numerous additional resources should readers require more information. A final source of consultation evaluation information is Chapter 11 of *Developing Consultation Skills*, by Richard Dean Parsons and Joel Meyers (1984). This chapter is informative and practical, and for convenience, includes a step-by-step model for implementing evaluation activities.

References and Suggested Readings

Anton, J. L. (1978). Studying individual change. In L. Goldman (Ed.), *Research methods for counselors: Practical approaches in field settings* (pp. 117–147). New York: Wiley.

Bardon, J. (1985). On the verge of a breakthrough. *Counseling Psychologist, 13*(3), 355–362.

Barlow, D. H., Hayes, S. C., & Nelson, R. O. (1984). *The scientist practitioner: Research and accountability in clinical and educational settings.* New York: Pergamon Press.

Beer, M., & Spector, B. (1993). Organizational diagnosis: Its role in organizational learning. *Journal of Counseling and Development, 71,* 642–650.

Bell, C. R., & Nadler, L. (Eds.). (1979). *The client-consultant handbook.* Houston, TX: Gulf Publishing.

Bloom, M., & Fischer, J. (1982). *Evaluating practice: Guidelines for the accountable professional.* Englewood Cliffs, NJ: Prentice-Hall.

Brown, D., Kurpius, D., & Morris, J. (1988). *Handbook of consultation with individuals and small groups.* Alexandria, VA: Association for Counselor Education and Supervision.

Brown, D., Pryzwansky, W., & Schulte, A. (1991). *Psychological consultation: Introduction to theory and practice* (2nd ed.). Boston: Allyn & Bacon.

Brown, D., Pryzwansky, W., & Schulte, A. (1995). *Psychological consultation: Introduction to theory and practice* (3rd ed.). Boston: Allyn & Bacon.

Campbell, D. T., & Stanley, J. C. (1963). *Experimental and quasi-experimental designs for research.* Chicago: Rand McNally.

Caplan, G. (1970). *The theory and practice of mental health consultation.* New York: Basic Books.

Cline, H. F., & Sinnott, L. T. (1981). What can we learn about change in organizations? In S. Bell (Ed.), *Assessing and interpreting outcomes* (New Directions for Program Evaluation No. 9, pp. 1–19). San Francisco: Jossey-Bass.

Cooper, S. E., & O'Connor, R. M., Jr. (1993). Standards for organizational consultation assessment and evaluation instruments. *Journal of Counseling and Development, 71,* 651–660.

Dougherty, A. M. (1990). *Consultation: Practice and perspectives.* Pacific Grove, CA: Brooks/Cole.

Dougherty, A. M. (1995). *Consultation: Practice and perspectives in school and community settings* (2nd ed.). Pacific Grove, CA: Brooks/Cole.

Dustin, D. (1985). On Brown's training and supervision of consultants. *Counseling Psychologist*, *13*(3), 436–440.

Froehle, T., & Rominger, R., III. (1993). Directions in consultation research: Bridging the gap between science and practice. *Journal of Counseling and Development*, *71*, 693–699.

Fuqua, D., & Newman, J. (1985). Individual consultation. *Counseling Psychologist*, *13*(3), 390–395.

Gallessich, J. (1982). *The profession and practice of consultation: A handbook for consultants, trainers of consultants, and consumers of consultation services*. San Francisco: Jossey-Bass.

Gallessich, J. (1985). Toward a meta-theory of consultation. *Counseling Psychologist*, *13*, 336–351.

Goldman, L. (1978). *Research methods for counselors: Practical approaches in field settings*. New York: Wiley.

Hansen, J. C., Himes, B. S., & Meier, S. (1990). *Consultation: Concepts and practices*. Englewood Cliffs, NJ: Prentice-Hall.

Harrison, M. (1987). *Diagnosing organizations: Methods, models, and processes*. Newbury Park, CA: Sage.

Head Start Resource and Training Center. (1994). *The Consultant On-Site Evaluation Form*. College Park, MD: Author.

Heller, K. (1984). Consultation: Psychodynamic, behavioral, and organizational development perspectives. In K. Heller, R. Price, S. Reinharz, S. Rigor, A. Wanderoman, & T. D'Aumno (Eds.), *Psychiatry and community change* (pp. 229–285). Homewood, IL: Dorsey Press.

Katzer, J., Cook, K. H., & Crouch, W. W. (1982). *Evaluating information: A guide for users of social science research* (2nd ed.). Reading, MA: Addison-Wesley.

Kerlinger, F. N. (1973). *Foundations of behavioral research* (2nd ed.). New York: Holt, Rinehart & Winston.

Kiresuk, T. J., & Sherman, R. E. (1968). Goal attainment scaling: A general method for evaluating community mental health programs. *Community Mental Health Journal*, *4*, 443–453.

Kurpius, D., Fuqua, D., & Rozecki, T. (1993). The consulting process: A multidimensional approach. *Journal of Counseling and Development*, *71*(5), 601–606.

Lazarus, A. A., & Davison, G. C. (1971). Clinical innovation in research and practice. In A. E. Gergin and S. L. Garfield (Eds.), *Handbook of psychotherapy and behavior change* (pp. 196–213). New York: Wiley.

Levine, V. (1981). The role of outcomes in cost-benefit evaluation. In S. Bell (Ed.), *Assessing and interpreting outcomes* (New Directions for Program Evaluation No. 9, pp. 21–40). San Francisco: Jossey-Bass.

Lockwood, D. L., & Luthans, F. (1980). Multiple measures to assess the impact of organization development interventions. In J. W. Pfeiffer & J. E. Jones (Eds.), *The 1980 annual handbook for group facilitators* (pp. 233–246). San Diego, CA: University Associates.

Parsons, R. D., & Meyers, J. (1984). *Developing consultation skills*. San Francisco: Jossey-Bass.

Patton, M. Q. (1987a). *Creative evaluation* (2nd ed.). Newbury Park, CA: Sage.

Patton, M. Q. (1987b). *How to use qualitative methods in evaluation*. Newbury Park, CA: Sage.

Paul, S. C. (1979). Consultation evaluation: Turning a circus into a performance. In M. K. Hamilton & C. J. Meade (Eds.), [VOL. TITLE??] (New Directions for Student Services No. 5, pp. 33–46). San Francisco: Jossey-Bass.

Perloff, R., & Perloff, E. (1977). Evaluation of psychological service delivery programs: The state of the art. *Professional Psychology*, *8*(4), 379–388.

Phillips, J. J. (1991). *Handbook of training evaluation and measurement methods* (2nd ed.). Houston, TX: Gulf Publishing.

Robinson, D., & Robinson, J. (1989). *Training for impact: How to link training to business needs and measure the results*. San Francisco: Jossey-Bass.

Scriven, M. (1967). The methodology of evaluation. In R. Tyler, R. Gagne, & M. Scriven (Eds.), *Perspectives of curriculum evaluations* (American Education Research Association Monograph Series on Curriculum Evaluation, pp. 39–83). Chicago: Rand McNally.

Smith, P. C., Kendall, L. M., & Hulin, C. L. (1969). *The measurement of satisfaction in work and retirement*. Chicago: Rand McNally.

Spitzer, D. R. (1986). *Improving individual performance*. Englewood Cliffs, NJ: Educational Technology Publications.

Swartz, D., & Lippitt, G. (1979). Evaluating the consulting process. In C. Bell & L. Nadler (Eds.), *The client-consultant handbook* (pp. 215–233). Houston, TX: Gulf Publishing.

Sze, W. C., & Hopps, J. C. (Eds.). (1978). *Evaluation and accountability in human service programs* (2nd ed.). Cambridge, MA: Schenkman.

Van Maanin, J. (1979). Reclaiming qualitative methods for organizational research: A preface. *Administrative Science Quarterly, 24*, 520–526.

Verhonick, P. J., & Seaman, C. C. (1978). *Research methods for undergraduate students in nursing*. New York: Appleton-Century-Crofts.

Weiss, C. H. (1972). *Evaluation research: Methods of assessing program effectiveness*. Englewood Cliffs, NJ: Prentice-Hall.

◆ CHAPTER FIVE

Resistance and Reactance to the Consultation Process

◆ For the purpose of this chapter, we define the term **organization** as an interdependent human system, *whether that system is an individual, a family group, a program, an agency or institution, an industry or business, or an entire community.* Hence, the obstacles to consultation that we address here are not limited to large organizations. As pointed out in Chapters 1 and 3, the consultant's initial contacts often come from administrators of agencies or institutions who are seeking assistance with the identification or resolution of problems they do not have the time, interest, or skills to address comfortably. While some of the presenting problems are organizational, the majority are not. Rather, they call for the consultant to work with individuals, families, and small groups served by the agency or institution, or with the agency's or institution's staff (teachers, counselors, therapists, or others). The focus of the consultees may be diagnostic assistance, individual or group therapy, special skills training, dealing with real or anticipated crises (the reaction of a group of students to the death of a classmate, for example), or an appropriate combination of these needs. Each consultation involves resistance and reactance. **Resistance** is defined as active or passive opposition, and **reactance** is understood as action taken in response to the threat of change or other action. Regardless of the consultee-group makeup, the resistance and reactance that consultants encounter are much the same, varying primarily in degree and complexity.

Experienced consultants are very much aware that resistance and reactance to the consultation process are inevitable. They are also aware that consultee resistance and reactance are the primary causes of failure for inexperienced consultants. It would be naive for consultants to think that an established human system (whether case, family, group, program, or organizational consultation) will submit passively to change, even when its members are aware that change is needed. Though people may accept the need for change in others, they quickly assume the attitude, "Don't tread on me or mine," when they are expected to change their attitudes or behavior. Their defensive stance to change takes many forms. Power structures unite, vested interests are protected, and defensive postures range from withdrawal and denial to open hostility and rebellion.

The consultation process involves the consultee's total professional identity and work environment as a network of human reactions. Resistance is a natural reaction to any threat to that identity or environment. In large organizations psychological consultants are often required to draw on all of their knowledge, skills, and experience, or for that matter, to work in areas new to them. Even the most experienced psychological consultants encounter unfamiliar forms of consultee resistance and reactance. However, because of the nature of consultation, experienced consultants are seldom surprised (Caplan, 1970; Gallessich, 1982; Hughes & Falk, 1981). Veteran consultants understand that resistance and reactance to the consultation process will differ significantly for external and internal consultants.

External Versus Internal Consultation

Once consultees decide to seek the services of a consultant to assist them with a perplexing problem area, they are faced with the decision of whether to search internally or externally for the most qualified person or consulting team. Their choice is difficult. The ongoing debate over the comparative efficacy of external and internal consultation remains unsettled. Both positions have definite advantages and disadvantages.

Advantages of the External Consultant

The external or outside consultant has the distinct advantages of independence and tran-sience (Caplan, 1970; Gallessich, 1982; Brown, Pryzwansky, & Schulte, 1987; Hansen, Himes, & Meier, 1990). As an outsider, the **external consultant** is independent of the organization's hierarchy and status system. Detached financially, socially, and emotion-ally from the consultee's system, the outside consultant is free to take needed risks in both expression and action. The external consultant also brings a fresh perspective and may be able to identify "games" that the consultee was unable to recognize.

Because the outside consultant's relationship to consultees is temporary, voluntary, and egalitarian, he or she is in a position to negotiate and, if necessary, to reject any con-tract containing adverse conditions. Adverse conditions that might be considered unre-alistic are unreasonable stipulations in relation to the organization's resources, unethical requirements beyond the consultant's perceived competencies, or the expectation that the consultant would serve as a cover for the consultee's hidden agenda. In theory at least, the outside consultant enters consultation with less bias than an internal consul-tant, is in a position to be more objective in the assessment and diagnostic stages of the consultation process, and is free to offer new perspectives and paradigms for action.

Advantages of the Internal Consultant

The **internal consultant** possesses the advantage of an effective working knowledge of the organization that can only be acquired by working in it. The internal consultant is aware of the existence of sensitive records and data; therefore, members of the organi-zation are less likely to withhold this information. Through experience, the inside con-sultant has prior knowledge of the organization's history, social structure, power structure (overt and covert), communication channels (formal and informal), politics, and local customs and beliefs in the organizational community. In addition, the internal consultant has command of the organization's language—the **jargon** (favorite terms and phrases unique to the organization) that must be learned by the outside consultant if much of the data gathered during the assessment stage is to be accurately interpreted.

Disadvantages of the External Consultant

While independence and transience are characteristics that contribute to the external consultant's objectivity, these same characteristics can be barriers for people within the organization. They mark the external consultant as an outsider, an individual who is nei-ther a part of the organization's history nor a participant in the organization's future. Nonacceptance of the external consultant as "part of the team" may be a source of en-mity between the consultant and members of the organization.

Those working for the organization, especially long-term staff who are entrenched in and identified with the system, are likely to be satisfied with the status quo and threat-ened by any idea of change. They may adopt the attitude, "This, too, shall pass," and simply decide to wait out the external consultant's transient tenure. Those who are in power positions in the organization may react to the consultation process with either covert or overt hostility.

Unlike the inside consultant, the outside consultant is usually unfamiliar with the physical and financial resources of the organization. The external consultant must rely on assumptions, experience, and "quick study" to learn the social and leadership structure, the language, customs, and beliefs of the organizational staff.

Disadvantages of the Internal Consultant

Internal consultants have a natural tendency to share a similar view of problems with most members of the organization because of organizational acculturation. But in contrast to external consultants, internal consultants may be granted less status because of previously existing relationships within the organization, particularly with the consultee. Conoley and Conoley (1982) suggest two important entry questions for the internal consultant to ask the consultee: "Why work on this problem now?" and "Why am *I* being asked to do it?" (p. 113). The consultee's responses may provide the very information the consultant needs in his or her decision to accept or reject the consultation project.

As a professional staff member of the organization, the internal consultant faces considerable personal risk. Not only may the internal consultant feel that the consultation assignment cannot be refused without negative consequences, but he or she has established numerous work and personal relationships that are nearly certain to conflict with the consultant role. There is also the very real possibility that friendships can end, or worse, turn into adversarial relationships when special favors are asked that must be refused.

The inside consultant may experience greater difficulty convincing both the professional and clerical staffs of the organization that safeguards to ensure confidentiality have been built into the assessment and diagnostic stages. Without assurance of this confidentiality, people are usually hesitant to make critical statements that could cause them problems in the future.

Sanctioned authority (authority granted by the senior administrator of the organization) may be unacceptable to the internal consultant's peers, especially when they believe that they are equally or better qualified than the person selected to serve as the internal consultant. Unlike the external consultant, who completes the activities outlined in the consultation contract and leaves, the internal consultant is often expected to be involved with the implementation of interventions that come out of the consultation process. There is also always the risk that the internal consultant will be held accountable for the success or failure of recommended interventions.

Consultee and Staff Resistance to the Consultation Process

The consultant role is complex, and consultation relationships typically begin in a strained atmosphere. As pointed out earlier, while consultee and staff resistance to the consultation process appears to be a natural phenomenon and is anticipated, it manifests itself in numerous and often-subtle ways. Intraorganizational forces emerging from a web of complex relationships are always shifting in emphasis, and a change in one affects all. Some degree of consultee uncertainty and ambiguity is inevitable. Professional consultants, therefore, are required to spend a comparatively large amount of their physical and psychic energy relieving tension and overcoming consultee resistance. Proven methods for doing this are:

1. Early focus on relationship-building skills
2. Working toward egalitarian relations
3. Being approachable, available, and helpful to all who request assistance
4. Clarifying the goals of the consultation process
5. Informing both consultees and concerned staff of the consultant's commitment to confidentiality
6. Observing the organization's written (and unwritten) behavioral norms
7. Avoiding all judgmental remarks, whether positive or negative, about specific consultees, staff members, and clients
8. Modeling a rational problem-solving approach
9. Recommending small steps and a gradual pace for change interventions
10. Holding to an unwavering belief in both the efficacy and value of the consultation process

Conflicts Between Consultant and Consultee

For some consultees, the decision to seek outside consultation for assistance with a difficult problem can be traumatic. The decision-making consultee may perceive this action as an admission of personal weakness or failure. When the decision to enlist a consultant arrives in the form of a directive from a senior administrator or the board of directors of the organization, it may be viewed as a lack of confidence in the abilities of the consultee.

The consultee may see his or her role as demeaning. Gallessich (1982) reminds consultants to keep in mind that they "may be more invested in being consultants than consultees are in being consultees" (p. 293). While the consultant role is the primary identity of the consultant, the consultee and the professional staff members of the organization "have other more pervasive and positive identifications" (p. 294). They often prefer not to think of themselves as consultees, a term they perceive as indicating lower priority and status than their professional identities.

Wallace (1966) makes the point that the consultant must also be mindful that he or she is asking the consultee to assume the risk of opening the organization to a comprehensive assessment. To be more specific, the consultant is stating that, when consultation requires an assessment of considerable proportions, it must be conducted properly so that the results are to be meaningful. The physical and organizational facilities and the records considered essential to accurate assessment must not be withheld. Members of the professional staff are to respond fully to all relevant questions. After being interviewed, staff members are not to discuss the questions or the nature of inquires with others so that the last member of the staff to be interviewed by the consultant can respond as spontaneously as the first. In return for this openness, the consultant offers the consultee the following assurances:

1. Every effort will be made not to interfere with or disrupt the work of the staff.
2. The assessment study will be designed to respect the confidence of all respondents.
3. At regular intervals the consultant will review the progress of the assessment with the consultee.
4. The consultant is committed to the presentation of results in a manner that, though factual, will reward rather than punish the professional staff for the trust and confidence they place in him or her and in the value of the assessment.

In brief, the consultant is asking the consultee to assume the greatest portion of the risk inherent in the consultation process.

Resistance Motivated by Mismatching   Professional consultants must learn to accept the fact that a service relationship is characterized by multidirectional forces. Different individuals and groups will perceive the role of consultants differently. A series of conflicts about the consultation roles and expectations may occur. Consultants must expect and resist the constant pressures to behave the way others believe they should behave.

Different people in the same organization may have different perceptions of what constitutes a successful consultation project. For example, a test personnel managers believe will screen out unqualified applicants may be perceived by the Equal Employment Officer as designed to improve the organization's equal employment opportunity profile. Not only is the consultant unknowingly placed in a no-win situation in the organization, but he or she may be faced with ethical or legal difficulties.

External consultants may also encounter resistance from peer specialists inside the organization who believe they are more qualified than the external consultant and, therefore, should have been selected for the job. To justify their perception, the consultant's peer specialists may intentionally, though covertly, subvert the efforts of the external consultant.

Resistance Stemming from Hidden Agendas   Consultees do not always share with the consultant all of their reasons for desiring consultation. Beneath their presenting problem may lie hidden agendas or covert expectations. Should it become known or carried out, the consultee's agenda could jeopardize the legitimacy of the consultation and possibly damage the consultant's reputation. Consultees may, for example, hire consultants for such covert reasons as impressing a committee evaluating the organization's grant or loan proposals; relieving the tension created by a dissatisfied public or powerful pressure group by demonstrating that the consultees are taking their demands seriously enough to hire an outside consultant; frightening troublesome or incompetent staff into leaving the organization; or supporting the consultees' predetermined plan to reorganize the organization or to restructure the organization's services, employee benefits, or salary schedule.

The presenting problem of a teacher seeking consultation with the school psychologist was the need for assistance with an especially disruptive student in the classroom.

The teacher's hidden agenda, however, was to obtain consultant verification that the teacher had already attempted all possible corrective alternatives, that the student remained a hopeless case, and that the only viable solution was to remove the student from the classroom. The hidden agenda became evident to the consultant when the teacher's response to every suggestion was some variation of "I've already tried that, and it didn't work."

Another example involves consulting with a counselor experiencing difficulty with a couple whose presenting problem was to salvage their marriage but who resisted all the counselor's efforts. One of the authors of this book suggested to the counselor that perhaps the couple had a different agenda than the one they presented. The consultant recommended that the counselor gently confront his clients with his confusion. "I'm really confused. You tell me that your reason for coming to me is to salvage your marriage, but you don't really seem interested in working toward that end. Is there something you're not telling me?" In a later session with the consultant, the counselor reported that, after a brief silence, the couple looked at each other, nodded in agreement, then told him that they had already decided that divorce was the only logical alternative. However, they knew that their parents would be terribly upset, especially over their fear of losing their grandchildren, whom they loved very much. To "prove" to their parents that they had "tried everything to salvage their marriage, even counseling," they had decided "to go to a counselor for six months." Once they shared their hidden agenda with the counselor, it became their presenting problem, the focus of counseling changed, and the counselor was able to help them work out ways to assure their parents and their children that a divorce was not a divorce of parents and children, or of grandparents and grandchildren. The counselor later reported that, during the divorce proceedings, arrangements for visitation rights included both the parents and grandparents.

Hidden agendas are not limited to consultees. Consultants also have been known to enter contractual agreements with covert expectations. They may promote their own products (such as assessment instruments, diagnostic surveys, training packages, seminars, workshops, and books), or attempt to convince the consultees of the superiority of the consultant's personal philosophy or favored theory.

As we pointed out in Chapter 2, experienced psychological consultants are always alert to the possibility of hidden agendas. During the entry stage, they will frequently request meetings with all involved constituents in the organization to make certain that the *presenting* problem is *the* problem, that there are no hidden agendas. At this time it is important to affirm that all persons involved, including the consultant, agree to the expectations of the consultation process. The consultant continues to be alert for signs of vested interest in any existing programs, particularly if that interest is of someone at a high level of management and the existing programs are among those to be evaluated by the consultant. The ultimate goal is for all who are involved to be in clear agreement about the purpose of the consultation process and to meet the needs of the organization.

Resistance Created by Unrealistic Expectations   Expected outcomes of the consultation process are not always realistic. Coyne and O'Neil (1992) warn consultants that consultees "can hold tenaciously to the position of the consultant as a 'problem fixer' where they expect consultation to take place somehow outside their involvement and without their investment" (p. 186). The initial contact with prospective consultees is the first test of the consultant's knowledge of his or her personal abilities, skills, values, and biases. Before entering the consulting relationship, consultants should assess their own readiness and ability to work with the presenting problem areas and with the organizational consultees. "They must work hard with consultees to convert their expectancies into achievable goals while mobilizing consultee efforts productively, even as resistance and complexity swirl around them" (Coyne & O'Neil, 1992, p. 186).

Caplan (1970) suggests that even when the consultant feels confident in his or her personal abilities and the consultee's expectations, a good way of beginning the consultation is with an informal contract for an exploratory phase of the consultation process. Usually this initial phase takes the form of an exchange of letters, which can later be reviewed and revised. "The written word is," according to Caplan (1970), "an excellent way of revealing misunderstandings, which may be obscured or omitted in verbal discussions" (p. 65). Caplan further recommends that the contents of these letters clearly specify the expectations of both the consultant and the consultee. Both informal and formal contracts should contain a clause dealing with systematic review and revision when unexpected changes take place (for example, a change of a key consultee or a modification of sanction). See also Chapter 11, Box 11–2, for topics to be addressed in an initial letter of understanding.

It is important to stress that the consultant must be fully aware of his or her personal competencies and limitations when deciding whether to undertake the consulting task. Promising more than one is capable of delivering is not only unwise but also unethical. Moreover, such a promise can lead to litigation.

Resistance Resulting from Theme Interference   **Theme interference** is a term coined by Caplan (1970) to describe the consultee who anticipates a disastrous outcome because of an unresolved personal past defeat or failure. According to Caplan (1970), the consultee has unconsciously created a disaster syllogism: When A (the theme derived from an unresolved defeat in the past) is present, B (disaster) is predicted as the inevitable outcome. An extreme sense of urgency and a high degree of anxiety are characteristics of the consultee experiencing theme interference. The consultee is absolutely convinced the situation is hopeless—as long as A exists, B is certain.

Caplan (1970) developed procedures for dealing with theme interference—**theme interference reduction**. First, in contrast to the consultee's anxiety and excitement, the consultant must model a calm, rational, problem-solving demeanor and approach. Second, the consultant accepts the consultee's syllogism but persuades the consultant that the disastrous outcome is *not* inevitable. Persuasion results from considering other possible outcomes. The consultee is persuaded to look at the present situation more realistically through a thorough examination of the facts. The goal of theme interference reduction is to reduce the strength of the theme. The consultant may relate personal experiences with a similar case or situation that illustrates that the consultee's feared inevitable outcome is not always the result. It should be noted that, while the consultant's personal experience must reflect the consultee's theme, it should differ from the consultee's prediction of a disastrous outcome. If the consultant is successful, the theme that interfered with the consultee's problem-solving approach is invalidated, and the consultee's feelings of competency and skills in problem solving return. The consultant then leaves the consultee to solve the problem.

Greiger (1972) disagrees with Caplan's theme interference reduction approach. He recommends that the consultant follow the rational-emotive approach of Albert Ellis's Rational Emotive Therapy and assist the consultee in recognizing and disputing the irrational ideas contained in the theme. Hughes and Falk (1981) argue that Greiger's suggested approach often results in even greater threat and resistance on the part of the consultee. They favor **paradoxical injunctions**, an approach developed by Haley (1963), which they claim utilizes the theme interference constructively. For example, if the consultee believes that staff members who are not constantly and closely supervised will *always* take advantage of the organization, the consultant may encourage the consultee to drop *all* supervision efforts for a specified period. When all staff members do not take advantage of the organization, the consultee's prediction of disaster is not verified, and the theme is reduced. Indeed, if even a few of the staff members act responsibly without any supervision during the specified period, the consultee may discover that time once spent on constant and close supervision can be used more productively and pleasantly for other activities.

Another example is the teacher who is convinced that when certain early childhood behaviors are evident (for example, copying a homework assignment, cheating on a test, or not telling the truth), the child will *always* become a delinquent adolescent and a criminal adult. Here again, the consultant may accept the teacher's syllogism, but offer facts (research studies and personal experiences) that clearly show that young children who manifested these behaviors grew to become productive, healthy adults. As in the theme reduction methods of Caplan and Greiger, the paradoxical injunction is a consultant technique designed to demonstrate that the consultee's predicted disaster is not inevitable.

Conflicts Between Consultant and Consultee's Staff

The initial perceptions of organizational staff members regarding the purposes of the consultation process can have a significant impact on the consultant's planning and behavior during the early stages of consultation. Often the consultant encounters numerous negative and inaccurate perceptions on the part of staff members, particularly when they were not involved in the decision to bring in an expert to assist with solving a crucial problem or problems. This is often the case when the organization is experiencing a crisis situation. Indeed, even when the consultee (for example, the director of the organization, a department head, or a board of directors) has discussed with the staff the need to seek outside assistance, the consultant is likely to encounter doubt and suspicion regarding his or her legitimacy, purpose, and role.

Resistance Created by the Fear of Change   For many of the organizational staff the consultant is a threat. He or she may be viewed as an unwelcome guest, invited by senior administrators or supervisors to discover and report their weaknesses, to point to errors they have made in the past, or to uncover the informal channels of communication they would prefer remain hidden and private. At the very least the consultant is a symbol of change. To the more insecure members of the organization, the consultant is viewed as the key to Pandora's Box that will release chaos at every level of the organization, deprive them of their sense of permanence and continuity, and force them to build new identities and roles. Even staff who are dissatisfied with the present situation have adapted to it and developed some degree of comfort in their established roles and status. They are painfully aware that change will demand the hard work of undoing a status quo that they have worked hard to create. Change may require them to exceed their abilities and make them feel like beginners again. Change may push their limits and call for resources that they do not believe they possess. Change could mean the loss of their present status and authority. Their response to the threat of change is directed to maintaining the status quo. They try to create or sustain the use of orderly and predictable procedures. In any change there is the threat of the unforeseen, and the reaction to threat is defense.

Defensive postures within an organization can take many forms. The first and most obvious of these is questioning the consultant's legitimacy—critically considering the consultant's credentials and experiential background. The consultant must be prepared to respond to questions with **latent content** (hidden intent or meaning). If the organization is a family, for example, the question might be, "How many children do you have?"; if an elementary school, "When were you last penned up in a room for five hours with 30 eight-year-olds?"; if a prison, "How long have you been with the federal prison system?"; if veterans' affairs, "Where did you see combat?"; if an industry, "What is your managerial experience?" Presenting cases with latent content is another common attempt of threatened staff members to check the qualifications of the consultant. Behind all their questions and case presentations is a single latent meaning: "Who are you to tell us how to do our jobs?"

There appears to be a direct and proportional relationship between the threat of change and the defensive stance taken within the organization. In short, people in the organization attempt to defend themselves from anticipated attacks by using manipulation. They are likely to be concerned about how they look to others, how they may win favors, and how they may dominate peers and impress their supervisors. As they become more defensive, threatened individuals are less able to perceive accurately the motives, values, emotions, and communications of others. In turn, their defensive postures elicit similar defenses within the consultation process, including the inexperienced or insecure consultant.

The consultant who understands the behavior of those threatened by the consultation process is less inclined to perceive their fear, anger, or resentment as a personal attack. Rather, the knowledgeable and experienced consultant responds to resistance by minimizing the defensiveness and establishing a cooperative orientation. The consultant does this by being open about the purposes of the consultation, being attentive to the staff members' ideas, and by expressing a genuine interest in their concerns. Perhaps Coyne and O'Neil (1992) offer the soundest advice to consultants:

> Treating people with respect, involving them, doing what you say you will do, behaving ethically and morally, hearing and responding to painful feelings and issues, sharing yourself appropriately, demonstrating concern, searching for valid information, giving credit where it is due, and clearly defining responsibilities are all part of this process. (p. 187)

Resistance Precipitated by Multiple Cultural Contexts   In the organizational context, **behavioral norms** are those implicit and/or explicit boundaries of acceptable group or organizational behavior. These boundaries define the cultural norms of the organization. The **cultural norms** of an organization are based on shared philosophies, ideologies, values, beliefs, and assumptions, especially about the "proper" way to approach problems and arrive at decisions. Cultural norms are usually limited to behavior related to the accomplishment of organizational goals and limited to the ability of the organization to maintain itself over time. Members in all levels of the organizational structure are aware that deviating from the organization's cultural norms has consequences. Consequences may come in the form of a mild warning or more severe censure. The more relevant the deviation to the purposes and tasks of the organization, the greater the pressures to conform and the stronger the pressures toward uniformity in task performance.

Expectations are also shaped in large part by an organization's cultural norms and may vary significantly from one organization to another. Caplan (1970) strongly advised consultants to familiarize themselves quickly with an organization's cultural norms. Just as strongly, he warned them to demonstrate their respect for the organization's behavioral norms by being careful not to violate them or to interfere with normal work schedules and procedures. A consultant's ignorance of an organization's cultural norms is likely to be viewed by members of the organization as reason enough to question the consultant's qualifications and competencies. Should the consultant's ignorance be interpreted as intentional ignoring of or, worse, disregard for widely held organizational values and beliefs, members of the organization may, in turn, refuse to cooperate in the consultation process and the implementation of the consultant's recommended organizational innovations.

Schein (1985) complicates the consultant's task of learning an organization's cultural norms further when he informs us that because culture is learned at the group level, organizations often develop multiple sets of behavioral norms. The implication of this for the organizational consultant is that different divisions of an organization will not always share a common set of norms. Indeed, the cultural norms for behavior of different groups within the same organization may vary significantly in such areas as perception of time (for example, punctuality), achievement orientations, participation, gender-role perceptions, reaction to confrontation or competition, and use of language.

Experienced consultants have learned, for example, not to generalize across the organization's cultural contexts when assessing the organization's readiness for change. The fact that one of the organization's cultural groups expresses a strong desire for change is not assurance that the other cultural groups in the organization share the same readiness for change. Indeed, because of the reciprocal relationship of different cultural groups in a single organization, change in any one group will affect to some degree all others, and that impact will require them to make cultural changes.

Cultural norms are not easily changed. Patience on the part of a consultant encountering multiple and divergent cultural norms within an organization that requests his or her assistance proves not only to be a virtue but a necessity as well.

Resistance Resulting from Poor Communication   Communication holds the potential to be either a significant variable in effective problem solving or a major source of organizational difficulty. Caplan (1970) reminds his readers: "Distorted messages and blocked or inadequate channels and flow of communication are among the commonest causes of administrative difficulty or inefficiency" (pp. 287–288). The consultant's communication effectiveness is improved when members of the organization have a clear understanding of the behaviors expected of them in the assessment stage. Congruent verbal and nonverbal messages aid in effective communication. The consultant's communication skills are enhanced even further when he or she is aware of the effects of his or her personal characteristics (that is, personal style, values, competencies, gender, and age). When the consultant asks for feedback concerning the way his or her messages are understood, communications improve.

If the consultant arrives at the invitation of the senior administrator, the consultant may be perceived by staff members as the administrator's agent whose purpose is to spy or to follow some prearranged and secret agenda. Such a feared agenda might include the elimination of individual positions, departments, or programs; reclassification of job descriptions; revision of salary schedules; or reduction of benefits. Distorted perceptions can often be avoided or negated by the consultant who effectively communicates the purpose of the consultation and the safeguards of confidentiality that are built into the consulting process.

Resistance Motivated by Reactance and Rebelliousness   Consultees who believe that they must always be in control and free to do whatever they believe is necessary may perceive the consultant and the consultation process as encroachments on their freedom of choice and self-direction. Even when these consultees invite the consultant to assist them with their problems and believe that the consultant is competent and sincerely motivated to help them, they may resist because of reactance and willfully rebel against the consultant's efforts. They may insist, for example, on acting as the intermediary between the consultant and the organization's staff members and on monitoring the consultant's work by making their presence felt at all meetings conducted by the consultant. Consciously or unconsciously the consultee's intent is to prohibit open staff discussion with the consultant and to weaken staff confidence in the consultant and the consultation process (Gallessich, 1982).

The experienced consultant will demonstrate to rebellious consultees that he or she will not take part in their reactance power games and will not suffer from their rebellious actions or feel defeated if they successfully resist the consultation process. Though rebellious consultees are entitled to resist change in any manner they choose, they (not the consultant) must accept the consequences of their rebellious behavior. Veteran consultants assure consultees in reaction that they are not interested in either coercion or manipulation, that all consultees will be involved in formulating intervention strategies, and further, that as consultees they are free to decide for themselves which, if any, of the alternative solutions and interventions offered by the consultant they will implement.

Ellis (1985) is convinced that willfully resistant consultees "almost invariably have decidedly irrational Beliefs that spark their self-defeating willfulness, and you [the consultant] can quickly show them their [irrational Beliefs] and scientifically dispute them" (p. 156). He, like the Adlerians, also recommends paradoxical intention to demonstrate irrational thinking (see "Resistance Resulting from Theme Interference," this chapter). Caplan (1970) makes use of interpretation as the major technique to facilitate the consultee's understanding of his or her unconscious motives for resisting the consultation process. Both Ellis and Caplan recommend the judicious use of humor. Hughes and Falk (1981) offer a social psychological theory of reactance as a framework for minimizing consultee resistance and for utilizing consultee rebellious behavior for beneficial change.

Practically all major therapeutic approaches warn therapists not to become involved in the reactance games of the resisting client. This warning should be heeded by consultants working with rebellious consultees.

Summary

The purpose of the consultant is to help individuals, family groups, agencies, businesses, industries, and communities solve problems. This chapter presented some of the obstacles that consultants are likely to encounter. Advantages and disadvantages of the external and internal consultant were also discussed. Significant obstacles that the consultant must face include consultee and staff resistance and reactance. Various forms of resistance and reactance to the consultation process were reviewed. While there are no right or wrong answers to dealing with the obstacles that threaten the efficacy of the consultation process, consultants may anticipate resistance and reactance to some extent in each consultation. The consultant with a clear set of goals who is skilled in human relations, experienced with different consultation models and problem solving, and realistically aware of his or her own strengths and limitations is more likely to be successful than the consultant who lacks these qualities.

A major weakness of the consultation literature—and of this chapter—is that insights into resistance and reactance to consultation are based almost entirely on anecdotal accounts of individual practitioners. In short, there is a distinct lack of empirical research. While descriptive accounts alert consultants that consultee resistance and reactance are natural reactions to the threat of change and, therefore, to be expected by the consultant, Randolph and Graun (1988) caution both practicing and training consultants that "the strategies for preventing and dealing with resistance have not been subject to empirical test" (p. 184). They further caution that consultants do not have empirical backing as they attempt to "determine which types of resistance are most likely to occur in certain consultation settings" or "the degree of effectiveness of various strategies . . . for dealing with specific forms of consultee resistance." They also have an inadequate basis for determining "whether some variables pertinent to the individual consultant are related to the occurrence and amelioration of consultee resistance" (p. 184).

It is not our intention to denigrate or discourage the reporting of anecdotal accounts or case studies by practitioners in the field. Indeed, it is from their descriptive reports that consultants have become alerted to the urgent need for specific research studies and additional training for consultants. If consultants are to learn to deal successfully with consultee and staff resistance and reactance, they must not only learn to recognize manifestations of this behavior but also to develop the necessary skills and strategies for dealing successfully with them.

GLOSSARY

Behavioral norms   In an organizational context, the implicit or explicit boundaries of acceptable group or organizational behavior.

Cultural norms   Behavior based on shared philosophies, ideologies, values, and assumptions, especially about the "proper" ways to solve problems and arrive at decisions.

External consultant   A consultant employed outside the general boundaries of the consultee's organization.

Internal consultant   A consultant employed within the same general setting or organization as the consultee.

Jargon   Favorite terms and phrases unique to the organization that must be learned by the external consultant if much of the data gathered during the assessment stage is to be accurately interpreted.

Latent content   Hidden intent or meaning.

Organization   A group of people working together to achieve some goal or purpose; an organization requires cooperation among people to perform work activities prescribed by established policies and procedures.

Paradoxical injunction   A theme reduction technique where the consultant persuades the consultee anticipating a disastrous outcome to behave as if the disaster were not inevitable and, by so doing, helps reduce or invalidate the strength of the theme (see **theme interference reduction**).

Reactance   Action in response to another action (for example, the threat of change).

Resistance   Active or passive opposition to the real or anticipated changes accompanying consultation.

Sanctioned authority   Authority granted the consultant by a senior administrator in the organization. Unlike line authority (authority of position), sanctioned authority requests staff cooperation and clearly specifies personnel and records that are to be available to the consultant in the assessment and diagnostic stages of the consultation process.

Theme interference   A term coined by Caplan (1970) to describe a consultee who anticipates a disastrous outcome because of an unresolved personal past defeat or failure.

Theme interference reduction   Persuading the consultee that the disastrous outcome of theme interference is *not* inevitable (see also **Paradoxical injunction**, a technique employed by the consultant to reduce theme interference).

ANNOTATED BIBLIOGRAPHY

We strongly recommend that those of you who wish to pursue the subject of this chapter further begin by reading two classic reference works, Caplan's *The Theory and Practice of Mental Health Consultation* (1970) and Gallessich's *The Profession and Practice of Consultation: A Handbook for Consultants, Trainers of Consultants, and Consumers of*

Consultation Services (1982). Although these books are somewhat dated and limited in scope by today's standards, few books include more thorough discussions of obstacles to the consultation process than those presented by Caplan and Gallessich. Moreover, you will find their presentations of consultee and staff resistance and reactance relevant enough today to compel attention and forceful enough to provoke thought. In addition to addressing the many and varied forms of resistance and reactance, both Caplan and Gallessich present techniques and strategies the consultant may employ to reduce the threat of consultation and, hence, the intensity of defensive actions and reactions. We are convinced that both Caplan's and Gallessich's books have earned a place on the bookshelves of all consultants and prospective consultants.

In their book *Psychoeducational Consultation: Definition-Functions-Preparation,* Kurpius and Brubaker (1976) summarize what they consider the essential research literature on resistance to change. Again, though the studies are dated and represent common knowledge to many experienced consultants, this book is recommended to those of you unaware of the earlier research studies that address the impact of obstacles to consultation. Of particular interest to the consultant in training are the lengthy lists (pp. 53–55) of "Conditions Producing Greatest Change" and "Conditions Producing Least Change," which remain as relevant today as when they were published.

Although Robert Kelly's *Consulting: The Complete Guide to a Profitable Career* (1981) does not address consultee resistance and reactance to consultation directly, it does have an entire chapter on the consultant's initial efforts to create an accepting interpersonal relationship that can reduce the anxieties of both consultee and consultant. Anxiety, Kelly asserts, leads to consultant and consultee traps that block consulting projects, particularly in the initial stages of the consultation process. Not only does Kelly label and describe potential traps, he also presents preventive measures the consultant can take to avoid them.

Although directed primarily to business management consultation, Lawrence Tuller's *Cutting Edge Consultants: Success in Today's Explosive Markets* (1992) thoroughly examines current and predicted realities that every consultant must face, and presents the most effective ways to solicit and serve clients. He also introduces his readers to eight general areas of knowledge that, he contends, are vital to consultants, regardless of the market they choose to serve. In addition, Tuller shares his view of the future of consulting in a changing world and covers such topics as education, state and federal certification and licensure, the changing structure of business, government controls, and financial systems. He emphasizes the need for consultants to adopt a global viewpoint if they are to retain a competitive edge.

Psychological consultants can also profit from reading Peter Drucker's *Management: Tasks, Responsibilities, Practices* (1973). The material in this book is relevant to all managers and, therefore, consultants of managers, regardless of functional area and size of organization. Drucker focuses on the manager *as a person.* He attempts always to integrate people and tasks. Because this book and its approach have been developed and tested in more than 30 years of teaching and consulting, it is read widely by managers in the field and is highly recommended to both professional consultants and students preparing for the consulting profession.

REFERENCES AND SUGGESTED READINGS

Brown, D., Kurpius, D., & Schulte, A. (1991). *Psychological consultation: Introduction to theory and practice* (2nd ed.). Boston: Allyn & Bacon.

Brown, D., Pryzwansky, W. B., & Schulte, A. (1987). *Psychological consultation: Introduction to theory and practice.* Boston: Allyn & Bacon.

Caplan, G. (1970). *The theory and practice of mental health consultation.* New York: Basic Books.

Conoley, J. C., & Conoley, C. W. (1982). *School consultation: A guide to practice and training.* New York: Pergamon Press.

Coyne, R. K., & O'Neil, J. M. (Eds.). (1992). *Organizational consultation: A casebook.* Newbury Park, CA: Sage.

Drapela, H. M. (1983). *The counselor as consultant and supervisor.* Springfield, IL: Thomas.

Drucker, P. F. (1973). *Management: Tasks, responsibilities, practices.* New York: Harper & Row.

Ellis, A. (1985). *Overcoming resistance: Rational-emotive therapy with difficult clients.* New York: Springer.

Fine, M. J., Grantham, V. L., & Wright, J. G. (1979). Personal variables that facilitate or impede consultation. *Psychology in the Schools, 16*(4), 533–539.

Gallessich, J. (1982). *The profession and practice of consultation: A handbook for consultants, trainers of consultants, and consumers of consultation services.* San Francisco: Jossey-Bass.

Greiger, R. M. (1972). Teacher attitudes as a variable in behavioral modification consultation. *Journal of School Psychology, 10,* 279–287.

Gutkin, T. B., & Bossard, M. D. (1984). The impact of consultant, consultee, and organizational variables on teacher attitudes toward consultation services. *Journal of School Psychology, 22,* 83–91.

Haley, J. (1963). *Strategies of psychotherapy.* New York: Grune & Stratton.

Hansen, J. C., Himes, B. S., & Meier, S. (1990). *Consultation: Concepts and practices.* Englewood Cliffs, NJ: Prentice-Hall.

Hare, C., & Wyatt, J. (1986). Meeting the needs of federal workers: How can OD practitioners become active? *Organization Development Journal, 4*(2), 57–60.

Hollway, W. (1991). *Work psychology and organizational behavior.* Newbury Park, CA: Sage.

Hughes, J. M., & Falk, R. S. (1981). Resistance, reactance, and consultation. *Journal of School Psychology, 19*(2), 134–142.

Kelly, R. E. (1981). *Consulting: The complete guide to a profitable career.* New York: Charles Scribner's Sons.

Kilmann, R., Saxton, S., & Serpa, R. (Eds.). (1985). *Gaining control of the corporate culture.* San Francisco: Jossey-Bass.

Knoff, H. M. (1984). The practice of multimodal consultation: An integrating approach for consultation service delivery. *Psychology in the Schools, 21,* 83–91.

Kolb, D. M., & Bartunek, J. M. (1992). *Hidden conflict in organizations: Uncovering behind-the-scenes disputes.* Newbury Park, CA: Sage.

Kurpius, D. J., & Brubaker, J. C. (1976). *Psychoeducational consultation: Definition-functions-preparation.* Bloomington: Indiana University Press.

Lanning, W. (1974, May). An expanded view of consultation for college and university counseling centers. *Journal of College Student Personnel,* 171–176.

Mannino, F. V., MacLennan, B. W., & Shore, M. F. (1975). *The practice of mental health consultation.* New York: Gardner Press/Wiley.

Piersel, W. C., & Gutkin, T. B. (1983). Resistance to school-based consultation: A behavioral analysis of the problem. *Psychology in the Schools, 20*(3), 11–20.

Randolph, D. L., & Graun, K. (1988). Resistance to consultation: A synthesis for counselor-consultants. *Journal of Counseling and Development, 67,* 182–184.

Schein, E. (1985). *Organizational culture and leadership.* San Francisco: Jossey-Bass.

Tuller, L. W. (1992). *Cutting edge consultants: Success in today's explosive markets.* Englewood Cliffs, NJ: Prentice-Hall.

Wallace, W. A. (1966). A formulation of a concept of the fully-functioning office of admissions in a large urban university (Doctoral dissertation, Wayne State University, 1966). *Dissertation Abstracts, 27*(3), 67-10,496.

◆ PART TWO

Consultation Settings

Now that you have read the introductory chapters of this book, you have a basic knowledge of consultation as it is generally practiced. As we have seen, most consultants, both novice and experienced, apply their skills in all types of settings, including large organizations, small human service agencies, community action programs, and family systems. Although the opportunity to serve in diverse settings is, indeed, one of the attractive features of consultation, the unique cultures, structures, philosophies, and work-related difficulties characteristic of various organizations present major challenges.

Part II includes four chapters. Each highlights the specific issues and processes that pertain to consultation in a particular setting. Note that as you review Chapters 6 to 9, you may encounter the conceptual issues discussed in earlier chapters in a somewhat different form because of the specific dynamics of each consultation setting. A chapter-by-chapter overview follows.

CHAPTER SIX
Consultation in Educational Settings

Chapter 6 examines the consultation issues and practices common to educational settings. The chapter is divided into two major parts: consultation in higher education settings and consultation in public school settings. For each setting, we highlight the specific issues and processes consultants must consider.

CHAPTER SEVEN
Consultation in Child Development Settings

Chapter 7 focuses on psychological consultation in child development settings. The unique challenges presented by these settings form much of the discussion. The chapter also identifies various child development programs that seek consultation, as well as the problems and interventions that exist in these settings. A key feature of the chapter is the discussion of consultation situations that relate to children, parents, and staff.

CHAPTER EIGHT
Consultation in Health Care Settings

This chapter provides information about an emerging and challenging type of consultation. The health care setting, though replete with opportunities for psychological consultants, is one in which consultation is less formally developed. We discuss the problematic aspects of psychological consultation and provide suggestions for beginning consultants. Existing as well as new and potentially useful forms of consultation are examined as well.

CHAPTER NINE
Consultation in Business and Industrial Settings

In business and industry, psychological consultation enjoys a long and rich history. Chapter 9 details the involvement of psychology in these settings with specific implications for the psychological consultant. The consultant's roles as a human resource professional, employee assistance program specialist, and organizational development specialist represent the major topics of this chapter.

CHAPTER SIX

Consultation in Educational Settings

Summary

Glossary

Annotated Bibliography

References and Suggested Readings

 Internal consultants are found in college and university settings as well as at all levels of public schools. These consultants are often selected from numerous student personnel specialists, including psychologists, counselors, social workers, learning resource specialists, and career planning specialists. Not only are these specialists likely to know the system intimately and view it from a developmental framework, they are also most likely to possess the qualifications and expertise in interpersonal relationships, behavior, and group dynamics. With these skills and knowledge the consultant may be well equipped for effecting change in individuals, groups, and institutions. Further, as full-time, staff members, these professionals are most likely to have acquired extensive information about students' personal, academic, and social concerns. They can also be given greater freedom of movement than staff responsible for regular classroom instruction.

Although many of these professionals are involved in testing, diagnosis, and individual and small-group counseling of individuals in crisis, they also see the need for greater emphasis on preventing problems before they reach the crisis stage. To achieve this goal they seek alternative techniques, strategies, and interventions to promote the full participation and personal development of all students in the educational setting through more active involvement in the educational process.

Consultation in Higher Education

Effective interventions in higher education depend on the consultant's understanding of the particular setting in which decision making occurs. Many variables influence the decision-making process in educational settings, including individual and group needs and desires, available resources, rewards and sanctions, group norms, and informal influence patterns. Consultants "have failed to initiate even routine change because they have not accounted for the system" (Dinkmeyer & Carlson, 1973, p. 44; see also Kotter & Heskett, 1992; Sarason, 1971). Hansen, Himes, and Meier (1990) strongly advise the outside consultant "to allow time to assess and evaluate the system" and the inside consultant "to step back and gain a more objective perspective" (p. 75). Internal consultants are too often prone to assume that, because they work in the system, they have full knowledge of system and cultural variables. Kotter and Heskett (1992) warn that this assumption may not be warranted: "When cultures are our own, they often go unnoticed—until we try to implement a new strategy or program which is incompatible with their central norms or values. Then we learn, first hand, the power of culture" (p. 3).

Psychological consultants in the educational setting must be acutely aware of the numerous and diverse system and cultural variables that can have a positive or negative impact on the consultation process. External system variables that directly define consultation opportunities and constraints in educational settings encompass federal and state government bodies and existing laws, political and economic climates, unions, advocacy groups, and accreditation standards. Examples of internal system variables include formal and informal power structures, cultural values and rules, the administrative hierarchy, role clarity, decision patterns, and the system's formal and informal communication systems. In short, the conditions for consultation innovations in educational institutions are set by the complex matrix of system and cultural variables.

Internal System and Cultural Variables in Higher Education

One of the first lessons for psychological consultants in a college or university environment, particularly external consultants, is that they are working in a bureaucratic setting. Colleges and universities must adhere to objectives and standards set by federal and state governments and national and state accrediting bodies, as well as an institutional mission statement.

Public college and university presidents are accountable to the state's higher education governing boards (a board of regents or board of trustees), whose members are usually appointed by the governor. Presidents of private schools likewise are accountable to a governing board, often elected from among influential alumni. Vice presidents and deans (in most instances, *all* administrators, including chairpersons) hold their offices "at the will and pleasure" of their president in both public and private organizations. Though the department chairpersons may, in some instances, be nominated by department faculty, final approval ultimately rests with the college dean, academic vice president or provost, the president, or even the governing board.

Many college and university presidents, once recruited and selected for distinguished records of scholarship, are often chosen today for their managerial, business, fundraising, and political skills. Indeed, many of today's college and university presidents acquired their expertise outside the educational profession. The experiential backgrounds of vice presidents in charge of such specialized function areas as finance, administration, fundraising, personnel, public relations, and research are often business, industry, economics, or politics. As a result, more and more deans and even department chairs are selected for their managerial talents, not for their scholarship abilities.

External System Variables in Higher Education

In addition to having to cope with bureaucratic constraints, psychological consultants in higher education find themselves in a system under attack. Higher education has always had its critics. Today, however, education is the subject of congressional investigations and scathing editorials in the media and is an easy target for candidates campaigning for political offices, including the presidency of the United States. Although voicing the concern of educators more than two decades ago, Sarason (1971) could be writing for today's psychological consultants in educational settings:

> We are now in an era when more people spend more time than ever before planning and executing educational programs and changes. And those who neither plan nor implement spend a portion of their leisure time criticizing those who do. (p. 7)

Sarason further asserts that many of the planners and implementers of change in the schools "have little or no basis, either in theory or experience, for understanding the social structure of the school, its traditions, and its usual ways of accommodating to change" (p. 8).

Classroom innovation in higher education, when it occurs, is typically the result of individual motivation and effort and is only occasionally supported by the administration. Curriculum change is also often the result of individual innovation. Discouragement results from insufficient financial resources to support innovative effort over the long term. Failure of campus administrators to provide leadership stifles innovative change. Other roadblocks that detour positive change in higher education include the lack of detailed strategies for definitive responsibilities and activities, extreme decentralization where only one person assumes responsibility for quality effort, and reluctance to relinquish leadership in existing programs to colleagues who will champion new programs.

Obstacles to Consultation in Higher Education

Psychological consultants in higher educational settings are often forced to confront obstacles that would impede their performance. Because internal consultants are employees and external consultants work at the discretion of educational setting administrators, the consultation process must overcome many barriers relative to power structures, role and rule constraints, and organizational inertia.

Formal and Informal Power Structures

As a bureaucracy the educational system's formal power structure is normally hierarchical and, for public institutions, set by law. There is no question about who has the authority to make decisions and direct activities. However, the formal power structure is not always strictly observed. There may be informal and conflicting power structures at all levels of the organization. Such informal power structures give influence to individuals or groups who have acquired authority and the ability to sway others because of their position in the union or faculty senate subsystem levels. Other examples of power structures working beyond the formal organization are (1) individuals who have access to people who hold formal decision-making status, (2) a person with recognized expertise that those in power positions lack and respect, and (3) people who benefit from their social position or status in the community or state. External groups, such as parents, business and industrial leaders, community officials, and dominant cultural groups, may also wield influence outside the official power structure.

While the psychological consultant in the educational setting must observe the formal power structure, he or she should also be alert for informal levels. Hansen, Himes, and Meier (1990) recommend that the consultant assess power "by observing communication patterns, such as the flow of communication—who speaks to whom, and who listens, is very beneficial" (p. 77). The consultant's assessment of the educational set-ting must examine the institution's mission, policies, programs, and activities to learn if they are attainable or pure rhetoric. Professed values and goals are not always prac-ticed. Are there clear priorities? Are results related to promises and expectations? How are decisions made? How are policies formulated and administered?

Authority relations in complex educational settings are sometimes blurred, am-biguous, and shifting, but they do exist, and the consultant should be aware of them (Baldridge, 1971). While Drucker (1985) insists that "authority is an essential dimen-sion of work" and "inherent in the fact of organization," he also reminds his readers that "fear is altogether incompatible with the production of knowledge. It may produce ef-forts and anxieties. It will not produce results" (p. 241). Indeed, the pervasive informal constraints found in today's colleges and universities are often even more inhibiting to innovation. North (1990) defines **informal constraints** as the "extensions, elaborations, and modifications of formal rules; socially sanctioned norms of behavior; and internally enforced standards of conduct" (p. 40).

Role and Rule Constraints

In the higher education environment, the role of consultation is stifled by archetypical paradigms that define the roles of counselors and psychologists as student advocates, campus advisers, service providers, and therapists. Student development or student af-fairs counselors, for example, most often conform to prescriptive and service-oriented job definitions that fail to include the need for systems consultation, data-based con-sultation, mental health support for faculty and staff, and innovative student-oriented consultation.

Unwritten rules may restrict the potential for success of internal or external consul-tation. *These rules may be judged faulty when assessed in terms of objective reality.* Ex-amples of such unwritten rules are:

1. For those having the potential to provide psychological consultation, their un-mistakable domain is student-oriented. Systems or faculty consultation is a mat-ter for others.
2. Faculty and staff are professionals responsible for their own departments or pro-grams. As capable teachers and administrators, they can resolve problems with-out collaboration with others.
3. Mental health problems are not widespread in the higher education environment. Moreover, because administrators, faculty, and staff have most often achieved high visibility and status, they will not participate in consultation interventions.
4. Departments are closed in terms of external input or problem-solving consulta-tion. They prefer to manage their own frustration, morale problems, and work overload.

As employees in the educational system, internal consultants are often limited by their role definitions outlined in job descriptions, by administrators, and by institutional, state, or federal policy. The impact of consultants may also be limited because they owe their position to supervisors, directors, or administrators who empower their actions and evaluate their worth to the organization.

External consultants are restricted by authority figures in the system who (1) acknowledged the need for outside consultation services, (2) selected or approved a particular consultant for the position, and (3) most important, set the consultation parameters. In addition, these authorities may retain the right to define the problem, guide the consultant's actions, and make the final decision on whether to accept the consultant's recommendations for intervention and organizational change. Indeed, it is often difficult for organizational staff to perceive the external consultant as an objective specialist divested from the authority of organizational leaders.

When staff and professionals within an organization are not invited to participate early in the consultation process, the external consultant is suspect. He or she is viewed as an outsider brought into the organization to present changes the administrators have already decided are needed but are hesitant to present themselves. All too often their suspicion is justified.

Organizational Inertia

Psychological consultants must also be aware that "most organizations have an inertia which enables them to resist any effort to examine themselves or change" (Dinkmeyer & Carlson, 1973, p. 44). Kotter and Heskett (1992) refer to the tendency of a system to revert to old habits and familiar roles as that "spring resistance quality." Sarason (1971) warns: "Another factor too lightly passed over by those involved in planning and change is that many of those who comprise the school culture do not seek change or react enthusiastically to it" (p. 8). Rather, they view consultation services as an intrusion in the educational setting—a threat to their territory, their privileges, and their time. Finally, plans for restructuring an educational system require financing, the removal of barriers to innovation, faculty development, and, perhaps most difficult of all, role changes and role clarity.

History and Need for Faculty Development Programs

McKeachie (1991) traced the emergence of the faculty development movement in the United States to the 1960s. While there was some progress in the 1960s and 1970s, significant growth in the need, interest, and demand for faculty development programs occurred during the two decades that followed. Programs for the personal development of faculty are even more recent. Though brief, its history is rich. ERIC/CUE via CD-ROM listings from 1982 to 1993 included 2608 abstracts of publications and conference presentations on the subject of faculty development. Despite the progress of the past two decades, the next few years may be crucial. To quote McKeachie (1991):

> We have gained a lot of practical wisdom. We are less naive about the ability of any one
> approach to solve problems of teaching and learning, and we have a substantial body of
> theory, research and practice on which to build during the 1990s. (p. 7)

Faculty Development Programs for Improved Instruction

More colleges and universities are establishing new offices of faculty and instructional development. Nemko, an independent consultant, and Simpson, from the University of California, report in a 1991 publication:

> The stage has been set for increased commitment to teaching. **AAHE (American Association of Higher Education)** national conferences have emphasized instruction, and lawmakers and college guide writers have indicted research-driven institutions for paying insufficient attention to teaching. The presidents of Harvard and Stanford have recently urged increased emphasis on teaching, and other college presidents are jumping on the bandwagon. (p. 83)

Experienced consultants, however, are aware that "jumping on bandwagons," though often tempting, can be high-risk behavior.

If called on to improve the teaching skills of university faculty, educational consultants are well advised to assess the university's incentive and reward system for faculty *before* accepting the assignment. A key aspect that must be determined is the importance and reward of quality teaching when faculty face tenure and promotion opportunities. Does the quality of teaching have comparable importance with research and publication? Should the consultant determine that a marked incongruence exists between the university's stated values and actual practice, he or she can expect that even the best faculty development program to improve instructional skills stands little chance of faculty acceptance.

Annual awards for teaching excellence may camouflage a devaluing of instructional abilities. Annual awards recognize only two or three faculty members each year and have no long-term impact on compensation. Incentives and rewards for teaching must be more than rhetoric.

Further complications are indicated if the consultant's assessment reveals an increasingly restricted access to tenure track positions, a growing number of part-time and adjunct faculty appointments, and special consideration given to successful grant writers. Another problem that the consultant's assessment may uncover is lengthy probationary periods for promotion, despite the time frame for promotions within university faculties outlined by the American Association of University Professors. With decreasing budgets, all these practices are fairly common among administrations in higher education, and they will adversely affect faculty acceptance of development programs for instructional improvement.

Eble and McKeachie (1985) warn that when faculty have little or no involvement in determining the need or content of faculty development programs, they may perceive the program "as an indication that the administration thinks the faculty is so inadequate that it needs special help to improve" (p. 208). The success of faculty development programs depends ultimately on the faculty members, and they prefer to be collaborators rather than targets. If faculty are to perceive themselves as collaborators, educational consultants must realize that their involvement is essential from the inception of the program planning. Representatives from faculty groups can assist in need assessment, participant selection, goal formation, financing, program planning, and scheduling.

Comprehensive faculty development programs may target faculty members who are required to improve instructional skills. Such remedial consultation may be extended at the discretion of faculty members who wish to assess existing skills or "re-tool" obsolete instructional tactics. Despite their resistance to skill-building consultation, some faculty members can be referred to the teacher consultation process by department chairpersons or college deans. The teacher consultation model encompasses a broad range of evaluation and feedback activities designed to improve instructional quality. To assess the faculty member's instructional abilities and deficiencies, teacher consultants may observe classroom teaching performance, review student evaluation ratings, and consult with the academic leaders regarding their evaluation methods and instruments. In addition, videotaping is a popular method that allows a faculty member to observe his or her own classroom performance.

Mentoring Programs

Nearly all colleges and universities have developed induction or orientation programs for newly appointed faculty. However, the quality and comprehensiveness of these programs vary considerably. Many induction programs in the not-too-distant past were limited to a brief welcome, introduction to other faculty, and the distribution of a faculty handbook that spelled out administrative policies and job requirements. In short, rules, roles, and regulations were the agenda for the day. Induction was based on a deficit model (the assumption that new faculty lacked specific knowledge and skills to do their jobs and, therefore, required remedial assistance to correct necessary knowledge gaps and problem areas).

Early induction programs were also conducted in one or two days before the first day of classes. They usually consisted of a quick review of required administrative tasks to be completed during the first week of the school term—items to be included in course syllabi, attendance policies, course requirements, and outside readings and class assignments, for example. From that point, new faculty were left on their own. After a brief review of earlier induction and orientation programs, Runyan and Buche (1991) observed that "education is one of the only professions where first year personnel are expected to assume the full duties [of experienced faculty] the first day on the job" (p. 12).

The more fortunate new faculty are those who find an experienced, sympathetic colleague or a department chair who, aware of his or her own critical first years, is unwilling simply to stand back and watch the newest member of the department sink or swim without adequate instruction or assistance. Research indicates that successful first-year faculty often attribute their survival to supportive, nonjudgmental mentors who not only listened to their professional and personal concerns but also helped them evaluate their expectations, some of which were unrealistic (Boice & Turner, 1989; Boice, 1991; Fink, 1984; Gmelch, 1993; Runyan & Buche, 1991).

Only recently have colleges and universities revised their philosophy toward newly appointed faculty. As a result, the time frames of induction and orientation programs have been extended, many for as long as two or three years. Emphasis today is on both personal and professional development, and the initial focus is on the individual concerns and problems of faculty. Research indicates that one of the most common and effective induction programs sponsored by **faculty development centers (FDCs)** for new faculty are formal **mentoring programs**, in which voluntary veteran faculty are selected and trained, then assigned to new faculty during their critical first years of appointment (Boice, 1991; Boice & Turner, 1989; Runyan & Buche, 1991). Research also indicates that well-written policies for the methods and criteria to be used in the selection and training of mentors are critical factors. In addition to years of experience, close proximity, and time available, characteristics of successful mentors include:

- A willingness to commit to the program
- A positive attitude
- Success as a teacher
- The same discipline area
- Compatible philosophy
- A separation from the formal evaluation system of the institution (Runyan & Buche, 1991, p. 48)

Consultants are also learning that planning for mentoring programs should include such issues as:

- Time involvement
- Mandatory, voluntary, or elective participation of newly appointed faculty
- Compensation for both participants and mentors
- Administrative involvement and support
- Needs assessment methods
- Periodic review and evaluation of the program

Faculty Development Programs to Alleviate Stress

Faculty in higher education are confronted with stressful situations daily. Most have learned to cope with minor stresses. However, there are occasions when the interaction of a series of even minor stresses becomes synergistic and explosive (see Box 6.1 for an example).

Because stress is idiosyncratic and can be traced to multiple sources, psychological consultants must be aware that no single corrective or preventive program for dealing with stress will benefit all faculty. Indeed, as Keyes (1991) points out, a time management program designed for the Type B personality could prove harmful for the rigid Type A personality. Time management techniques, which may help Type B personalities become more disciplined and make better use of time, will often only make Type A personalities even more clock-conscious, more determined to control time, and more likely to continue to add tasks to an already hectic schedule without first eliminating old ones. Rather than planning *time,* Type A personalities must learn to plan their *lives;* to weed out ruthlessly those activities that do not enhance the achievement of life goals; to schedule some time for solitude and reflection, personal matters, and family obligations; and finally, to give up the fantasy that there is one best way for everyone to manage time. Only with clear purpose in mind can they choose what must be done and

---

Box 6.1
Interaction of minor stresses can become synergistic and explosive.

Professor X makes it a practice to sit down with his pocket secretary every Sunday evening and plan his activities for the coming week. He reviews his calendar carefully and blocks out periods of time to work on a book chapter due in three weeks. He plans to begin his week and his work on the chapter by arriving at his office two hours before his regularly scheduled office hours.

As he puts his key in the door Monday morning, the telephone rings. While X is still on the phone with a student who wants an appointment as soon as possible for advising, a colleague enters to discuss problems he is experiencing with "an extremely difficult class."

The telephone rings again. This time it's the department chair asking if X can meet a class of another member of the department faculty who has just reported that he is ill and unable to make it in. Though X doesn't have the time, he feels obligated and says he will do it. Meanwhile, his colleague is still sitting in the office waiting for X to listen to his problems, and standing just outside the door is a student who has missed the last two classes of a course that is to meet at 1:00.

The phone rings for the third time. Feeling trapped in a sudden major stress reaction, Professor X storms past his colleague and the waiting student. Without a word to either, he rushes down the hall seeking to escape all the interruptions.

---

what can be ignored. In short, they must first become convinced that they *can* learn to say no, and then be given the assertiveness training to help them say it.

Some higher education settings have adopted an **employee assistance program (EAP)** model to help stressed faculty and staff members. The EAP concept, originally developed within business and industrial settings, addresses the problems of distressed workers by providing referral or treatment opportunities, along with incentives for overcoming maladaptive behaviors or emotions. EAP policies are grounded in the philosophy that: (1) Faculty or staff members are valuable human resources and overcoming their stress problems is a cost-effective measure, and (2) higher education organizations have a humanistic commitment to promoting both the renewal and well-being of their members. Further, most comprehensive EAPs extend preventive, educational opportunities for stress management and health promotion.

Even a cursory review of the literature reveals both need and opportunity for educational consultants skilled in alleviating academic stress in higher education. Today, academic stress is recognized as a national phenomenon that crosses all discipline boundaries (Seldin, 1987). While space limitations in a single chapter make it impossible to trace the literally hundreds of sources of academic stress, consultants need to be apprised of sources that appear repeatedly in the literature. Outside sources of academic stress are:

1. Economic crises
2. Political forces that criticize and prescribe for higher education
3. Government and business forces that tie research grants and equipment to patents, censored or delayed publications of research findings, and a role in personnel selection
4. Demographic changes in student and faculty populations

A major institutional stress source contributing to a shifting of academy norms is the replacement of collegiality with autonomous administrative systems that follow industrial and business models, impose formal relationships on professionals, retain final decisions in such areas as evaluation, advancement, compensation, institutional mission, organization, and policies, and set fiscal responsibility as the primary goal. Administrative economic strategies include: (1) hiring adjunct and part-time faculty at lowest market rates, with no benefits and no possibility of tenure, (2) increasing the probationary period and requirements (for example, a set number of publications) for tenure of full-time faculty, and, if all else fails, (3) retrenchment. Add to these sources the idealized professional and personal aspirations of both new and tenured faculty and the result is often stress saturation, or worse, burnout.

Senior Faculty   As a group, senior faculty report fewer work-related stressors in their lives. Still, significant numbers voice concern because they see themselves as being locked into a position with no chance of advancement and into a system with a stultifying reward structure. There are those, also, who believe administrators, board members, and legislators are making decisions that directly affect their lives without seeking their participation in the decision-making process. Indeed, many feel that the faculty role in institutional planning and governance is eroding, and they predict that it will continue to do so in the decade ahead.

New and Junior Faculty   New and junior faculty, in their attempt to balance their daily teaching assignments, keep current in their discipline, conduct research, publish, write grant proposals, attend committee meetings, perform institutional and community service, attend and make presentations at professional conferences, and still find time to meet family obligations, feel the tremendous stress of time and resource constraints. Keyes (1991) warns that bodies rebel when people experience an inordinately high degree of stress. Stress hormones suppress immune responses. New faculty often report physical symptoms, such as headaches, insomnia, irritable bowel syndrome, high blood pressure, chronic fatigue, reduced alertness, short-term memory loss, inability to concentrate, stimulant abuse, and irritability. Yet for new faculty members the stakes are high—their career possibilities. Teaching, research and publication, and service seem to require all their time. An unbalanced priority, granting one component of the three faculty tasks more energy to the point where it adversely affects the other two, can prevent tenure and promotion. Time extended in any one of these tasks takes time from all others or from time needed by the family or for personal matters. Stress increases for this group when stringent tenure and promotion policies are unclear and when evaluation methods of their performance are not shared by the chair or dean.

Junior faculty who take an institution's professed emphasis on teaching at face value are often confronted too late with the reality that research and publication will determine their tenure and promotion chances. After an extensive study of the reward structure of a representative sample of 480 colleges and universities, Fairweather (1994) concluded: "Except for community colleges, . . . faculty members who spent more time on research and who published the most were paid more than their teacher-oriented colleagues" (p. 53). Further, he discovered, research and publication were the major salary determinants of both nondoctoral and elite research universities. In both instances, teaching was either a neutral or negative factor in the reward systems of these institutions.

Despite the promised advances in instructional technology, consultants in higher education anticipate faculty shortages in the late 1990s and early 2000s for increasing numbers of academic disciplines. Administrators, concerned about the recruitment and retention of new faculty during the next decade, are establishing FDCs and charging the directors to conduct studies of the characteristics, concerns, and expectations of new faculty. Although there is still much to learn about new faculty, research in this area has increased, and consultants must be aware of the research literature.

Researchers concerned with the characteristics, expectations, attitudes, and needs of new faculty (Baldwin & Blackburn, 1981; Boice, 1991; Boice & Turner, 1989; Fink, 1984; Lee & Field, 1991; Stanley & Chism, 1991; Waldinger, 1985) recognize that faculty development programs must broaden their offerings to address a diversity of professional, organizational, and personal concerns. Further, they recognize the need for a strong relationship between key campus administrators (departmental chairs and deans particularly), the faculty, and FDCs to make both administrators and faculty more aware and understanding of their roles in the development and support of both new and experienced faculty.

Robert Boice (1991, 1989), director of the Faculty Instructional Office and professor of psychology at the State University of New York at Stony Brook, has contributed much to what is known about the experiences of new faculty on both teaching and research campuses. Of particular interest is Boice's (1991) longitudinal study, which covered the period 1985–1990 and clearly revealed the needs, concerns, and accomplishments of new faculty. Further, Boice's study indicates that many colleges and universities, possibly due to the value placed on autonomy, "tend to let new faculty 'sink or swim' on their own" and "tolerate the conditions that produce poor morale and the resulting low productivity" (p. 173). Finally, Boice suggests faculty development consultants could "learn something of value about how new faculty could develop as teachers from observing individuals who excel quickly" (p. 173).

Psychological consultants with faculty development experience are often sought from outside the university to assist in such areas as:

1. The initial assessment of new faculty
2. Their expectations and needs
3. The selection and training of faculty mentors
4. Faculty development program design
5. Follow-up study to evaluate the program's success

Part-Time Faculty   The major stressors for part-time faculty (reported by Gappa, 1987, to be 30% of all faculty in the 1980s and likely to reach 40% in the 1990s) are uncertainty and insecurity. Appointments are often semester by semester, depending entirely on enrollment figures. The prospect of termination is always present, particularly in times of budget crises or retrenchment. Compensation for part-time faculty is at best inadequate, and they are typically perceived by full-time faculty as less qualified. Part-time faculty are often given little administrative or supervisory support, and they are seldom asked to contribute to department and college decisions.

Faculty Renewal and Wellness Programs   For many years traditional "faculty renewal" programs were limited to sabbaticals, other leaves, and reduced teaching loads for research, special institutional and community service responsibilities, or temporary administrative assignments. Sabbaticals are usually scheduled for a single semester or quarter at full salary or for one academic year at half salary. Depending on the institution, sabbaticals may be awarded automatically to all faculty, selected on a competitive basis, or some combination of these traditional patterns.

Faculty renewal programs today have been expanded to include on-the-job workshops, seminars, and training sessions designed for such areas as:

1. Updating instructional methods
2. Integrating critical thinking into teaching methods
3. Improving awareness of changing demographics on campus
4. Acquiring new skills, assignments, or careers (for example, the use of computers for instruction, research, and networking)
5. Maintaining health and wellness
6. Planning for retirement

Summer research grants awarded for scholarly pursuits have also become fairly common, as have travel and housing stipends to assist faculty invited to make presentations at world, national, or regional conferences. After reviewing faculty development efforts in the literature and the results of personal research, Bowen and Schuster (1986) conclude: "On the whole, the many efforts toward 'faculty development' seem to us to have had a modestly favorable impact on overall trends in working conditions, though in some cases they have been spectacularly successful" (p. 135).

North (1990) describes **faculty wellness programs** as those "institutional efforts to promote and maintain the health and overall well-being of faculty" (p. 11). While some programs "concentrate on the physical aspect," North asserts, "a full wellness program will address other aspects of a person's life, such as career issues; work situation; family, social, and spiritual or meaning issues" (p. 11). All recognize the interrelationships among body, health, emotions, and work performance.

Consultation with Students

Although consultation aimed at student populations occurs in multiple forms, it is nearly always a helping process delivered through either organizational programs and activities or direct student contact. The role of consultation by student development specialists has expanded significantly during the past decade. Newman and Fuqua (1984) contend that student development professionals should practice organizationally centered consultation to help the college environment provide the best overall service to students. This is supported by Plato (1977), who believes that student affairs staff should acquire the necessary consultation and organizational skills to work effectively in the university setting. As organizationally minded consultants, student development specialists help the college organization design and implement programs and services that benefit students. Direct student consultation then occurs within special programs in a more traditional form of remedial training and problem solving.

Examples of campus programs grounded in consultation are:

1. *New-student orientation programs*   Student development consultants design and implement support programs that acquaint new students with the college or university setting. The goals of this type of consultation are to familiarize students with a range of information that will allow them to ease into the college environment.

2. *Residential programs*   The college setting represents a community of diverse individuals and groups who reside together in relatively close quarters. Indeed, the campus becomes the student's "home away from home." Student development consultants design residential programs that ease adjustment, teach life skills, and promote harmonious, cooperative living.

3. *Special needs of returning students*   Much has been written recently about the "returning student phenomenon" in modern college settings. **Returning students** are older, life-experienced adults who return to the college environment to begin a college career or "retool" for personal, career, or occupational demands. Because returning students represent a unique group with distinct interests and needs, student development consultants must prepare special programs designed specifically to meet their needs.

4. *Special services*   Today's college campuses are multidisciplinary settings that address the needs of diverse students. University and college personnel have come to recognize that students exhibit personal characteristics, developmental features, and learning styles that necessitate special approaches and remedial training. Indeed, because of students' physical or learning disabilities, educational background, and socioeconomic status, many special services are required to meet the challenges imposed by today's higher education centers.

Consultation in Public School Settings

Most pupil personnel specialists in the public schools today (elementary, middle, and secondary school counselors, school psychologists, school social workers, and learning resource teachers) agree that they need to reach greater numbers of students. The literature calls for an increased movement toward developmental and preventive approaches and interventions, including system interventions (Milstein, 1986). There appears also to be a rather strong conviction (though certainly not a consensus) that school counselors and school psychologists could maximize their impact and effectiveness in the school setting by focusing on the most significant adults in the students' lives (Milstein, 1986; Carlson, Splete, & Kern, 1975; Umanski & Halloway, 1984). One approach recommended repeatedly is to further develop their roles as consultants to parents, teachers, and administrators, and, when indicated, as system change agents. Dinkmeyer (1975), an early advocate for consultation in the elementary school, asserts: "The rationale for consultation proceeds from the belief that the objectives of elementary school guidance can be reached for all children only through an emphasis on consultation" (p. 67). Dinkmeyer is also a firm believer in the integration of the guidance function with the educational process and the curriculum.

Several factors can impede movement toward greater emphasis on consultation by student development specialists. One key factor is *lack of autonomy*. The administration of student development specialists in public schools falls under the auspices of the school principal, regardless of his or her background. Not only does the principal administer the special service programs and define the function of individual staff specialists, the principal also functions as supervisor and evaluates the specialists' professional competencies. Under this system, the counselor positions "fall into the category of technical arm of the administration" (Warnath, 1975, p. 166). Lacking autonomy from the administration, student development specialists cannot arbitrarily change their traditional roles. Another factor that stymies consultation for these professionals is *excessive workload*. In many public school settings, at least half the counselor functions are quasi-administrative duties. School psychologists face a backlog of diagnostic evaluations and reports. Social workers are unable to keep up with home visitations, agency referrals, and family education programs. Counselors, psychologists, and social workers have traditionally been removed from the teaching/learning process, and they usually have little input regarding curricula. For a student development specialist to step into areas considered by teachers and administrators to be outside his or her role could prove an invitation to censure or even nonrenewal of contract if the person is still in probationary status. Realizing these factors, it is clear that counseling professionals in public schools face many difficulties if they hope to serve as change agents.

Internal System Variables in the Public Schools

Public school systems are also bureaucratic systems. At the federal level there is the U.S. Department of Education, headed by the Secretary of Education. Each state has a Department of Education and a state superintendent of education. Each county has a superintendent and a board of education. Huelskamp (1993) warns: "The U.S. education system was built on the foundation of a combination of local control, state influence, and federal interest. The existence of more than 15,000 independent school districts nationwide attests to this concept" (p. 721).

These education governing bodies provide the financial support and decide how, when, and where all funds will be spent. These same governing bodies determine the minimum number of days school will be in session each year and what subjects will (and will not) be offered in the curricula. Though professional educators in the system may make recommendations, the final decisions on practically all educational matters will come from one of these three governing bodies. Bureaucratic decisions represent compliance with directives from superiors, and when the bureaucrat holds the power, the resulting conflict will prove difficult for the professional educator.

Internal consultants in the public schools are certified for their positions by the state. It is the state, then, that defines their roles and functions and prescribes to colleges and universities the minimum course of study for students preparing for these positions. To date, consultation is not included in either the role and functions of student development specialists or the states' prescriptions of minimal preparation standards.

External System Variables in the Public Schools

Because public schools are sociopolitical institutions, consultants will enhance their understanding of the environment in which they work by accepting the fact that priorities are often based on political rather than educational assessments. State and local boards may make decisions based on what they expect will win public support during an election rather than coming to decisions based on educational efficacy. Psychological consultants who fail to recognize the political nature of decision making in public schools and the bureaucratic nature of the organization run a high risk of failure. The consultant must also be aware that though the needs and desires of professional educators are great, **resources** (money, people, facilities, equipment, energy, and time) are limited, particularly "when the future holds the threat of retrenchment, and the present offers only the pressure to produce in a bureaucratic structure that offers neither inspiration nor motivation" (Lauter, 1986, p. 70).

In the public school system, accountability is a one-way street. Board members are accountable *by law* to their constituents, superintendents to their boards, principals to their superintendent, teachers to their principal, and students to their teachers. While this organization works well to maintain a disciplined compliance with rules, regulations, and directives (and these are numerous), it is not always conducive to creative change, innovative methodology, or quick response to changing needs.

Role and Rule Constraints in the Public Schools

As a sociopolitical system, public schools develop roles and rules. While some are formal and rather narrowly prescribed, others, the unwritten roles and rules especially, may not be so clearly defined. Neither formal nor informal roles and rules are immune to distortion; indeed, many informal communications on roles and rules are based solely on individual perceptions. Both formal and informal roles and rules can create faculty resistance to the consultation process. Examples of some of the more negative unwritten roles and rules that teachers in the public schools sometimes adhere to are:

1. The classroom is the teacher's domain; all others are outsiders and unwelcome, including other teachers, pupil personnel workers in the system, and consultants, whether internal or external.

2. The competent teacher should be able to deal effectively with *all* classroom learning and behavioral problems without outside assistance. Referring a student to the principal's office for discipline, for example, will be interpreted as a sign of the teacher's incompetence and likely result in a poor annual evaluation.

3. Collaborating with a consultant will be viewed as a sign of weakness, and the teacher who does so willingly will be evaluated and judged by veteran teachers and the principal as weak.

4. Parents are to be appeased regardless of the circumstances.

5. Like the classroom, teacher time is sacrosanct, and because of already overburdened time demands, teachers should not be expected to meet with a consultant before or after school hours.

6. A failure rate of more than 5% is unacceptable to the administration or, even stronger, "No student fails in this school."

7. Any negative statement about the system to those outside it, including outside consultants, will be interpreted by the administration, the board of education, and certain other teachers as an act of disloyalty and will be reflected in the principal's annual evaluation report.

Counselors in public school settings have complained vehemently that they are unable to meet students in face-to-face counseling interventions because of system priorities that demand that other duties come first. Indeed, the time constraints imposed on professional educators, prospective consultants included, can seriously restrict consultation and professional interactions (Brown, Pryzwansky, & Schulte, 1991). Academic scheduling, managing special student cases, and serving as the go-between with complaining parents are examples of responsibilities that impede consultants' availability to pursue more substantive consultation activities. Further, school psychologists are so integrally involved with specialized testing, advising placement committees, and adhering to legislated federal or state policies that they have little time to consult with teachers and administrators.

Consulting with Public School Teachers

For educational consultants who want to maximize their impact on the learning and behavioral needs of all students, consulting with teachers is a logical objective. First, teachers have more direct, daily contact with greater numbers of students than do any other professionals in the school system. Second, if teachers generalize what they learn in the consultation process to their work with future students, the consultant's potential impact on the lives of students over the long term is not only significantly increased, but also highly rewarding and motivating.

Reality dictates that teachers are often responsible for implementing the consultant's intervention strategies. They will ultimately determine the success or failure of any teacher consultation effort. This alone is reason enough for the psychological consultant in the educational setting to do everything possible to establish a collaborative relationship between two professionals, characterized by mutual trust and respect, open communication, and cooperative problem solving. In such a relationship, each professional is fully aware of and sympathetic to the role, rule, and time constraints imposed on the other by the school environment.

Effective communication between the psychological consultant and the teacher (the consultee) requires an awareness that the philosophical orientations of psychological consultants and teachers may differ significantly and hold the potential for divergent cognitive, emotional, and attitudinal perspectives on the teachers' presenting problem. For example, teachers are generally classroom-focused, while psychological consultants are generally focused on the total physical and psychological environment of all students. Knapp and Salend (1984) remind consultants who work with teachers that "successful programs require interpersonal skills and sensitivity to the concerns of the teacher" and further that "insensitivity is likely to be counterproductive, creating reactance—resistance to treatment" (p. 289).

Individual Case-Focused Consultation

While an individual case-focused consultation may eventually involve others (such as other teachers, administrators, parents, a case study team), it is based primarily on a one-to-one relationship between the consultant and consultee (teacher). The third party, who is often unaware that he or she is the subject of consultation, is usually a student or students whose behavior the consultee reports as disruptive or abnormal or who is experiencing learning difficulties. The consultee initiates the consultation process, in the form of a written request or, as is more often the case, a brief encounter during the day:

Teacher: I need to talk with you sometime soon about Johnny. He's a nice kid, but he's driving me crazy. I've tried everything I know, but nothing works. He constantly disrupts my class. It's reached the point where I'm so busy with him that I haven't time to teach.

Consultant: I can see where this is a problem. Let's set a time and place for our first meeting. What time is best for you?

During the first meeting, the consultant listens carefully to the teacher's description of the problem. The consultant's early responses are generally empathic, demonstrating understanding of the teacher's concerns and feelings and conveying attitudes of acceptance and genuineness. Later, the consultant may ask specific questions that are intended to generate alternative problem definitions and to convey to the consultee that problem solving is an essential aspect of the consultation process. The consultant's questions also communicate to the consultee that consultation is a collaborative effort and that the consultee is expected to participate actively in the consultation process.

- What are examples of specific behaviors you find disruptive?
- Can you describe specific events that you believe are typical of Johnny's actions?
- When did Johnny begin acting this way?
- What is Johnny's reaction when you correct him?
- If forced to guess at this point, what do you believe is motivating Johnny to behave as he does in your classroom? What do you think Johnny gains from his behavior?

- What is Johnny's behavior doing to you? To the other students in the classroom? To Johnny?
- What specific behavioral outcomes would you like to see result from the work we do?

Once the consultant and teacher agree on a limited number of preliminary problem definitions, they select one or two that they believe to be most reasonable, workable, and worth pursuing. They then direct their attention to assessment strategies to test their hypotheses (for example, observation in and out of the classroom setting, interviewing previous and present teachers, anecdotal records, family visitation, personal and medical histories, test records).

If their assessment confirms their problem definition, the consultant and consultee begin to plan intervention strategies to correct it. Here, again, mutual agreement is essential. Both must agree that the interventions are realistic and achievable. Both must be convinced that the consultee and the client (student or students) will benefit from the interventions chosen.

Progress evaluation, in collaboration with the consultee and based on the problem definition and desired outcomes, continues throughout the consultation process (see Chapter 2); however, evaluation is an essential step to termination and should not be ignored. A written, summative evaluation report, if agreed to by both parties, may serve as a termination of the consultation relationship.

Group Consultation with Teachers

School-based psychological consultants who possess the necessary knowledge, leadership skills, training, and experience in group dynamics and group work may elect to work with teachers experiencing similar concerns in small, structured issue or case study groups. Based on the research provided in the literature on Task-Oriented Groups (T-Groups), Dinkmeyer and Carlson (1973) developed experiential groups specifically for teachers that they called "C" Groups. The C in "C" Group represents the specific components facilitated by the consultant who serves as the group leader: collaborating, consulting, clarifying, communicating, being cohesive, being concerned, confronting, caring, being confidential, being committed, and being willing to change. The "C" group may take either an issue or a case study approach (Dinkmeyer & Carlson, 1973).

Faculty acceptance of the "C" Group approach to consultation is more likely to occur if participants in the first group report their group experience favorably. Selection of the first group, then, is crucial. Dinkmeyer and Carlson recommend the following selection procedure:

1. Select voluntary teachers with similar concerns or, when case-focused, who work with the same students.
2. From this group select teachers who are admired and respected by the majority of the faculty. A favorable report from this group will carry more weight with other faculty members.
3. By interview, narrow this group to five or six members of different ages, levels of experience, and teaching/learning approaches. Greater success is reported with heterogeneous groups.

4. During the interview, clarify goals of the group. Supply all members with written materials describing purposes, rationale, and benefits of the "C" Group experience.

5. With administrative approval and assistance, decide on a time and place for one-hour group sessions over a period of six to eight weeks. The "C" Group may also be conducted at a one- or two-day retreat away from the school setting. "C" Groups may employ structured experiential exercises, readings, work assignments, or contracts.

Consulting with Public School Administrators

When the central administration of a public school system calls on an educational consultant or a consulting team for assistance, the consultant or consulting team is often faced with a crisis situation that requires working with the entire system and most or all of the human resources of that system. Indeed, there are occasions when they may be required to work with individuals and groups outside the system. Examples of such crises are natural disasters (for example, floods, hurricanes, tornadoes that cause extensive damage and deaths), social crises that invade the system (racial tensions, gang wars, a sudden rash of teenage suicides, a sudden or inordinately high dropout rate), and organizational or system crises (organizational restructuring, a mass faculty exit, systemwide curricula revision, loss or probation of national accreditation status, sudden drop or loss of public confidence, a recognized need for faculty and/or administrative development and renewal programs). Although the ultimate beneficiaries of any educational consultation are the system's human resources—students, teachers, parents, and administrators—the client and chief focus of systems in crisis in some instances may be the system itself. Severe system crises call for highly trained, experienced consultants possessing a broad array of special knowledge, skills, and experiences.

Fortunately, most consulting with public school administrators is neither so urgent nor so complex as the examples listed above. Initial contact may be with a teacher, supervisor, assistant principal, or principal in one of the system's schools for assistance with a specific problem or program. The request for assistance may be as simple as an afternoon or evening workshop to address a specific topic or concern (for example, teaching critical thinking, improving teacher-constructed tests, stimulating classroom discussions) or a series of seminars or workshops to address such problems as student discipline in the classroom or Writing Across the Curricula. School administrators may also seek the assistance of an educational consultant when organizing for an accreditation association's requirement of a self-study or when preparing for an accreditation team's evaluation visit. Depending on the consultee's expectations of the consultant, such a consultation time frame could run as long as one or two years.

Regardless of how simple or complex the consultation request, Dinkmeyer and Carlson's (1973) advice to educational consultants more than a decade ago is still relevant: "The consultant never accepts an assignment in a school district unless he [or she] has had complete communication with central administration on a number of basic issues" (p. 36; see also Chapter 2).

Even a cursory review of the literature reveals that the most successful educational consultants whose consultees are school administrators are those able to establish collaborative, egalitarian consultant-consultee relationships—no small task when hidden agendas or ulterior motives are behind the consultation request (see Chapter 5). Keys to collaborative, egalitarian consultant-consultee relationships seem to be:

1. Finding an administrator/consultee "who is equally concerned with becoming a catalyst and who seeks to attack resistance" (Dinkmeyer & Carlson, 1973, p. 36)
2. Establishing a clear role and function agreement for both the consultant and consultee
3. Communicating clearly to the consultee how the consultant can and will help the consultee achieve his or her goals
4. Scheduling periodic meetings to review progress and evaluate how well both the consultant and consultee are living up to their contractual agreements

Only when these conditions are present is the consultee likely to give the consultation function high priority, to work with the consultant to formulate a successful consultation program, and to provide the program with adequate physical facilities, supplies, clerical assistance, and qualified staff.

All adults in the educational setting (mid-level administrators, classroom teachers and, where the occasion calls for it, parents) must perceive that the consultant has the full acceptance and support of the central administration and the administrator/consultee (the local superintendent or school principal). They must not believe that the consultant was brought into the system to endorse an administrative program formulated prior to the consultant's entry into the educational setting. The schism between administration and faculty naturally created by a bureaucratic system can be bridged if those affected believe they are truly an integral part of the consultation process, that their ideas, feelings, and beliefs are not only sought but also valued from the early entry and planning stage through termination, that they are not expected to be passive followers, that the consultant's study of the system or problem is objective, and that the interventions recommended will work if followed. In short, only when the consultative relationship is collaborative, egalitarian, and based on the trust of all involved can the consultation process work.

Consulting with Parents

"Practically every theorist [of personality development] acknowledges the importance of the early years on personality formation" (Wallace, 1993, p. 542). Though there is disagreement on the specific roles that significant adults play in the lives of children, none of the theorists ignores the influence of parents or parent surrogates. Indeed, Carl Gustav Jung, an early psychoanalytic theorist and founder of a system of psychotherapy, believed emotional disturbances in children were actually reflections of emotional disturbances in their parents. Alfred Adler, founder of Individual Psychology, thought the mother played the primary role in the child's conscious development of the predisposition for **social interest** (a term he considered synonymous with psychological health). Albert Bandura, who developed the Social-Cognitive Theory of personality development, identified parents as their children's earliest models. Even theorists who grant healthy adults functional autonomy consider the effects of childhood experiences and the immediacy of the present in their attempts to explain present human behavior. These theorists include Alfred Adler; Carl R. Rogers, founder of Person-to-Person Therapy; Abraham Maslow, who presented one of the first studies on self-actualization; George Kelly, an early cognitive theorist who gave us the Theory of Personal Constructs; Albert Ellis, founder of the Rational-Emotive-Behavioral Theory of personality and psychotherapy; Rollo May, a renowned existential theorist; and Viktor Frankl, a Viennese psychiatrist and founder of Logotherapy.

Psychological consultants in educational settings, particularly those interested in serving all students over the long term, are certain to be called on to consult with parents. Teachers may ask the consultant to sit in on a parent-teacher conference. Parents experiencing difficulty with their child or children may request the assistance of the consultant. The **Parent Teachers Association (PTA)** may invite the consultant to work with a group of parents who have expressed interest in learning specific parenting skills (for example, improving communication between parent and child). Administrators may ask consultants to work with parents when a child (or children) has become a discipline problem. When these and similar requests are made, the psychological consultant must remember to inform those seeking assistance of the boundaries of parental consultation (Brown et al., 1991; see also Chapters 1 and 3, this volume).

While there are similarities, parental consultation differs significantly from family therapy, marriage counseling, and parent education. Brown et al. (1991) strongly advise the consultant not to be drawn into therapeutic or educational relationships, even when their degree specialty may be in one of these areas. Parental consultation is a triadic relationship—that is, a relationship between the consultant and consultee (parent or parents), with the third party identified as the child or student. The goal of consultation is to change the consultee in ways that will indirectly benefit the client (in this instance, the parents' child or children). Specifically, Brown et al. (1991) advise the consultant to differentiate parental consultation from **family therapy** ("a direct service to the entire family in which parent and children participate simultaneously with a therapist to correct problems in the family," p. 259), **marriage counseling** (a therapeutic approach to couples experiencing marital problems), and **parent education** (approaches designed to teach specific parenting skills; see Chapter 7). Unlike the usual triadic relationship of psychological consultation, where the consultant-consultee relationship is between two professionals (consultant-teachers, for example) trained in different disciplines and working together in a collaborative relationship for improved functioning of clients (students), the relationship of parental consultation is between a consultant and nonprofessionals.

Popular theoretical models for parental consultation include Caplan's (1970) mental health model, the Adlerian model (Dreikurs, 1972; Dinkmeyer & Carlson, 1973), Bandura's (1986) social-cognitive model, the systems theory model (Capra, 1982), and the behavioral theory model (Knapp & Salend, 1984). There are recent moves, also, toward the development of a number of eclectic models (Brown et al., 1991, for example). Regardless of the theoretical model the consultant employs, consultation generally follows certain stages, though not always in a linear fashion. Because the stages of consultation have already been discussed in some depth (see Chapter 2, this volume), they will not be repeated here. However, in parental consultation Brown et al. (1991) recommend the addition of another stage—an explanation of psychological principles. They believe that it is necessary for parents "to understand the *why* as well as the *what* of the intervention to be employed" (p. 252) for effective communication and understanding to occur. Once the consultant and consultees agree on the goals of consultation, the psychological principles to be followed in designing intervention strategies are explained in terms the parents can understand. Moreover, the consultant involves the parents in the explanation and encourages them to question the principles and to discuss ways they apply in their family. Only when it becomes evident that the parents fully understand the psychological principles behind interventions and are able to apply them to their particular family situation does the consultant permit the consultation process to proceed to a selection of strategies and goal attainment (Brown et al., pp. 262–263). Finally, parents are cautioned that if they encounter problems in the course of the intervention, "they should either call the consultant or discontinue the intervention until they have had an opportunity to discuss the problems they are experiencing with the consultant" (p. 264).

SUMMARY

Student personnel specialists most often attracted to psychological consultation and selected as psychological consultants were identified in the chapter. Their unique qualifications were listed, and areas in which they may need additional knowledge and experience were discussed.

Because psychological consultants' knowledge and understanding of the educational environment are critical to their success, internal and external system and cultural variables were presented in some depth. Psychological consultants must recognize that they are working in a bureaucratic setting organized to implement objectives and standards set by federal and state government bodies, judicial rulings, and national and state accrediting, credentialing, and licensing boards. It is equally, if not more, imperative that they become aware of and sensitive to the more subtle, informal aspects and issues that await them and that can, if ignored, adversely affect their efforts. In addition, this chapter addressed the need for consultant assessment of the pressures exerted on today's schools and colleges by numerous influential special interest groups.

Obstacles to consultation at all levels of education were also discussed in the chapter, including those unique to both internal and external educational consultants. Focus was placed on formal and informal power structures, written and unwritten role and rule constraints, and organizational inertia.

Various faculty development efforts were also covered to the degree possible in the limited space allotted to a single chapter. In particular, the chapter discussed faculty development programs for improved instruction, mentors for new, junior, and part-time faculty, the alleviation of faculty stress, and faculty renewal and wellness. Finally, consultation with students, teachers, administrators, and parents or families was covered briefly.

GLOSSARY

American Association of Higher Education (AAHE)   A national professional association for both administrators and faculty in higher education. The AAHE hosts a national conference and publishes a journal, in addition to providing other services.

Employee Assistance Program (EAP)   Initially found in business and industrial settings as a referral service for employees needing assistance with behavioral, physical, or psychological problems. EAPs were established in higher education settings to help faculty and staff overcome stress and stress-related problems. Their primary goal is to promote the renewal and well-being of faculty and staff.

Faculty wellness programs   Institutional programs to promote and maintain the health and overall well-being of faculty.

Family therapy   A direct service to the entire family in which parents and children participate simultaneously with a therapist to correct problems in the family.

Faculty development centers (FDCs)   Centers on college and university campuses whose goal is to make both administrators and faculty more aware of their roles in the development and support of both new and experienced faculty. FDC personnel are involved in research, program development, and follow-up evaluations.

Informal constraints   Extensions, elaborations, and modifications of formal rules, socially sanctioned norms of behavior, and internally enforced standards of conduct.

Intrasystem variables   Formal and informal power structures, normative structure, role clarity, decision patterns, formal and informal communication systems.

International Society for Technology (ITSE)   Now an affiliate of NCATE.

Marriage counseling   A therapeutic approach to work through marital problems. The counselor or therapist may work with either husband or wife or both.

Mentoring programs   Programs that provide new faculty with mentors—experienced faculty committed to helping them through their first year(s) on the job. Programs vary from one educational setting to another.

National Council for Accreditation of Teacher Education (NCATE)   The only body officially sanctioned by the U.S. Department of Education to accredit schools of education.

Parent education   Approaches designed to teach specific parenting skills.

Parent Teacher Association (PTA)   A volunteer organization devoted to the education, welfare, and protection of children and youths, founded in 1897 in Washington, D.C. Membership in a local unit includes membership in the state branch and in the National Congress of Parents and Teachers.

Resources   In educational settings, people, money, facilities, equipment, energy, and time.

Returning students   Older, life-experienced adults who return to the college environment to begin a college career or to "retool" for career or occupational demands.

Social interest: For Alfred Adler, social interest was synonymous with psychological health.

ANNOTATED BIBLIOGRAPHY

Seymour B. Sarason's book *The Culture of the School and the Problem of Change* (1971) is as timely today as when it was published, more than two decades ago. In short, it is must reading for both new and experienced psychological consultants who choose to practice in educational settings, particularly in the public schools. Although psychological consultants were not the primary targets of Sarason's book (he addressed his writing to all "agents of change" from within or outside the school culture), they will find his book instructive. Moreover, they will gain new conceptualizations that not only account for many failures in consultation but that also give rise to new modes of action and intervention. They will no longer view simple solutions as ends. They will become more aware of the realities of culture and the problems of change. They will be convinced, as was Sarason after ten years spent planning and directing the Yale Psycho-Educational Clinic, that "we know far less about the '*actual* functioning of schools and school systems' than we have realized" (p. 229). More important, they will encounter a level of conceptual understanding that, if taken seriously and further developed, may well lead to more appropriate and effective efforts at change.

Although Kotter and Heskett's *Corporate Culture and Performance* (1992) is aimed at those interested in the relationship between corporate culture and long-term economic performance, there is much in this book that could benefit psychological consultants working in educational settings. Indeed, we strongly recommend that you follow up on Sarason's 1971 work by reading *Corporate Culture and Performance*. Not only do Kotter and Heskett confirm many of the conclusions drawn by Sarason, but they offer strategies and practices that continuously respond to changing environments, reversing unhealthy cultures and making them more adaptive. Further, Kotter and Heskett's book is based on four empirical studies, conducted between 1987 and 1991, in more than 200 companies. They discuss in depth the hazards of attempting change in bureaucratic, political, conservative cultures that stifle initiative and innovation by clinging to once-successful, old and familiar values. Psychological consultants will be interested in Kotter and Heskett's descriptions of the subtle and covert ways that power structures attempted to thwart changes that might threaten their privileges, promote managers rather than leaders, discourage experimentation, decentralize decision making, and eliminate their traditions and methods of management. In addition to stressing the difficulties of changing unhealthy organizations, Kotter and Heskett also trace the roots of healthy organizational cultures that promote excellent performance over the long term.

For readers interested in the development of faculty and instructional development programs in higher education, we recommend *FACE to ECAF: A Sourcebook of Individual Consultation Techniques for Faculty/Instructional Developers,* edited by Lewis and Povlacs (1988). The material in the book was gathered by its editors with both the novice and veteran consultant in mind. Regardless of experience (or the lack thereof), readers are invited to "browse" and "to discover what is useful to [them]" (p. v). Readers are also invited to correspond with individual chapter authors for additional information or to contribute methods and strategies they use successfully and want to be considered for possible inclusion in a second volume.

REFERENCES AND SUGGESTED READINGS

Alpert, J. L., & Associates. (1982). *Psychological consultation in educational settings: A casebook for working with administrators, teachers, students, and community.* San Francisco: Jossey-Bass.

Armour, R. A., Caffarella, R. S., Fuhrmann, B. S., & Wergin, F. J. (1987). Academic burnout: Faculty responsibility and institutional climate. In P. Seldin (Ed.), *Coping with faculty stress* (pp. 3–11). San Francisco: Jossey-Bass.

Aubrey, R. F. (1978). Consultation, school intervention, and the elementary counselor. *Personnel and Guidance Journal, 56*(6), 351–354.

Baker, S. B. (1981). *School counselor's handbook: A guide for professional growth and development.* Boston: Allyn & Bacon.

Baldridge, V. J. (1971). *Power and conflict in the university.* New York: Wiley.

Baldwin, R. G., & Blackburn, R. T. (1981). The academic career as a developmental process: Implications for higher education. *Journal of Higher Education, 52,* 598–614.

Bandura, A. (1986). *Social foundations of thought and action: A social cognitive theory.* Englewood Cliffs, NJ: Prentice-Hall.

Benjaminson, P. (1990). Publishing without perishing. *Thought and Action, 6*(2), 27–119.

Berkowitz, M. I. (1975). *A primer on school mental health consultation.* Springfield, IL: Thomas.

Boice, R. (1991). New faculty as teachers. *Journal of Higher Education, 62*(2), 149–173.

Boice, R., & Turner, J. L. (1989). Experiences of new faculty. *Journal of Staff, Program, and Organization Development, 7*(2), 51–57.

Bowen, H. R., & Schuster, J. H. (1986). *American professors: A national resource imperiled.* New York: Oxford University Press.

Braucht, S., & Weime, B. (1992). The school counselor as consultant on self-esteem: An example. *Elementary School Guidance and Counseling, 26,* 229–236.

Brown, D., Pryzwansky, W., & Schulte, A. (1991). *Psychological consultation: Introduction to theory and practice* (2nd ed.). Boston: Allyn & Bacon.

Brown, D., Wyne, M. D., Blackburn, J. E., & Powell, W. C., (1979). *Consultation: Strategy for improving education.* Boston: Allyn & Bacon.

Brubaker, D. L., & Nelson, R. H., Jr. (1972). *Introduction to educational decision-making.* Dubuque, IA: Kendall-Hunt.

Caplan, J. C. (1970). *The theory and practice of mental health consultation.* New York: Basic Books.

Capra, F. (1982). *The turning point: Science, society, and the rising culture.* New York: Simon & Schuster.

Carlson, J., Splete, H., & Kern, R. (Eds.). (1975). *The consulting process* (APGA Reprint Series No. 7). Washington, DC: American Personnel and Guidance Association.

Conoley, C. W., Conoley, J. C., Ivey, D. C., & Scheel, M. J. (1991). Enhancing consultation by matching the consultee's perspective. *Journal of Counseling and Development, 19,* 546–548.

Conoley, J. C., & Conoley, C. W. (1982). *School consultation: A guide to practice and training.* New York: Pergamon Press.

Covey, S. R. (1989). *The seven habits of highly effective people.* New York: Simon & Schuster.

Curry, B. K. (1992). *Instituting enduring change: Achieving continuity of change in higher education* (Report No. 7). Washington, DC: George Washington University, School of Education and Human Development.

Deck, M. D. (1992). Training school counselors to be consultants. *Elementary School Guidance and Counseling, 25,* 221–228.

Dinkmeyer, D. (1975). The counselor as consultant: Rationale and procedures. In J. Carlson, H. Splete, & R. Kern (Eds.), *The counseling process* (APGA Reprint Series No. 7, pp. 65–72). Washington, DC: American Personnel and Guidance Association.

Dinkmeyer, D., & Carlson, J. (1973). *Consulting: Facilitating human potential and change processes.* Columbus, OH: Merrill.

Dinkmeyer, D. C., Pew, W. L., & Dinkmeyer, D. C., Jr. (1979). *Adlerian counseling and psychotherapy.* Chicago: Alfred Adler Institute.

Douglas, J. M. (1984). The labor relations issue. *Thought and Action, 1*(1), 151–159.

Downing, J., & Downing, S. (1991). Consultation with resistant parents. *Elementary School Guidance and Counseling, 25,* 296–300.

Dreikurs, R. (1972). *The challenge of child training: A parents' guide.* New York: Hawthorne Books.

Dressel, P. L. (Ed.). (1971). *The new colleges: Toward an appraisal.* Iowa City, IA: American College Testing Program.

Drucker, P. F. (1985). *Management: Tasks, responsibilities, practices* (Rev. ed.). New York: Harper & Row.

Duffy, G. G. (1994). Professional development schools and the disempowerment of teachers and professors. *Kappan, 75*(8), 596–601.

Duncan, C. F., & Pryzwansky, W. (1986). Consultation research: Trends in doctoral dissertations 1978–1985. *Journal of School Psychology, 26,* 107–119.

Dustin, D., & Ehly, S. (1992). School consultation in the 1990s. *Elementary School Guidance and Counseling, 26,* 165–175.

Eble, D. E., & McKeachie, W. J. (1985). *Improving undergraduate education through faculty development.* San Francisco: Jossey-Bass.

Fairweather, J. S. (1994). The value of teaching, research, and service. *The NEA 1994 Almanac of Higher Education* (pp. 39–58). Washington, DC: National Education Association.

Fink, L. D. (1984). *First year of college teaching.* San Francisco: Jossey-Bass.

Fulmer, D. W., & Benard, H. W. (1972). *The school counselor-consultant.* Boston: Houghton Mifflin.

Gallessich, J. (1985). Toward a meta-theory of consultation. *Counseling Psychologist, 13*(3), 336–354.

Gappa, J. M. (1987). The stress-producing working conditions of part-time faculty. In P. Seldin (Ed.), *Coping with faculty stress* (New Directions for Higher Education No. 29, pp. 33–42). San Francisco: Jossey-Bass.

Gardner, J. W. (1981) *Self-renewal: The individual and the innovative society* (Rev. ed.). New York: Norton.

Gilly, J. W. (1991). *Think about American higher education* New York: Macmillan.

Gmelch, W. H. (1993). *Coping with faculty stress.* Newbury Park, CA: Sage.

Gutkin, T. R., & Bossard, M. D. (1984). The impact of consultant, consultee, and organizational variables toward consultation services. *Journal of School Psychology, 22,* 251–256.

Hall, D. L., & Barker, L. W. (1985). Consultation to high risk families: A conceptual model. *West Virginia Mental Health Counselor Journal, 3*(2), 10–17.

Hansen, J. C., Himes, B. S., & Meier, S. (1990). *Consulting: Concepts and practices.* Englewood Cliffs, NJ: Prentice-Hall.

Hipps, G. M. (Ed.). (1982). *Effective planned change strategies* (New Directions for Institutional Research series). San Francisco: Jossey-Bass.

Huelskamp, R. M. (1993). Perspectives on education in America. *Phi Delta Kappan, 74*(9), 718–721.

Hughes, J. N., & Falk, R. S. (1981). Resistance, reactance, and consultation. *Journal of School Psychology, 9*(2), 134–142.

Idol, L., & Baran, S. (1992). Elementary school counselors and special educators consulting together: Perilous pitfalls or opportunities to collaborate? *Elementary School Guidance and Counseling, 26,* 202–213.

Keyes, R. (1991). *Timelock: How life got so hectic and what you can do about it.* New York: HarperCollins.

Knapp, S., & Salend, S. K. (1984). Maintaining teacher adherence in behavioral consultations. *Elementary Guidance and Counseling, 18,* 287–294.

Kotter, J. P., & Heskett, J. L. (1992). *Corporate culture and performance.* New York: Free Press.

Kuh, G. D. (1993). Appraising the character of a college. *Journal of Counseling and Development, 71,* 661–668.

Kurpius, D. J. (1985). Consultation interventions: Successes, failures, and proposals. *Counseling Psychologist, 13*(3), 368–389.

Lauter, P. (1986). University reform: Threat or opportunity? *Thought and Action, 2*(1), 5–22.

Lee, R., & Field, M. (1991). University faculty attitudes toward teaching and research. In K. J. Zahorski (Ed.), *To improve the academy* (Vol. 10, pp. 47–54). Stillwater, OK: New Forums Press.

Lewis, K. G. (Ed.), & Povlacs, J. L. (Assoc. Ed.). (1988). *FACE to ECAF: A sourcebook of individual consultation techniques for faculty/instructional developers.* Stillwater, OK: New Forums Press.

London, M. (1991). Practice in training and development. In D. W. Braw & Associates, *Working with organizations and their people* (pp. 67–94). New York: Guilford Press.

Maslow, A. H. (1959). *New knowledge in human values.* Chicago: Regnery.

Maslow, A. H. (1968). *Toward a psychology of being* (2nd ed.). Princeton, NJ: Van Nostrand Reinhold.

Maslow, A. H. (1970). *Motivation and personality* (3rd ed.). New York: Harper & Row.

Mathias, C. E. (1992). Touching the lives of children: Consultive interventions that work. *Elementary School Guidance and Counseling, 26,* 190–201.

McCellan, M. (1994). Why blame schools? *Research Bulletin, 12.* (Available from Phi Delta Kappa Center for Evaluation, Development, and Research, P.O. Box 789, Bloomington, IN 47402.)

McKeachie, W. J. (1991). What theories underlie the practice of faculty development? In K. J. Zahorski (Ed.), *To improve the academy: Resources for student, faculty, and institutional development* (pp. 3–8). Stillwater, OK: New Forums Press.

Melendez, W. A. (1986). Powerless Prof: From candle bearer to burnout. *Thought and Action, 2*(1), 5–22.

Metzger, R. O. (1993). *Developing a consulting practice.* Newbury Park, CA: Sage.

Meyers, J., Martin, R., & Hyman, I. (Eds.). (1977). *School consultation: Readings about preventive techniques for pupil personnel workers.* Springfield, IL: Thomas.

Miller, T. K., & Prince, J. S. (1976). *The future of student affairs.* San Francisco: Jossey-Bass.

Milstein, M. M. (1986). The future of consultation in public schools. *Urban Education, 21*(2), 149–168.

Nemko, M., & Simpson, R. D. (1991). Nine keys to enhancing campus wide influence of faculty development centers. In K. J. Zahorski (Ed.), *To improve the academy* (Vol. 10, pp. 13–87). Stillwater, OK: New Forums Press.

Newman, J., & Fuqua, D. (1984). Data-based consultation in student affairs. *Journal of College Student Personnel, 30,* 206–212.

North, D. C. (1990). *Institutions, institutional change, and economic performance.* Cambridge, England: Cambridge University Press.

Peters, T. (1988). *Thriving on chaos: Handbook for a management revolution.* New York: Knopf.

Plato, K. (1977). Student development as policy: Strategies for implementation. *Journal of College Student Personnel, 18,* 518–521.

Rosovsky, H. (1990). *The university: An owner's manual.* New York: Norton.

Runyan C. K., & Buche, J. R. (1991). *Developmental induction programs with the "mentorship" concept: A district teacher induction program.* Plano, TX: Lester, Allen and Sherrill.

Sarason, S. B. (1971). *The culture of the school and the problem of change.* Boston: Allyn & Bacon.

Schultz, D. (1977). *Growth psychology: Models of the healthy personality.* New York: Van Nostrand.

Schuster, J. H. (1989). The personal dimension: Faculty development. *Thought and Action, 5*(1), 61–72.

Seldin, P. (Ed.). (1987). *Coping with faculty stress.* San Francisco: Jossey-Bass.

Shaw, G. C. (1985). Debunking the myth of academe. *Thought and Action, 1*(2), 5–16.

Smith, D. K., & Lyon, M. A. (1985). Consultation in school psychology: Changes from 1991–1884. *Psychology in the Schools, 22,* 404–409.

Stanley, C. A., & Chism, N. V. (1991). Selected characteristics of new faculty: Implications for faculty development. In K. J. Zahorski (Ed.), *To improve the academy, 10,* 55–62.

Stark, D. K., & Lyon, M. A. (1985). The university goes to market. *Thought and Action, 1*(1), 9–21.

Subotnic, D. (1988). Wisdom or widgets: Whither the academic enterprize? *Thought and Action, 4*(1), 67–80.

Swick, K. (1987). *Student stress: A classroom management system.* Washington, DC: National Education of the United States.

Thomas, L. G., Taylor, H. G., & Knezek, D. G. (1993). National accreditation standards impact teacher preparation. *T.H.E. Journal, 20*(11), 62–64.

Umanski, D. L., & Holloway, E. L. (1984, March). The counselor as consultant: From model to practice. *School counselor,* 329–338.

Waldinger, R. (1985). New faculty members: Expectations and responsibilities. *ADFL Bulletin, 19*(3), 38–41.

Wallace, W. A. (1993). *Theories of personality: A basic issues approach.* Boston: Allyn & Bacon.

Warnath, C. F. (1975). The school counselor as institutional agent. In J. Carlson, H. Splete, & R. Kern (Eds.), *The counseling process* (APGA Reprint Series No. 7, pp. 202–208). Washington, DC: American Personnel and Guidance Association.

West, J. F., & Idol, L. (1993). The counselor as consultant in the collaborative school. *Journal of Counseling and Development, 71,* 678–683.

Westbrook, F. D., Kandell, J. J., Kirkland, S. E., Phillips, P. E., Regan, A. M., Medvene, A., & Oslin, Y. D. (1993). University campus consultation: Opportunities and limitations. *Journal of Counseling and Development, 71,* 684–688.

Wilcox, J. R., & Ebbs, S. I. (1992). *The leadership compass: Values and ethics in higher education* (ASHE-ERIC Higher Education Report No. 1). Washington, DC: George Washington University, School of Education and Human Development.

Zahorski, K. J. (Ed.). (1991). *To improve the academy: Resources for student, faculty, and institutional development* (Vol. 10). The Professional and Organizational Development Network in Higher Education. Stillwater, OK: New Forums Press.

◆ CHAPTER SEVEN

Consultation in Child Development Settings

America's commitment to children represents a national imperative, and indisputably, a substantial investment in our society's future. Indeed, our society acknowledges that the successful maturation of today's children will have a profound influence on tomorrow's world. For many children, however, the growth and development process signals a bleak or uncertain future. Even in stable and mentally healthy families, children must constantly adapt to an array of psychological and physical changes, complex family dynamics, and intense social demands. Add the frenzy of stressful environmental forces and changes that plague modern families and it is evident that the challenges to young children's development have never been greater.

The term **child development** refers to human growth in the first stage of life (through adolescence). Berk (1991) writes about the immense range of factors that the field of child development encompasses: "No branch of human behavior is broader in scope than the study of development, for every facet of the individual—physical, mental, social, and emotional—changes over time" (p. 1). The child development field is rooted in the belief that children progress through profoundly significant stages, with adaptation in each stage contributing to successful adjustment and well-being in later stages.

As a result of America's commitment to children, many children attend **child development programs** that help children up to the age of five years acquire the life skills essential to healthy physical and psychological growth. Although their titles and range of services vary, child development programs reflect the belief that the child's earliest years are usually the most important. Many of these programs, to best serve children's needs, exist within a comprehensive framework that emphasizes children's growth in multiple areas, including psychological, emotional, and behavioral development.

This chapter describes a new and expanding role for psychological consultants. Their growing presence in child-related programs is tied to the fact that social, emotional, and family problems often seriously impair young children's educational accomplishments (Mowder, Unterspan, Knuter, Goode, & Pedro, 1993; Nicoll, 1992). **Psychological consultation in child development settings** refers to a broad helping process in which child- and family-oriented consultants provide help to consultees (teachers, aides, social services staff, parents) relative to the psychological and developmental needs of young children.

Types of Child Development Programs

America's child care options have proliferated dramatically in recent years. According to Spodek, Saracho, and Davis (1987), "Federal, state, and local governments, industry, religious groups, parent groups, and private entrepreneurs all sponsor early childhood programs" (p. 35). We take a broad approach in defining child development programs in this chapter; of necessity, the examples we discuss are comprehensive programs that extend much more than custodial or physical child care. We describe a few representative child development program models in the section that follows.

Head Start Programs

Head Start programs are highly visible, federally funded programs that emerged in 1965 amidst unyielding social and political pressures (Valentine & Zigler, 1983). Responding to the needs of impoverished families, Head Start programs were developed to prepare three- to five-year-old children for future enrollment in public schools. Throughout their history, these programs have endured despite fervent economic and political changes, and fortunately for children and their families, these programs continue to thrive.

Head Start programs incorporate a range of child and family services that are conveniently integrated into multiple program components. Spodek, Saracho, and Davis (1987) provide a comprehensive list of the educational, social, and emotional goals that distinguish Head Start programs:

1. To improve the child's physical health,
2. To facilitate the child's emotional and social development,
3. To enhance the child's cognitive skills,
4. To establish patterns of success for the child,
5. To promote positive family-child interactions and relations,
6. To promote the child's and family's positive relationship with society in resolving their problems, and
7. To foster a sense of dignity and self-esteem within the child and family (p. 40)

Head Start programs, as Zigler and Styfco (1994) point out, include "preschool education, health screening and referral, mental health services, nutrition education and hot meals, social services for the child and family, and parent involvement" (p. 129). Among the many trends affecting these programs, the move to extend Head Start services to more families is most dramatic. Head Start has accepted other initiatives as well. Adult literacy programs, programs that facilitate children's transition to public school, and full-day programs are visible examples. Zigler and Muenchow (1992) describe an additional development relevant to the topic of this chapter:

> One promising development is that the American Psychological Association has recently established a network of 500 psychologists to volunteer their services at Head Start centers across the country. Psychologists will be called upon to screen and diagnose developmental disabilities, conduct parent support groups, and train project staff on dealing with such problems as substance abuse and family violence. (p. 219)

Parent and Child Centers

Evolving out of the Head Start philosophy and reflecting similar goals, the first Parent and Child Centers (PCCs) were opened in 1967 to address the early childhood needs of children in the age range birth to three years (Zigler & Styfco, 1994). Although PCC programs reflect many of the characteristics and philosophies of their Head Start predecessor, the equal attention to children and parents represents their most unique feature. PCC programs, for example, require parents to attend program activities with their children, participate in parent-centered program activities, and cultivate stronger parent-child relationships. The emergence of PCCs has been fueled by research findings that suggest that Head Start programs begin their interventions too late in children's lives. Having similar priorities to Head Start programs with respect to expansion, PCC programs are growing in number. Along with more programs come more services and larger enrollments.

Nursery Schools

Nursery schools are child care programs that support the mental and physical development of young children. Although these programs grew out of the need to nurture socioeconomically disadvantaged children in areas of physical care (Spodek, 1973), modern nursery schools expand their focus to integrate educational goals that encourage creativity and the arts. Comprehensive nursery schools focus on the needs of parents and families through the provision of parent training in home management (Spodek et al., 1987). Nursery schools are often sponsored within college or university settings as laboratory study programs.

Comprehensive Child Care Centers

Changing family roles, including dual-career parents and single-parent families, are significant factors that contribute to the need for comprehensive child care centers. The growth of child care centers as acceptable alternatives to daily child care is evidenced by the phenomenal number of parents who make use of such programs (Almy, 1975). Although the earliest child care centers were single-purpose day care programs primarily concerned with custodial care, many have evolved into comprehensive programs that provide a range of educational, social, and psychological services (Decker & Decker, 1984).

Program Referrals to Psychological Consultants

Child advocates agree that the problems of young children are increasing at an alarming rate (Thompson & Rudolph, 1988). There is also evidence that the types of problems that children are experiencing are multidimensional. That is, they often cross developmental, social, emotional, and family boundaries, inhibit the educational process, and prompt referrals to external psychological consultants.

Although child development program employees refer children to psychological consultants for multiple and often overlapping reasons, referral dynamics and etiologies fall within relatively predictable categories. Mowder, Unterspan, Knuter, Goode, and Pedro (1993), for example, following a study of the referrals common to Head Start settings, identified the major referral categories. Although derived from a cumulative study of Head Start referrals to psychological consultants, these groupings appear generalizable to other programs that enroll young children. Thus, consultants to child programs may anticipate referrals that stem from the following psychological issues (Mowder, Unterspan, Knuter, Goode, & Pedro, 1993, pp. 2–3):

1. *Problems in attention*   Referrals specific to this category include child problems associated with attention span, impulsivity, and activity.
2. *Developmental concerns*   Child characteristics that appear discrepant when compared to expected developmental performances (intelligence, maturation, and overall functioning) comprise referral issues in this category.
3. *Referrals that involve the child's family*   This category embodies child referral issues in which family dynamics appear as contributing or related factors (e.g., separation, poor attendance, and mistreatment).
4. *Physical health concerns*   The child's physical health and medical concerns are included in this category.
5. *Gross and fine motor issues*   This category is reserved for child concerns that incorporate psychomotor development and coordination.
6. *Disturbances related to social-emotional issues*   Child referrals with respect to the child's behavior and affective problems (e.g., socialization, self-esteem, and conduct).
7. *Communication skills*   Referrals in this category include matters of articulation, expressive, and receptive language.

One broad problem area that appears etiological with respect to the problems children experience is stress. The term *stress* describes the demands, problems, and pressures that afflict families. Of particular interest to child development programs and consultants are the effects of stressful conditions on children's development. Very young children are particularly vulnerable to stress because they not only lack a mature understanding of their problems, but the alleviation of stressful conditions is usually the responsibility of parents or other adults. Elkind (1981) was among the first writers to emphasize the pernicious effects of stress on children:

> Today's child has become the unwilling, unintended victim of overwhelming stress— the stress borne of rapid, bewildering social change and constantly rising expectations. The contemporary parent dwells in a pressure-cooker of competing demands, transitions, role changes, personal and professional uncertainties, over which he or she exerts slight direction. (p. 3)

While the cumulative sources of child stress are multifaceted and overlapping, many stressors reflect a range of familial and ecological conditions.

1. *Changing family roles*   By necessity or choice, modern families have seen fundamental changes in parental roles and responsibilities. Among the many transitions that affect families is the surging number of dual-earner parents, a trend reflecting the growing career orientation of mothers (Gilbert & Rachlin, 1987). Working mothers who take advantage of long-overdue opportunities for advancement and personal fulfillment often create a need for "role expansion," in which the family must shift responsibilities

and tasks (Gilbert & Rachlin, 1987, p. 13). Regrettably, as Gilbert and Rachlin (1987) contend, many families have failed to greet these new roles with appropriate changes in household and parenting obligations. When career-minded mothers continue to "shoulder the primary responsibility for the care of the home coupled with work responsibilities" (Thompson & Rudolph, 1988, p. 5), for example, the stress in the family often rises.

2. *Marital schism*   The current rates of divorce and separation are extremely high, and as a result, a parent's departure from the family mainstream represents a potentially serious stressor for each family member. Of concern, also, are the prospects that divorce often creates the "single-parent home" phenomenon that challenges families to adapt to new lifestyles and parenting responsibilities. Although this message is not intended as an indictment of the single-parent family model, single-parent arrangements do appear to involve extra challenges and transitions. Also not surprising are the statistics that suggest that many children enrolled in child development programs experience unique stress relative to their "blended" families (Powell, 1989, p. 15).

3. *Child abuse or inattention*   Child abuse and neglect have increased dramatically in recent decades (Takanishi & DeLeon, 1994), and as known episodes increase, so do fears that most occurrences of child mistreatment are unreported or undiscovered. Mistreatment of children threatens their emotional and physical well-being. Of concern, also, is the prediction that the psychological scars brought by abuse and inattention cycle into later adult disturbances.

4. *Substance abuse and addiction*   As substance abuse and addiction become more pervasive in society, the far-reaching, devastating effects ultimately extend into the family (Thompson & Rudolph, 1988). Substance abuse and addiction by parents appear related to many of the negative conditions that impair family harmony, including family violence, sexual abuse, marital discord, and unemployment. Psychological experts fear that these conditions often inflict spiraling and enduring damage on children.

5. *Poverty*   Many child development programs—Head Start programs and PCCs in particular—serve impoverished children. A steady stream of empirical investigations point to the ravaging effects of poverty on children's mental health and sense of security (Albee & Ryan-Finn, 1993; Bruner, 1972). Indigence creates a stressful culture in which the family's potential is restricted and the child's psychosocial development impaired. Bruner (1972) expresses concern that children who live in poverty encounter pervasive conditions that restrict intellectual promise, goal seeking, problem solving, language use, and socialization.

6. *Children with disabilities*   Child specialists acknowledge an increase in the number of preschool-age children with disabilities who attend early-childhood programs (Widerstrom, Mowder, & Willis, 1989). For these children and their parents, the stress is often enormous. Children, for example, learn firsthand that accomplishing developmental milestones requires constant adaptation. Parents, in addition to their concern for their child's well-being, must contend with the frustration brought by inadequate resources and facilities. Stress also results when children with disabilities require an assortment of ancillary services (for example, speech/language therapy, physical therapy, visual and hearing services, and rehabilitation), so that parents must routinely cross program boundaries to access services.

Delineating Processes

Although consulting in child development programs is similar to consulting in other settings with respect to methods and practices, several special features deserve attention. First, child development settings provide fertile ground for consultants who desire opportunities for **prevention-oriented consultation**. An obvious goal of prevention-oriented consultation is to prevent or reduce the occurrence of undesirable conditions affecting children. Prevention goals are served, also, when consultants implement interventions that enhance positive conditions for the family. Prevention goals guide the work of child specialists in child development settings, a point Barclay (1984) emphasizes:

> Embedded in the concept of prevention are some values about what constitutes effective human behavior in our society, such as responsibility in personal and social behavior. There is also the assumption that certain skill areas such as the development of academic and social skills must be nurtured and guided in their unfolding developmental and learning process. (p. 475)

Consultants to child programs must acknowledge the unique characteristics and needs of infants and preschool children. In exploring the role of school psychologists in preschool programs, Widerstrom et al. (1989) point out that "the areas of expertise expected of them by early intervention professionals are very different from the expertise expected of them in working with school age populations" (p. 245). Indeed, psychological consultants who work in preschool settings are required to deemphasize highly standardized, formal assessment methods and to give more attention to classroom- and home-based interventions.

Child development consultants must integrate their services into a network of community resources. That is, through the processes of networking, advocacy, and dialogue with the deliverers of community services, consultants supplement their range of human and social services. Since many child and family problems (for example, children with developmental disabilities, parental skill deficits, child psychopathology, dysfunctional family relations, and child abuse) require direct interventions that exceed the corrective influences of consultation, consultants must turn to community-based options. Knowledge of community resources and the ability to link children and families to these resources are important attributes of consultants. File and Kontos (1992) concur in their summary of consultation activities that pertain especially to children with disabilities: "Preliminary to the development of consultation services, much effort must be given to community-wide, interagency planning of the service delivery system" (p. 229).

As in other consultation settings, child development program consultants must acknowledge the rapidly expanding cultural diversity that exists in American society. Given the millions of children served by child care programs, the presence of diverse educational, familial, and social values is inevitable (Office of Human Development Services, 1988; Powell, 1989; Sale, 1988). Consultants should be aware that families naturally define mental health, childrearing practices, and family problem solving within the context of their culture. Consultants must become sensitive to cultural issues by exploring the values of the specific cultures they encounter (Jackson & Hayes, 1993).

Forging Consultant-Consultee Relationships

Problem solving in child development settings requires that consultants attend to key relational issues. Since child development consultants are usually external professionals who bring a range of unknown or unanticipated attributes to the consultation process, they represent unfamiliar visitors whose style, demeanor, and theoretical orientation are new to the child development setting. Consultants must also consider the unique qualities of those who work in child development settings. Because of deflated budgets and minimal salaries, for example, many programs rely on volunteers or paraprofessionals to meet educational, social service, and transportation needs (Spodek et al., 1987; Zigler & Styfco, 1994). Even in contemporary Head Start programs that strive to professionalize and train their staff, estimates suggest that less than half the teaching staff have had college-level training (Zigler & Styfco, 1994). Since staff members often lack formal expertise with regard to complex psychological concepts and interventions, they may prefer a consultee role marked by acquiescence, submissiveness, or defensiveness. These dynamics require consultants to place high priority on effective and harmonious relations with child development consultees. Although there are few assurances, adherence to several principles may serve this goal:

1. *Consultants should integrate egalitarian principles into the consultant-consultee relationship.* Consultants are professionals who bring formalized training and credentials to the consultation relationship and, although these attributes benefit the consultation process, these traits often threaten or intimidate less-qualified consultees. Thus, the consultant's task is to balance the responsibilities and power in the consultation relationship. Consultants should view consultees as partners throughout the consultation process and emphasize this status through communication, role descriptions, and decision making. Moreover, consultants must avoid actions (such as verbal messages, gestures, behaviors, or tactics) that suggest consultees are subservient or unimportant contributors to the consultation process.

2. *Consultants must emphasize the consultee's contributions and skills.* Despite the absence of highly formalized educational or psychological backgrounds, many child development staff acquire skills and insights through personal and work experiences. Years of dedication and caring for children amount to work experiences that contribute, at times invaluably, to consultation problem solving. Further, many comprehensive child programs institute staff development and continuing education efforts that emphasize the insights and skills necessary to solve work problems. Effective consultants further the purposes of consultation when they foster an atmosphere in which consultees are respected, encouraged, and motivated.

3. *The consultant's use of psychological language and concepts should match the consultee's understanding.* Psychological issues are often laden with unknown or confusing theoretical and conceptual information. Because consultees are often unschooled in psychology, consultants must avoid terminology or jargon that contains specialized psychological language or nomenclature. Consultants must communicate, explain, or interpret the relevant psychological principles that underlie child problems and associated interventions. Further, consultants should avoid actions that communicate superiority

(for example, "talking down" to consultees or denigrating their efforts and ideas). In short, if psychological information is to be useful, consultees must be able to relate to it.

Assessing the Characteristics of Young Children

Formal consultation in child development settings most often requires consultants to engage in the assessment of child and family dynamics. Assessment as it relates to consultation in child development settings involves a broad range of activities that contribute to the body of information needed for curriculum development, the provision of special services or behavioral interventions, and the impetus for referrals to community services.

Assessment in early childhood settings includes a range of methods; given the behavioral and developmental characteristics of very young children, certain practical and theoretical factors shape the process. For example, assessment in these settings is subject to definite limits. Since consultants play a temporary, indirect role, clinically sophisticated or highly formalized assessment activities are rarely feasible. Further, many consultants may lack the clinical skills necessary for psychometric or standardized testing. Within the context of consultation to child development programs, therefore, consultants must select assessment methods that are time-limited and less direct or intense, and must ultimately rely heavily on inferences that describe children's traits or problems.

Consultants must also acknowledge that assessing the behavior and development of preschool-age children requires methods that differ from the assessment of older children (Fantuzzo & Polite, 1990; Mowder et al. 1993; Salmon & Lehrer, 1989). While each young child responds to problems in a unique way, most are unable to verbalize or conceptualize their feelings and behaviors. As a result, consultants must rely on their understanding of developmental and behavioral theories to discern important clues to the child's psychological status. Infants in particular have characteristics that limit the type of assessment to observational data on cognitive and general developmental factors (Martin, 1988).

Certain conceptual limitations restrict the consultant's ability to generalize assessment data on the problems of very young children. For example, the child's rapid growth in early life affects the validity of assessment outcomes over time (Martin, 1988). That is, while assessment results are valid at one point, their usefulness erodes as the child's development progresses. An important consideration, also, is the reality that many child-age tests are normed according to an invariable sequence of developmental achievements that children follow. Although most children indeed follow a developmental progression, the age at which they accomplish developmental milestones often varies considerably. Thus, comparing a child's test results to standardized norms may present a false picture of a child's developmental status.

Since many referrals to psychological consultants entail social and emotional concerns (Mowder et al., 1993; Widerstrom, Mowder, & Willis, 1989), assessment processes must examine children's problems within the context of behavioral learning and environmental factors (Martin, 1988). Such processes require consultants to assess young children through methods that target multiple levels. Most consultants apply a range of assessment strategies situationally.

Consultant-Consultee Dialogue   Many child assessment methods begin with inquiries offered through dialogue between consultants and the adults responsible for child care. The opinions and observations of those who know the child best can be synthesized into substantive psychological hypotheses on the child's problems and needs. Such early diagnostic impressions set the course of consultation and guide decisions about subsequent assessment methodologies.

Review of Relevant Records   Most comprehensive child development programs maintain formal and informal documentary records that chronicle the child's status. Such records provide cumulative information about the child's history, medical status, general development, and psychosocial history. Some records include family-related data that reveal information about the needs and characteristics of the home environment. In addition, records often include evaluative measures that have been completed by earlier professionals who serve the child development program.

A helpful source of information is the program's or consultee's **anecdotal records** (brief, narrative, handwritten records maintained at the discretion of a staff member to document samples of a child's behavior). Such records, written by teachers, staff members, program supervisors, or visiting professionals, can provide rich details on the child's behavior over time (Beaty, 1986). Consultants, however, should keep in mind that anecdotal records can be highly subjective; that is, they often include intuitive or observational impressions that lack formal psychological foundation and evaluation.

Child Observation   In child development settings, observing infants and young children is an established assessment practice (Beaty, 1986). Within the conceptual framework of psychological consultation, assessment data based on observational tactics provide a foundation for understanding the behavior and development of the child. **Observation** refers to a systematic process in which psychological consultants view the behavior and development of children in order to understand their problems and prescribe a course of helpful interventions.

Consultants should acknowledge that observation is much more than simply watching children from a distance. As Beaty (1986) contends in her comprehensive guide to observing young children: "In systematic observation, there is a specific purpose for gathering the information about the children, as well as a particular method for collecting and recording" (p. 5). Observations that include behavioral checklists or rating scales, for example, allow consultants to document impressions as they occur.

Observational assessment processes should be organized and purposeful. Adhering to a relatively standard set of guidelines will enhance the validity of observational processes:

1. Consultants should observe children within a natural setting in which behavior is authentic and representative.

2. Since young children will likely react to the consultant's presence, consultants must diminish the potential threat or distortion they bring to the child's environment.
3. Children must be observed over time so that various samples of behavior can be assessed.
4. Consultants must utilize a valid and reliable method of observation that entails recordkeeping and documentation.
5. Observational processes extend beyond the child; that is, they should acknowledge the range of environmental influences (teacher, peers, physical environment) that potentially influence the child's behavior.

Consultant-Child Interaction   Face-to-face interaction with children often provides the basis for the consultant's assessment judgments. Interactional methods require child development consultants to seek and implement structured or unstructured activities, often spontaneously and informally, that afford dialogue and observation. Consultants often interact with children during play and learning activities, including storytelling, books and literature, games, art, and puppetry.

The interaction approach gives the psychological consultant general data on the child's physical, cognitive, behavioral, and social development. Such information can be collected as mental notes that add to information derived from other assessment tactics. Essential to the consultant's interaction with children is the ability to establish rapport and defuse the anxiety or fear brought on by the consultant's presence.

Examination of Ecological Factors   Environmental determinants unquestionably have an impact on the behavioral problems of young children (Neisworth & Bagnato, 1988). Children's emotions and behavior are constantly under the influence of **ecological factors**, including the entire psychosocial field within which the children's problems have emerged. For the ecologically minded consultant, the multiple points of reference include the classroom environment, peer affiliations, parent-child relations, family characteristics, and neighborhood dynamics.

Although ecological factors encompass a broad range of influences, parental and other family dynamics appear to the most prominent influences on the child's early life (Allen & Goetz, 1982). The consultant's examination of relevant family characteristics, influences, and interactions often reveals dynamics that contribute to the emotional and behavioral problems of the child. Martin (1988) emphasizes the importance of family influences: "One set of data that will generally prove essential for mental health professionals who work with children is the nature of the psychological climate in the home and some characteristics of the relationships between the family members" (p. 186).

Within the framework of consultation, consultants are rarely authorized to administer formal assessment methods to families. Rather, they must draw inferences from the information obtained from consultees, professional observations, or brief parent conferences. Through consultant-parent dialogue, consultants form intuitive impressions of children's problems and make diagnostic inferences from such information. They may seek answers to a range of questions:

- What is the composition of the child's family?
- What factors create stress in the family?
- What are the parental influences on the child?
- Is the family a blended, single-parent, or dual-parent family?
- What are the resources in the family?
- What are the relationships in the family (parent-parent, parent-child, child-child)?
- Are dysfunctional conditions present in the family (for example, abuse or neglect, substance abuse, violence)?
- Who serves as important models in the family, and what behaviors are demonstrated?
- How do parents respond to the child's maladaptive or undesirable behavior?
- Are parents sensitive to their roles as parents?
- In what sort of neighborhood does the family live?

Consider the example of a three-year-old child who suddenly exhibits aggressiveness and defiance in the classroom. In a brief conference with the child's mother, the consultant learns that the child's father (the primary authority figure in the family) has separated from the mother and a divorce is pending. Knowing these family dynamics, the consultant hypothesizes that the child's aggression and acting-out behaviors could be consequences of family discord.

In addition to exploring family dynamics, consultants should consider the potential contributing effects of a range of program and classroom factors. Room and furniture arrangements, number of children in attendance, program schedules, peer relations, the ratio of adults to children, and staff-child relations are examples of classroom characteristics that contain strong psychological implications. Although these factors alone may not be the sole contributing factors to the problems of young children, they can prolong or exacerbate existing disturbances.

A small classroom with limited floor space and overcrowded conditions, for example, is likely to contribute to an overactive child's failure to adapt to classroom rules and structured activities. The arrangement of furniture may also create conditions that promote inappropriate running, jumping, climbing, or hiding. Curricular offerings and schedules that fail to stimulate the interest of young children may create boredom and disinterest, conditions that often lead to behavioral problems (Spodek et al., 1987). Staffing patterns that require child development staff to monitor large numbers of children create conditions in which individual attention is difficult. Withdrawn and socially isolated children, for instance, may not have their needs met should teachers and staff have time for only the more active and verbal children.

For the child development staff teacher and aide: "The tone you set and the way you arrange your classroom can contribute to a child's mental health by encouraging her to be self-aware and independent" (Office of Human Development Services, 1988, p. 18). The creation of a positive atmosphere is essential. How discipline is applied and verbal and nonverbal commands or reprimands are administered are matters of concern. These points are supported by Spodek et al. (1987), who write: "Consistency, firmness, and patience are essential in working with young children" (p. 128).

Consultation at Multiple Levels

Although the child is the ultimate beneficiary of psychological consultation in child development settings, consultants address child problems at multiple levels. For example, they often engage teachers and child care staff, volunteers, parents, or the child development organization as a whole. At each level, consultation interventions are tied to the belief that positive changes in children depend largely on changes in the adults and organizations that care for them.

Consulting with Child Development Staff   During the course of consultation in child development settings, consultants most often seek problem-solving strategies that involve teachers and other staff members who fill specific roles relative to children and families. Despite the range of practices and interventions available, the format for staff consultation is most often connected to three general modalities: case-oriented consultation, consultant-staff teams, and psychological education.

1. *Case-oriented consultation*   **Case-oriented consultation** refers to an approach in which consultants and consultees engage in problem-solving dialogue and action relative to the needs and characteristics of a specific child, or case. The general format of case consultation resembles the structural and philosophical characteristics of Caplan's (1970) *client-centered case consultation* described in this volume (see Chapter 3). In child development settings, the process of case-oriented consultation requires consultants to address problems by consulting with the deliverers of child services. For example, consultants and consultees assess the child's behavioral or developmental status, synthesize assessment information into intuitive impressions, and design and implement relevant interventions. Emerging from case-oriented dialogue is a comprehensive plan that explains how the child's behavioral or emotional problems can be corrected (see Chapter 6 for a more detailed discussion of case-oriented consultation).

Although several consultation models provide useful interventions that address the child's needs in school and child settings, case-oriented consultation appears especially well suited for behavioral applications in consultation (Reynolds, Gutkin, Elliott, & Whitt, 1984). Behavioral interventions are grounded in a view of the child's behavior based on objective data and scientific learning principles (see Chapter 3). Although techniques based on behavioral principles are applicable to all children, Allen and Goetz (1982) point out that they appear especially helpful to teachers and consultants who wish to address maladaptive or deviant behaviors (for example, aggression, tantrums, defiance, verbal abuse, and withdrawal). Incorporating behavioral approaches into consultation presupposes that home and school environments are significant determinants of learning and that they must respond to interventions if a child's behavior is to change. A major advantage of behavioral principles is that child development staff find these principles relatively easy to conceptualize and apply (Allen & Goetz, 1982).

2. *Consultant-staff teams*   The team approach to problem solving is an organized method of bringing together child development staff and the consultant in a forum of collaboration, problem solving, and planning. The team is a useful medium through which staff, in groups, identify problems and plan interventions. The team concept has the advantages of multiple contributors, collective expertise, mutual problem solving,

and efficiency. The team approach fosters communication and the exploration of a variety of services with the "least amount of duplication" (Mathias, 1992, p. 194). In child development programs, problem-solving teams allow a centralized approach that seeks open dialogue and understanding of children's needs (see Chapter 6).

3. *Psychological education* In traditional educational settings, educational and curricular objectives almost exclusively target the child's cognitive processes and academic achievement. While such objectives are indisputable priorities within programs serving young children, child development specialists contend that the child's emotional and psychological development are essential goals (Beaty, 1986). Indeed, since the child's formative years appear indelibly linked to future emotional well-being and stability, child development programs must emphasize the child's affective and psychosocial growth.

Psychological consultants, cognizant of the behavioral and affective needs of young children, can be invaluable to child development staff designing and implementing a **psychological education** curriculum (curriculum components that foster self-esteem, emotional development, and psychosocial competence). The argument that psychological education experiences promote positive outcomes for children is supported in the professional literature (Briggs, 1970; Ivey & Alschuler, 1973; Sprinthall, 1973).

Kersey (1986), writing about the importance of parents in helping children manage stress, could be advising child development teachers and consultants about the goals of psychological education:

> Your goal should be to give your children inner skills and strengths, so they can handle the challenges ahead. We know that our children will trip and fall at times, but we want to teach them how to pick themselves up, how to turn problems into opportunities, and stumbling blocks into stepping stones. (p. 7)

Such innovative and preventive educational approaches attempt to connect curriculum content to the psychological growth of young children. Growth-oriented exercises, including storybooks, games, exercises, and art and music activities, are based on the scientific and theoretical knowledge of child psychology.

Consultants can help child development staff implement and evaluate a range of activities and exercises that have clear psychological goals. Examples include the published curricula *Developing Understanding of Self and Others* (Dinkmeyer & Dinkmeyer, 1982) and the *As I Am* program (Office of Human Development Services, 1988), which introduce a psychological curriculum into traditional classroom offerings. A third and more recent option is the *Responding to Children Under Stress* program (Head Start Bureau, 1994), in which classroom teaching personnel learn "practical strategies for working with children who live in multistressed environments" (p. iii).

Although the *As I Am* model was developed for Head Start and related programs (Office of Human Development Services, 1988), its goals are applicable to other child development settings:

1. *Developing self-awareness* Self-awareness activities and exercises are designed to help children learn who they are and develop a sense of "being" (p. 17).
2. *Learning about feelings* Child development staff plan and implement curriculum activities that teach children about their emotions.

3. *Relating*   The importance of communicating and maintaining meaningful relationships with others is emphasized through curriculum exercises, games, and activities.
4. *Thinking*   This category includes goals that emphasize competence in cognitive skills, imagination or creativity, and language expression.
5. *Experiencing literature*   Curriculum offerings emphasize the use of literature in promoting children's general understanding, imaginativeness, and language skills.

Parent Consultation   Consistent with the emphasis on young children's education and development is the attention child development programs give to the parents of enrolled children. Parental and family dynamics are consistently examined as factors that contribute significantly to the adjustment of young children (Nicoll, 1992). Indeed, the focus on parental involvement is rooted in the assumption that the total family's involvement advances the child's academic, social, and emotional growth (Shelton & Dobson, 1973). With many programs, interventions target the parents' competencies as parents and as persons. In **parent consultation**, psychological consultants engage parents as consultees with respect to the behavior and development of their children. Consulting with parent populations is stressed in the professional literature as a strategy for alleviating family and child problems (Brown, Pryzwansky, & Schulte, 1991; Cobb & Medway, 1978; Parker, Piotrkowski, & Peay, 1987). Among the best-known benefits is the potential of parent consultation to strengthen parents' psychological well-being and sense of competency (Parker et al., 1987). Some programs, such as Head Start and PCC programs, so strongly value parent consultation that they have integrated clear parent participation guidelines into their standards (Piotrkowski, Collins, Knitzer, & Robinson, 1994).

Not everyone agrees that parent consultation is desirable. Some question whether the consultation structure should be triadic in this case. Caplan (1970), for example, excluded parents as prospective consultees in his early writings; that is, he restricted the consultant-consultee relationship to "two professional persons" (p. 19). Since Caplan's influence in the field of consultation is widespread, others have also been led to de-emphasize the role of laypersons (including parents) in mental health consultation (Brown et al., 1991). However, most contemporary consultation specialists defend parent consultation as a useful way of addressing family and child problems (Altrocchi, 1972; Bacon & Dougherty, 1992; Brown et al., 1991; Mathias, 1992).

Special Features   Consulting with parents and families requires the consultant to study the persuasive influences of several unique conditions. First, because many child problems do not occur in isolation from the family, the consultant must consider remedies that incorporate a family systems framework. Though there are obvious exceptions, a common hypothesis is that parent and family disturbances are the direct or indirect cause of problems for children. Just as etiological factors spread through the family system, so too will solutions. That is, as consultants consider child change strategies, they must anticipate the systems implications that remedial actions have for the entire family system. What impact, for example, will a parent's new discipline tactics have on other family members? What about the actions of grandparents who are long-term members of or occasional visitors to the family system? An example of a family systems influence on a child's behavior is presented in Box 7.1.

Second, since parents are often unaware of the succinct purposes and strategies attached to consultation, they often confuse the consultant's role with that of a therapist. Consultants must anticipate this logical assumption since consultation problems are often indelibly linked to parents' mental health needs. Parents often reveal personal or intrapsychic issues that, though related to the child's needs, are best addressed in more direct interventions (Brown et al., 1991), and indeed, consultants risk legal or ethical complications when they allow consultation to evolve into therapy. As a matter of routine practice, Brown et al. (1991) advise consultants to remain focused on consultation goals, redirect parents' thinking toward the child, and ultimately, terminate consultation should these tactics fail (see Box 7.2). These tactics cannot be generalized to all situations, however. Working with parents who exhibit acute emotional disturbances in which they or their children are at risk, for example, requires consultants to handle the crisis appropriately. Consultants should rely on therapy or crisis intervention skills to deal with the immediate situation and provide referrals to appropriate sources of counseling and therapy.

Third, consulting with parents draws on the consultant's relational skills as mechanisms for promoting cooperation and collaboration. Since many parents view the field of psychology and mental health with suspicion and hesitation, they often resist the consultant's proposals. Thus, relationship building is a critical feature of successful parent consultation. To help this cause, consultants should possess effective relational skills and should try to dispel myths or stereotypes about mental health issues.

Fourth, consultants must emphasize collaborative, empowering processes rather than advice-giving strategies. Since parents usually perceive consultants as psychological experts, they tend to expect consultants to provide immediate or advice-oriented solutions. But consultation should focus on mutual problem solving (Brown et al., 1991), joint ownership of consultation goals, and valuing the parent as an integral contributor to the consultation process.

Fifth, consultants must avoid insinuating that parents deserve blame for the child's problems. While parenting styles, without question, strongly influence children's behavior, consultants must take a problem-solving approach rather than making accusatory remarks that threaten the consultee's cooperation and confidence (Caplan, 1970). Further, consultants should explain to guilt-ridden parents that parenting is a difficult process, one for which most parents are often unprepared and, indeed, an experience full of trial-and-error learning. Moreover, consultants must help parents recognize that children's behavior often results from an array of biological and environmental influences and that rarely is there a single, isolated cause.

Alternative Frameworks   As consultants interact with parents, they choose from a range of processes, techniques, and strategies that are implemented in assorted frameworks. Three of the most common frameworks are highlighted in the present discussion: consultant-parent conferences, parent education/training, and parent support groups.

Box 7.1
The family systems influence

A child psychologist, according to the terms of a contract with a Head Start program, is asked to observe a four-year-old boy who exhibits disruptive behavior in the classroom. According to the consultant's observations and assessment, the child is disorganized and undersocialized. He is undisciplined and seems to have no understanding of consequences. The consultant, following several conferences with the child development teacher, decides that a meeting with the boy's parents may help explain the disruptive behavior. The meeting includes the following dialogue:

CONSULTANT: I'm pleased that you're able to meet with me this morning. I'm the Head Start program mental health consultant.

MOTHER: Nice to meet you.

CONSULTANT: I want to talk to you about Jimmy. I've observed him in the classroom and he appears disruptive. He just doesn't seem to concentrate on one activity at a time; he runs when he should walk, interferes with classroom activities, and fights with other children.

MOTHER: He's like that at home. I'm afraid he doesn't get enough food because he wants to play so much. He won't cooperate with any rules. When he is with me, I try to reprimand him for not obeying, but when he stays with his father, he just runs wild.

CONSULTANT: You and the boy's father are separated?

MOTHER: Yes, we've been divorced for the last two years. Also, when Jimmy visits his father, his grandparents watch him and they don't seem to care one way or the other. Then he comes home and I have to go to work on weekends and my sitter just watches television all the time. Good babysitters are hard to find, you know.

CONSULTANT: It seems that the child is cared for by several people. Do you suppose they all have different ways of disciplining him?

MOTHER: Well, I guess. But how can I get all of them to do the right thing?

CONSULTANT: It isn't easy, but perhaps a good start is to arrange a meeting with everyone to discuss the problem.

In child development settings that advocate a "parents as partners" philosophy, the psychological consultant is a key resource for parents. The consultant's presence offers a convenient opportunity for parents to seek information needed to resolve child-related matters through **parent conferences**. Such meetings bring the consultant and parent together in a private, nonthreatening environment. The parent conference is unique in

---

Box 7.2
Consultation versus therapy

A social work professional, with a specialty in consulting with families, is asked by the family services director in a child development program to discuss the behavior of a three-year-old child in a Head Start program. The child has suddenly exhibited difficulty separating from his mother each morning and spends much of the day crying or whining. The consultant decides that a meeting with the mother is necessary to assess contributing factors. The following dialogue describes the meeting:

CONSULTANT: Good morning. I'm pleased that you agreed to meet with me.

MOTHER: Hello.

CONSULTANT: I want to talk to you about your son. It seems that he has difficulty when he leaves you at the bus stop each morning and continues to cry throughout most of the day.

MOTHER: Well, I know he has a tough time. It's just that his father and I have recently argued all the time and he has left home. I have been so depressed about this. I've been thinking about talking to someone, you know, a therapist or someone.

CONSULTANT: You've been upset lately?

MOTHER: Yes, I can't sleep and seem to worry about myself more than my children.

CONSULTANT: I understand that feeling down or worrying about the marriage can be very upsetting. What effect do you think this has on your son?

MOTHER: I guess my worries are getting to him too! But I just want to talk to someone about how badly I feel.

CONSULTANT: I will suggest someone who is really very experienced with the kind of problems you have, but for now, let's talk about how your situation causes your son to cry and not want to go to school.

---

several respects. First, parents' relationships with their children are different from the typical consultee-client relationship. Consultants encounter resilient habits, parenting styles, and beliefs about the parenting process. Often, such rigid patterns have prevailed for years and blocked the changes necessary to resolve problems.

Further, parent conferences provide face-to-face encounters in which parents are without question major influences on the success of planned interventions. Consultants often have little control over parents' commitment to change strategies and their implementation. Usually, the interventions that emerge from consultant-parent dialogue must occur in the privacy of the home, limiting the consultant's role to that of a hopeful supporter.

With the increasing emphasis on parents, consultants to child development programs are often asked to provide parent education and training opportunities. **Parent education** refers to the general approach in which consultants interface with parents in a teaching or instructional format. Spodek et al. (1987) summarize the broad purposes of parent education:

> [Programs] range broadly from programs that help parents develop positive self-concepts to programs designed for unwed teenage mothers. No one parent education program can meet the needs of all parents. Each teacher or school should develop programs that reflect the specific needs and interests of their parents. (p. 146)

Some authors distinguish parent education from consultation on the basis that parent education is more structured, involving the use of established teaching strategies and predetermined curriculum materials (Brown et al., 1991; Brown, Wyne, Blackburn, & Powell, 1979). Although valid in a strict sense, this assertion appears overly restrictive. It is difficult to create any parent education program without at least fragments of consultation dialogue with respect to the specific needs of individual parents. Some preschool parent training programs are broad, multifaceted programs that emphasize much more than simply teaching parents about children. Spodek, Saracho, and Davis (1987), for example, conceptualize parent education as opportunities to help parents develop positive self-esteem. Bacon and Dougherty (1992) discuss the benefits of parent education and training in preventing future problems and unhealthy family interactions. Daniel and Hyde (1975) write about the comprehensive goals of a parent education approach for high-risk parents: "The Parent Education Program is aimed at helping parents acknowledge and use their strengths in order to better meet their personal needs and increase their awareness and ability to meet the needs of other family members" (p. 23).

We regard parent education and training as important components of the broader process of consultation. Despite the tendency of some writers to differentiate parent education from consultation, we think that parent training programs are viable mechanisms for helping parents strengthen parenting competencies and insights. In the role of parent trainer, the consultant works as a knowledgeable professional "who possesses information or skills that the consultees need and transmits that knowledge in one or more of the roles of adviser, educator, or trainer" (Bacon & Dougherty, 1992, p. 26).

In response to the need for parenting skill-building programs, several popular parent education models have emerged through the years. *Parent Effectiveness Training* (PET), developed by Gordon (1975) during the 1970s, is a popular training model that emphasizes the efficacy of parents in resolving parent-child conflicts. Further, Dinkmeyer's (1976) *Systematic Training for Effective Parenting* (STEP), based on Adlerian principles, is a widely used and highly visible model that guides parents through a series of steps for resolving parent-child problems. Other well-known approaches include the *Active Parenting* program (1983) and family systems perspectives on parenting (Getz & Dunn, 1988).

Parent education consultants are often frustrated by the lack of opportunity to focus on parents' individual needs and interests (Bacon & Dougherty, 1992). These dilemmas often result from preplanned parent education curricula designed for large groups. Consultants who wish to avoid these limitations may prefer to serve parents in small groups that allow consultants to attend more specifically to family and child issues (Carlson, 1969). A small-group format adds the benefit of support and encouragement with respect to the specific issues and problems that concern parents. Moreover, small groups have the potential to create an ambience of trust in which parents explore anxieties, uncertainties, and parental weaknesses as they relate to children's problems. Although the dynamics of a particular setting may alter the consultant's actions, a parent-group format should generally conform to the following guidelines:

1. Parent groups should be promoted as supportive and educational opportunities.
2. Participant numbers should be limited to a size that allows individualization, support, and participation.
3. Consultants begin the parent group by focusing on the group process dynamics that facilitate parental comfort and cooperation.
4. Elements of parent education, problem solving, and support underscore the goals of the parent group.
5. The consultant individualizes the group's agenda by considering the questions, issues, or parental circumstances of each participant.
6. Discussions of sensitive or intimate parental concerns that cannot be addressed through the parent-group format should be avoided.
7. Consultants should end each parent consultation by suggesting an action plan to be reviewed at subsequent meetings.

Organizational Consultation   Some consultants extend program-centered consultation to address the organizational issues that surround child programs. Child programs, like most organizations, often encounter the need for program-centered interventions that address systems concerns (for example, the need for strategic planning, staff development, expansion, or downsizing). The roles of consultants as organizational specialists may include the following:

1. *Training and development*   Most child development programs are committed to enhancing the competencies and insights of their staff. The emphasis on training is fueled by financial and program limits that restrict programs' abilities to employ educators with highly specialized backgrounds. The need for training is also heightened when new interventions, educational philosophies, and psychological concepts as well as unique child problems appear relevant to the delivery of quality services (Whitebook, Howes, & Phillips, 1989).

2. *Technical assistance*   Many child development programs operate according to performance, accreditation, or licensure standards. In most cases, programs that fail to satisfy the operating criteria demanded by governing or funding bodies cannot survive. The need to develop quality standards or comply with existing standards prompts comprehensive child development programs to rely on supportive guidance and consultation. One example is the **technical assistance (TA)** service model. TA is a consultation approach whose purpose is to help programs assess their services, identify areas of noncompliance, and implement new or remedial strategies that bring program improvement. A novel example involves Head Start and related programs, in which TA

consultants are retained by regional Head Start offices and affiliated support centers. More specifically, the Head Start Resource and Training Center (1993) in Region III has developed an "expert consultants' pool" in which consultants are assigned to Head Start programs to help with a broad range of performance issues.

3. *Management consultation*   Rapid change, expansion, the need for specialization, and fluctuating environmental demands have created a need for child development program leaders to focus on organizational planning and problem solving. Consultants—specifically those trained in organizational theory and practice—help program leaders focus on organizational weaknesses and on increasing their organization's readiness for the future. Such consultation is delivered in large and small groups or in an individual consultation framework.

An innovative organizational consultation model is the Creating and Managing Effective Organizations (CAMEO) program designed and implemented through the collaborative efforts of the Region III Administration for Children and Families (ACYF) and the Head Start Resource and Training Center. CAMEO is a novel consultation-based program in which organizational consultants collaborate with Head Start program management teams to identify emerging program demands and prepare a strategy to move into the future (Head Start Resource and Training Center, 1993). CAMEO consultation, extended over time, emphasizes skill building in the areas of leadership, strategic planning, team building, and conflict resolution. The highlight of the CAMEO project is a five-day seminar that affords program leaders opportunities for small- and large-group participation.

SUMMARY

Even in healthy environments and stable families, a child's development is complicated by dramatic and far-reaching conditions. The stress that results appears critically related to the psychosocial development of young children and can become a priority issue in child development settings. As we have seen, modern society relies heavily on a broad range of child care programs and other options situated outside the family. A large number of children are enrolled in comprehensive child development programs in which interventions are directed at their physical, cognitive, behavioral, and social development. In addition, most programs extend their attention to a multitude of family dynamics and priorities that influence the children's development.

In this chapter, we have described consultation in child development settings as a professional helping process that includes a broad array of strategies and interventions. We have given special attention to the various options consultants pursue in their work with child development teachers, child care workers, aides, and parents. A growing number of comprehensive child development programs (for example, nursery, preschool, and early childhood education programs) rely on external psychological consultants to help with complex behavioral and developmental concerns. This chapter has provided an introduction to the role of consultants in such settings as well as an overview of their work.

GLOSSARY

Anecdotal records   Often handwritten, informal records maintained at the discretion of a child care staff member to document a child's behavior.

Case-oriented consultation   A consultation practice in which consultants and consultees engage in collaboration relative to the needs and characteristics of a specific child.

Child development   The range of physical, cognitive, and emotional factors that comprise the child's sequential growth.

Child development program   A broad description of child care programs that target the child's cognitive, physical, and emotional growth.

Ecological factors   Within the context of child assessment, the physical, social and psychological dynamics that surround the child.

Observation   A systematic process in which psychological consultants view the behavior and development of children in order to understand and find solutions to their problems.

Parent conference   A face-to-face meeting or interview between a psychological consultant and parents that focuses on the problems or needs of a child or family.

Parent consultation   A consultation format in which consultants interact with parents as consultees regarding the needs and problems of children.

Parent education   A multifaceted intervention that has an instructional focus. Parent education has the implicit purpose of improving parents' childrearing competencies while enhancing certain personal attributes associated with the parenting process.

Prevention-oriented consultation   Consultation interventions designed to prevent the occurrence or recurrence of undesirable conditions affecting children.

Psychological consultation in child development settings   A broad helping process in which child- and family-oriented consultants provide help to consultees (teachers, aides, social services staff, parents) relative to the psychological and developmental needs of young children.

Psychological education   The cumulative processes in which child development programs implement curricula that educate children in the areas of emotional development, self-esteem, and psychosocial competence.

Technical assistance (TA)   A consultation approach in which consultants help child development programs assess their services, identify weaknesses, and propose remedial strategies that conform to published operating standards.

ANNOTATED BIBLIOGRAPHY

Consultants who need published literature explaining the consulting process in child development settings will find their search difficult. Specific practical information on consultation in these settings appears sparse. Consultants must rely on related or peripheral readings instead. To begin, psychological consultants should acquire a thorough background in the child growth and development field. The literature on child development is extensive; a representative work is *Learning and Growing: A Guide to Child Devel-*

opment, by Laurie Braga and Joseph Braga (1975). This book outlines the child's development across key physiological and behavioral categories. A second source is Laura Berk's 1991 book *Child Development.* This volume provides a comprehensive, meticulous analysis. For information on stress as it affects child development, David Elkind's *The Hurried Child: Growing Up Too Fast Too Soon* (1981) is a classic that merits serious attention.

Consulting with child development programs is enhanced when consultants are familiar with the general nature and structural elements of the programs they serve. Moreover, an awareness of the distinct goals and programmatic features associated with early childhood education is essential. Some especially useful publications describe the psychological characteristics of children in consultation settings. A few examples include the books *Early Childhood Education: Special Problems, Special Solutions,* by K. Eileen Allen and Elizabeth M. Goetz (1982), and *Foundations of Early Childhood Education,* by Bernard Spodek, Olivia N. Saracho, and Michael D. Davis (1987). In addition, Bernard Spodek's 1973 book *Early Childhood Education* provides a historical perspective on early childhood education. Collectively, these works orient consultants to the fundamentals of early childhood education, child development program characteristics, and other special issues.

A series of articles in the February 1994 (volume 49) issue of *American Psychologist* highlight the special characteristics of Head Start programs. Specifically, consultants should read the article by Edward Zigler and Sally J. Styfco titled "Head Start: Criticisms in a Constructive Context." Another useful article is "Strengthening Mental Health Services in Head Start: A Challenge for the 1990s," by Chaya S. Piotrkowski, Raymond C. Collins, Jane Knitzer, and Ruth Robinson. Since it is apparent that Head Start and related programs are expanding and will perhaps require more external consultation, consultants to such programs will benefit from studying these sources.

Working in child development settings will inevitably bring opportunities to consult with parents. Although parent consultation appears to lack formal, empirically supported ideologies, a few sources outline practical parent consultation strategies and processes. Duane Brown, Walter Pryzwansky, and Ann Schulte, for example, include a full chapter in their book *Psychological Consultation: Introduction to Theory and Practice* (2nd ed., 1991) that describes consultation practices in detail. These authors provide a practical discussion of the dynamics and processes inherent in consulting with families (pages 247–276). A second source that contains numerous relevant articles is *The Consulting Process,* edited by Jon Carlson, Howard Splete, and Roy Kern (1975). Chapter 7 of this volume reviews a series of articles that can help consultants gain insight into parent and family consultation processes. In addition, interested readers may wish to turn to several articles that describe consultation with parent and family populations. Representative of these articles is Martin H. Ritchie and Ronald L. Partin's "Parent Education and Consultation Activities of School Counselors" (1994). William G. Nicoll's 1992 article, "A Family Counseling and Consultation Model for School Counselors," is also helpful. A third article, written by Carlabeth E. Mathias, is "Touching the Lives of Children: Consultative Interventions That Work" (1992). In addition, Ellen Bacon and A. Michael Dougherty's 1992 article, "Consultation and Coordination Services for Prekindergarten Children," provides relevant and useful information.

References and Suggested Readings

Active Parenting. (1983). *Active parenting discussion program*. Marietta, GA: Active Parenting Publishers.

Albee, G., & Ryan-Finn, K. (1993). An overview of primary prevention. *Journal of Counseling and Development, 72*, 115–123.

Allen, K. E., & Goetz, E. M. (1982). *Early childhood education: Special problems, special solutions*. Rockville, MD: Aspen Systems Corporation.

Almy, M. (1975). *The early childhood educator at work*. New York: McGraw-Hill.

Altrocchi, J. (1972). Mental health consultation. In S. E. Golann & C. Eisdorfer (Eds.), *Handbook of community mental health* (pp. 477–508). New York: Appleton-Century-Crofts.

Bacon, E., & Dougherty, M. (1992). Consultation and coordination services for prekindergarten children. *Elementary School Guidance and Counseling, 27*, 24–32.

Barclay, J. (1984). Primary prevention and assessment. *Personnel and Guidance Journal, 62*, 475–478.

Beaty, J. (1986). *Observing development of the young child*. Columbus, OH: Merrill.

Bergan, J. R. (1977). *Behavioral consultation*. Columbus, OH: Merrill.

Berk, L. (1991). *Child development* (2nd ed.). Boston: Allyn & Bacon.

Brack, G., Jones, E., Smith, R., White, J., & Brack, C. (1993). A primer on consultation theory: Building a flexible worldview. *Journal of Counseling and Development, 71*, 619–628.

Braga, L., & Braga, J. (1975). *Learning and growing: A guide to child development*. Englewood Cliffs, NJ: Prentice-Hall.

Briggs, D. (1970). *Your child's self-esteem*. Garden City, NY: Doubleday.

Brown, D., Pryzwansky, W., & Schulte, A. (1991). *Psychological consultation: Introduction to theory and practice* (2nd ed.). Boston: Allyn & Bacon.

Brown, D., Wyne, M. D., Blackburn, J. E., & Powell, W. C. (1979). *Consultation: Strategy for improving education*. Boston: Allyn & Bacon.

Bruner, J. (1972). Poverty and childhood. In R. Parker (Ed.), *The preschool in action: Exploring early childhood programs* (pp. 7–33). Boston: Allyn & Bacon.

Bundy, M. L., & Poppen, W. A. (1986). School counselors' effectiveness as consultants: A research review. *Elementary School Guidance and Counseling, 20*(3), 215–222.

Caplan, G. (1970). *The theory and practice of mental health consultation*. New York: Basic Books.

Carlson, J. (1969). Case analysis: Parent group consultation. *Elementary School Guidance and Counseling, 4*(2), 136–141.

Carlson, J., Splete, H., & Kern, R. (Eds.). (1975). *The consulting process*. Washington, DC: American Personnel and Guidance Association.

Cobb, D. E., & Medway, F. J. (1978). Determinants of effectiveness of parental consultation. *Journal of Community Psychology, 6*, 229–240.

Daniel, J. H., & Hyde, J. N., Jr. (1975, November-December). Working with high-risk families: Family advocacy and the parent education program. *Children Today*, 23–25.

Decker, C., & Decker, J. (1984). *Planning and administering early childhood programs* (3rd ed.). Columbus, OH: Merrill.

Dickinson, D., & Bradshaw, S. (1992). Multiplying effectiveness: Combining consultation with counseling. *School Counselor, 40*, 118–124.

Dinkmeyer, D. (1976). *Systematic training for effective parenting*. Circle Pines, MN: American Guidance Service.

Dinkmeyer, D., & Dinkmeyer, D., Jr. (1982). *Developing understanding of self and others* (Rev. ed.). Circle Pines, MN: American Guidance Service.

Elkind, D. (1981). *The hurried child: Growing up too fast too soon.* Reading, MA: Addison-Wesley.

Fantuzzo, J. W., & Polite, K. (1990). School-based behavioral self-management: A review and analysis. *School Psychology Quarterly, 5*(3), 180–198.

File, N., & Kontos, S. (1992). Indirect service delivery through consultation: Review and implications for early intervention. *Journal of Early Intervention, 16*(3), 221–231.

Getz, H., & Gunn, W. B. (1988). Parent education from a family-systems perspective. *School Counselor, 35,* 331–336.

Gilbert, L. A., & Rachlin, V. (1987). Mental health and psychological functioning of dual-career families. *Counseling Psychologist, 15*(1), 7–49.

Gordon, T. (1975). *Parent effectiveness training.* New York: New American Library.

Head Start Bureau. (1994). *Responding to children under stress: A skill-based training guide for classroom teams.* Washington, DC: DGK & Co.

Head Start Resource and Training Center. (1993, June). *Creating and managing effective organizations* (seminar workbook). College Park, MD: Author.

Hymes, J., Jr. (1991). *Early childhood education: Twenty years in review.* Washington, DC: National Association for the Education of Young Children.

Ivey, A. E., & Alschuler, A. S. (1973). An introduction to the field. *Personnel and Guidance Journal, 51*(9), 591–597.

Jackson, D., & Hayes, D. (1993). Multicultural issues in consultation. *Journal of Counseling and Development, 72,* 144–147.

Kassebaum, N. (1994). Head Start: Only the best for America's children. *American Psychologist, 49,* 123–126.

Kersey, K. (1986). *Helping your child handle stress.* Washington, DC: Acropolis Books.

Martin, R. (1988). *Assessment of personality and behavior problems: Infancy through adolescence.* New York: Guilford Press.

Mathias, C. E. (1992). Touching the lives of children: Consultative interventions that work. *Elementary School Guidance and Counseling, 26,* 190–201.

Mowder, B., Unterspan, D., Knuter, L., Goode, C., & Pedro, M. (1993). Psychological consultation and Head Start: Data, issues, and implications. *Journal of Early Intervention, 17,* 1–7.

Neisworth, J. T., & Bagnato, S. J. (1988). Assessment in early childhood special education: A typology of independent measures. In S. L. Odom & M. B. Karnes (Eds.), *Early intervention for infants and children with handicaps: An empirical base* (pp. 23–49). Baltimore, MD: Brooks.

Nicoll, W. G. (1992). A family counseling and consultation model for school counselors. *School Counselor, 39,* 351–361.

Office of Human Development Services. (1988). *As I am* (DHHS Publication No. [OHDS] 88–31542). Washington, DC: U.S. Government Printing Office.

Parker, F. L., Piotrkowski, C., & Peay, L. (1987). Head Start as a social support for mothers: The psychological benefits of involvement. *American Journal of Orthopsychiatry, 57*(2), 220–233.

Parsons, R. D., & Meyers, J. (1984). *Developing consultation skills.* San Francisco: Jossey-Bass.

Piotrkowski, C. S., Collins, R. C., Knitzer, J., & Robinson, R. (1994). Strengthening mental health services in Head Start: A challenge for the 1990s. *American Psychologist, 49,* 133–139.

Powell, D. (1989). *Families and early childhood programs.* Washington, DC: National Association for the Education of Young Children.

Reynolds, C. R., Gutkin, T. B., Elliott, S. N., & Whitt, J. C. (1984). *School psychology: Essentials of theory and practice.* New York: Wiley.

Ritchie, M. H., & Partin, R. L. (1994). Parent education and consultation activities of school counselors. *School Counselor, 41,* 165–170.

Sale, J. (1988). Promoting mental health: A parent/child care provider partnership. In S. Goldston (Ed.), *Promoting mental health in early childhood settings* (pp. 3–19). Los Angeles: University of California, Neuropsychiatric Institute.

Salmon, D., & Lehrer, R. (1989). School consultation's implicit theories of action. *Professional School Psychology, 4*(3), 173–187.

Shelton, J. E., & Dobson, R. L. (1973). FICS: An expanded view of counselor consultation. *Elementary School Guidance and Counseling, 7*(3), 210–215.

Spodek, B. (1973). *Early childhood education.* Englewood Cliffs, NJ: Prentice-Hall.

Spodek, B., Saracho, O. N., & Davis, M. D. (1987). *Foundations of early childhood education.* Englewood Cliffs, NJ: Prentice-Hall.

Sprinthall, N. (1973). A curriculum for secondary schools: Counselors as teachers for psychological growth. *School Counselor, 20*(5), 361–369.

Swick, K. (1983). Parent education: Focus on parent needs and responsibilities. *Dimensions, 11*(3), 9–12.

Takanishi, R., & DeLeon, P. (1994). A head start for the 21st century. *American Psychologist, 49,* 120–122.

Thompson, C., & Rudolph, L. (1988). *Counseling children* (2nd ed.). Pacific Grove, CA: Brooks/Cole.

Valentine, J., & Zigler, E. (1983). Head Start: A case study in the development of social policy for children and families. In E. Zigler, S. Kagan, & E. Klugman (Eds.), *Children, families, and government* (pp. 266–280). New York: Cambridge University Press.

Whitebook, M., Howes, C., & Phillips, D. (1989). *Who cares? Child care teachers and the quality of care in America* (Final report, National Child Care Staffing Study). Oakland, CA: Child Care Employee Project.

Widerstrom, A., Mowder, B., & Willis, W. G. (1989). The school psychologist's role in the early childhood special education program. *Journal of Early Intervention, 13*(3), 239–248.

Zigler, E., & Muenchow, S. (1992). *Head Start: The inside story of America's most successful experiment.* New York: Basic Books.

Zigler, E., & Styfco, S. J. (1994). Head Start: Criticisms in a constructive context. *American Psychologist, 49,* 127–132.

◆ CHAPTER EIGHT

Consultation in Health Care Settings

The focus on health care has increased dramatically in recent years, making the provision of adequate medical care a high-profile issue demanding attention from government leaders as well as medical professionals. Interest in health care is fueled by the recognition that the level of medical treatment available to each citizen can have far-reaching implications not only for the individual but for society as a whole. The health care system, however, appears in a state of flux. Because of exorbitant costs and inaccessible medical treatment, major reforms loom on the health care horizon (Frank, 1993). Although the result is likely to be more accessible and less costly health care, the reform process will undoubtedly involve major changes in the way medical services are delivered.

One facet of the health care system that merits emphasis in times of reform is the role of psychology in medical settings. Mental health has long been a significant part of health and, because of this close connection, psychological specialists now realize a greater presence in health care settings. Lucignano and Lee (1991), for example, point out that "it is estimated that over 10% of the American Psychological Association (APA) members work in medical settings, with an increase of 200 to 300 each year" (p. 55). Schenkenberg, Peterson, Wood, and DaBell (1981) add that "psychologists have become increasingly involved in medical education, in medical research, and in providing health services" (p. 309). These and similar statements reveal the momentum with which opportunities for psychological specialists in health care are expanding.

This chapter examines a necessary and growing role for psychological consultants. **Psychological consultation in health care settings** comprises the consultation processes and actions, delivered from a psychological or mental health perspective, that help medical authorities provide comprehensive care to patients. Implicit in this definition is the assumption that health integrates biological, psychological, social, and environmental factors.

The roster of psychological consultants who work in health and medical settings is as broad as the services they provide. Thus, in this chapter, psychological consultants are assumed to include, but are not restricted to, psychologists (health, clinical, and counseling), counselors (health, mental health, and rehabilitation), and social workers (social service and psychiatric).

Types of Health Care Settings

Americans in both urban and rural regions rely on an array of services and facilities to satisfy their health and medical needs. Services range from prevention and general health care to inpatient medical treatment. Though traditional medical care focuses on preventing and treating organic illness, many programs augment conventional medical care with psychological interventions. Elaborating in detail on all the health and medical settings would be an enormous task—one that is beyond the scope of this chapter. We describe only a few representative models here.

1. *General hospital* The general hospital is a multifaceted and comprehensive health care institution and is the most recognizable health care facility. According to Robinson (1984), "The general hospital is an institution providing health services

which include diagnostic tests, medical treatment, surgical intervention, and rehabilitative care" (p. 1). Some hospitals are connected to large universities; though medical care remains a key activity in university hospitals, teaching and education are also central functions. In addition to the assortment of medical treatment services provided by general and university hospitals, many settings include psychiatric and specialized inpatient programs that apply psychotherapeutic interventions for psychiatric disturbances (for example, psychotic, mood, eating, and substance-related disorders).

2. *Primary health care clinics*   The driving force behind primary health care clinics is the need to provide timely health and medical interventions "close to the places where people work and live" (Hylbert & Hylbert, 1979, p. 26). The variety of medical interventions delivered in primary care settings reflects the range of disorders that occur most frequently in society. A salient feature of the primary clinic is the presence of front-line generalists who must be skilled in an array of interventions, including mental health. Patients in such settings often present with psychologically laden symptomatologies that require liaison with more specialized programs. Issacs (1975), for example, points out that "a strong linkage with mental health services and educational facilities, including consultative services, is essential if the primary care practitioner is to provide optimal mental health care along with other health services" (p. 183).

3. *Public health services*   The public health model of health care has "long been concerned with the prevention of disease" (Albee & Ryan-Finn, 1993, p. 115). Public health facilities are community-based entities that respond to the need to immunize citizens from illness in the short term and eradicate disease in the long term. Although public health officials conventionally address the prevention of physical disease, their view has broadened over the years to incorporate prevention-oriented programs as they relate to the mental health arena (Albee & Ryan-Finn, 1993).

4. *Family practice settings*   This medical specialty emerged during the late 1960s "to meet the needs of those physicians who followed general practice and who did not choose to enter a more circumscribed area" (Hylbert & Hylbert, 1979, p. 22). The family practice environment affords diagnosis and treatment for a range of general medical conditions, some complicated by the presence of psychological problems and subsequent referrals to mental health agencies (Thorne, 1993). Although referrals to outside agencies are accepted options, patient resistance or complacency may inhibit subsequent mental health treatment. Thorne proposes an alternative model in which psychological specialists integrate their services into the family practice setting as employees or consultants. The immediate presence of psychological consultants affords a wider array of treatment provisions while increasing "the capacity of the physician to deal with psychosocial aspects of medical care" (Thorne, 1993, p. 1367).

5. *Rehabilitation programs*   Rehabilitation services for citizens with disabilities and physical injuries exist in a large number of private and public agencies nationwide. Rehabilitation programs are found in hospital settings, comprehensive rehabilitation centers, or private clinics, with each program having the goal of restoring patients to optimal functioning. While rehabilitation patients may seek rehabilitation services to address physical dysfunction, their presenting problems are usually only a part of the necessary treatment (Jaques, Kauppi, Steger, & Lofaro, 1979). Krusen's (1971) definition highlights the multiple realms served by comprehensive rehabilitation programs:

"Rehabilitation involves the treatment and training of the patient to the end that he may attain his maximal potential for normal living physically, psychologically, socially and vocationally" (p. 1). Many rehabilitation programs employ psychological professionals who address the psychological ramifications of physical impairment. Although these programs provide restorative psychotherapy as an adjunctive service (Fox, 1994), one function that connects psychological treatment to physical care in large rehabilitation programs is consultation (Bronson, Butler, Thoresen, & Wright, 1967; Hylbert & Hylbert, 1979; Wright & Fraser, 1975).

Psychology and Health: An Enduring Connection

The close relationship between health and psychology encourages the movement of psychological consultants into the health care arena. The convergence of medical and psychological groups is now closer to a reality than in any other period. As Ballou, Fetter, Litwack, and Litwack (1992) point out, for example, "The health professions feel, suggest, propose, and claim that their services and academic domains should include the mental health and psychological well-being of individuals being served" (p. iii). Some mental health proponents believe the health field is in the midst of a paradigm shift in which modern health professionals are paying more attention to systemic or organic principles (Liese, 1986; Nicholas, Gobble, Crose, & Frank, 1992; Seaward, 1994). Organic views reflect the assumption that human beings, as whole entities, are influenced by interconnected and mutually interdependent factors. These beliefs underscore the implementation of **holistic interventions** in medical settings that treat the human organism as a complex, systemic being, comprised of a diverse ensemble of divisions and subparts. According to the holistic framework, any organic factor or division exerts a potentially significant influence on the wellness of the whole organism—even such psychological phenomena as lifestyle, cognitive elements, and psychosocial factors.

The contribution of psychology to illness, as we have indicated earlier in this chapter, requires much attention (Liese, 1986). Brannon and Feist (1992) agree: "Psychology has been involved with people's physical health almost from the beginning of the 20th century" (p. 13). Indeed, the role of psychological factors in physical illness is multidimensional, complicated, and often unpredictable. For instance, some disorders, despite their presentation as physical disorders, are psychological in origin (an example would be conversion disorders). Conversely, many organic disease processes, though they have clear physical etiologies, are exacerbated by the psychological stress accompanying the illness. Despite their origin and dynamics, VandenBos (1993) asserts that "all are painful, and they cause psychological dysfunction, behavioral disruption, and somatic difficulties in varying degrees and combinations" (p. 287).

Evolving out of the newer holistic philosophies are several fields of study grounded in the assumption that psychological factors mix with biological factors to produce illness. Though they have separate areas of emphasis, these fields often share similar views and ideological foundations. They have given rise to a range of specialized programs that require the joint efforts of medical and psychological personnel. Certain features of consultation, including collaboration and interdisciplinary dialogue, help to link medical and psychological staff. We describe a few relevant models in the section that follows.

Psychosomatic Medicine

A field that has long considered the relationship between physical and mental factors in the production of disease is psychosomatic medicine. **Psychosomatic medicine** "encompasses the view that physical illnesses have emotional and psychological components and that psychological and somatic (physical) factors interact to produce disease" (Brannon & Feist, 1992, p. 21). This approach has broad implications for medical and psychological specialists alike, and of necessity, brings a collaborative approach to medical treatment. Psychosomatic medical treatment programs appear to have been the early forerunners of behavioral medicine programs.

Behavioral Medicine

The link between behavior and illness is the primary concern of psychological specialists who work in behavioral medicine settings. Dating from the late 1970s, **behavioral medicine** programs are inspired by research indicating the powerful role of behavioral elements in physical disease. According to Schwartz and Weiss (1978),

> Behavioral medicine is the interdisciplinary field concerned with the development and integration of behavioral and biomedical science knowledge and techniques relevant to health and illness and the application of this knowledge and these techniques to prevention, diagnosis, treatment, and rehabilitation. (p. 250)

The field of behavioral medicine employs a range of psychological specialists in large medical facilities or highly specialized outpatient centers. Nicholas, Gerstein, and Keller (1988) point out that "the expertise of mental health professionals that is most relevant to behavioral medicine pertains to the mental health correlates and consequences of physical illnesses" (p. 82).

Health Psychology

Society's emphasis on wellness exerts pressure on health programs and practitioners to maximize health in ways that prevent illness (Brammer, Abrego, & Shostrom, 1993). This emphasis, fueled by the theoretical and practical successes of the field of psychology, has generated the modern profession of **health psychology**. This expanding field is the area of psychology that applies psychological principles to the health arena in order to maximize good health and challenge unhealthy lifestyle habits. Matarazzo (1984) describes the field of health psychology as the aggregate of the specific educational, scientific and professional contributions of the discipline of psychology to the promotion and maintenance of health, the prevention and treatment of illness, and the identification of etiologic and diagnostic correlates of health, illness, and related dysfunction. (p. 815)

Adler, Cohen, and Stone (1979) point out that the term *health psychology* distinguishes the field on two counts. First, since the term includes *health,* not *medicine,* it emphasizes wellness. Second, the term specifically emphasizes the involvement of psychology as an area germane to the field. Brannon and Feist (1992) cite the various responsibilities of health psychologists; some of these responsibilities have clear consultation implications:

> Health psychology . . . encompasses the various contributions of the field of psychology to the enhancement of health, the prevention and treatment of illness, the identification of health risk factors, the improvement of the health care system, and the shaping of public opinion with regard to health. (p. 19)

Potential Barriers to Consulting in Medical Settings

Despite the noticeable presence of psychological specialists in health and medical settings, their work emphasizes the clinical activities of treatment and diagnosis. The integration of formalized consultation practices into mainstream medicine lags behind these more established psychological roles. Even when practiced in the health care environment, consultation is often conceptually fragmented and seems to lack a practical foundation. Moreover, as consultants interface with medical professionals, turf problems become common. Some believe the work of psychological consultants in health care settings represents a curious paradox. While their potential contribution to medical treatment is promising on the one hand, their presence in medical settings often meets with resistance and controversy on the other (Hansen, Himes, & Meier, 1990). Part of the sluggish maturation of psychological consultation in health-related settings has to do with the newness of psychological consultation in medical environments and the inevitable growing pains that parallel its development. Indeed, the presence of nonpsychiatric consultants in health institutions is a somewhat novel idea that has received attention in the professional literature only recently (Gabinet & Friedson, 1980).

Although resistance to psychological interventions in health settings stems from multiple sources, the contributing factors include the philosophical differences that divide psychology and medicine. Medical practitioners, for example, adhere to the **biomedical model**, a stringent orientation within medical settings that interprets illness as the unequivocal consequence of biological anomaly, defect, or viral invasion. This model prescribes a rigid philosophical mission for the health delivery system, and without doubt, is a dominant influence on the conceptual outlook of medical personnel. Thoresen and Eagleston (1985), mindful of the dramatic and far-reaching biomedical influence, write: "Health care in the United States is based primarily on treating acute, well-advanced (and often terminal) disease processes (often in hospitals), using an infection/disease paradigm" (p. 17). Brannon and Feist (1992) add: "The biomedical model uses molecular biology to identify bacteria, viruses, and other microorganisms as the invading agents" (p. 10). Since the biomedical view defines and underscores almost all forms of medical treatment, medical care appears dominated by physiological practices (Brammer, Abrego, & Shostrom, 1993). A not-so-surprising consequence of this strict biomedical orientation is the devaluation of psychological and mental health ideologies.

The presence of psychological specialists in health care environments also stirs controversy inside these settings. One difference stems from the accepted rule in medical settings that medical authorities direct and dictate all regimens of patient care (Altmaier, 1991; Good, 1992). Altmaier (1991), for instance, is concerned that the medical setting is an arena in which the "physician-led model prevails" (p. 345). Altmaier argues that this hierarchy creates an ambience in which physicians have undue influence on the interventions of other health care constituents, even those not under their immediate supervision. In offering a similar warning, Good (1992) describes the "medical hierarchy" in which physicians are the guardians of medical treatment, generate the most income, and receive the greatest recognition (p. 69). The inadvertent result is a "second-class" status for psychological consultants that leads to isolation and professional distance between medical and psychological professionals (Good, 1992, p. 72). In a strong statement, Good draws an interesting conclusion: "Counseling psychologists in the medical setting, much like the imperiled Zorro, had best learn to parry and spar the challenges to their profession, identity, role, services, and personhood" (p. 67). Although these points are not intended to blame physicians or devalue their vital role in health care, professional differences do represent potential barriers with which new consultants must contend.

Psychological consultants in health care settings also confront the very real concern that, as medical and psychological groups work together, opposing standards of patient care evolve. This confrontation prompts Altmaier (1991) to write: "Medical settings, and problems of health, impose a unique set of standards that on occasion, collide with those of psychology" (p. 358). One example is that in medical settings, psychologists commonly encounter ethical values that conflict with their own (Altmaier, 1991; Lucignano & Lee, 1991; Nicholas et al., 1988). Ethical conflicts, for instance, emerge when psychologists are expected to implement treatment paradigms that exceed professional competencies (Altmaier, 1991). Further, psychological specialists in health settings may be pressured to adhere to a medical model without consideration of behavioral or environmental factors (Lucignano & Lee, 1991). Still other ethical confrontations stem from differences with respect to patient confidentiality and informed consent issues. Regrettably, ethical conflicts represent only one class of differences that divide psychological and medical professionals. Others include diagnostic practices, theoretical orientations, treatment methodologies, and professional preparation standards.

Some barriers emerge inside the disciplines of those who wish to become consultants in medical settings. Fox (1982), for example, expresses concern that the psychology profession has become narrowly focused and single-minded:

> At a time when society needs a broad-gauged profession able to take on its most pressing health needs (which are behavioral in nature), psychology has become a narrow specialty with an arcane and largely invisible delivery system. We have defined ourselves, and are seen by others, as merely a mental health specialty. (p. 1052)

Similar barriers exist in other professional disciplines. Mental health counselors, for instance, have yet to enter the health care picture with much success. Their integration into medical settings has not only been sluggish, but their presence within health care settings must confront ambiguous boundaries and indecision (Ballou et al., 1992). Not only do a profession's identities and missions restrict where its members subsequently work, they also prescribe the content of professional preparation programs. Most programs fail to include exposure, either in core courses or program specializations, to mental health interventions as they relate to medical settings. Without the frame of reference provided by training, graduates are reluctant to seek employment in such settings.

Gaining Acceptance in Medical Settings

Despite the conditions that may discourage would-be consultants in medical settings, psychological specialists have the potential to offer a broad range of valuable health-related services. Now is the time for them to enter the health care picture, since there appears to be a growing receptivity to their presence (Liese, 1986). An important first step, especially for consultants new to the medical setting, is to achieve recognition, to be professionally appreciated, and to gain acceptance from medical peers. Consultants can further their cause by adhering to several strategic initiatives.

Develop Competencies

The medical setting is a unique setting that requires specialized performance from all, including those from nonmedical disciplines. Though psychological professionals bring valuable diagnostic and treatment skills to the medical forum, acceptance by medical authorities may be more a function of the competencies they acquire once inside the health setting. To further their cause, psychological consultants should engage in continuing education, broadened job experiences, introspection, and ongoing dialogue with medical authorities. A part of their expertise centers on the relationship between physical and psychological factors. Gabinet and Friedson (1980) offer this advice: "Psychologist consultants in the general hospital also must adapt to their particular environment by learning the mechanisms whereby physical disturbances can produce psychological changes and the psychological manifestations of organic dysfunction" (p. 944).

Cole and Lacefield (1975) point out that social work and medical groups can weave a net of trust and acceptance by recognizing the characteristics these groups share. To the benefit of patients, for example, both parties possess observational, inference, interpersonal, research, and flexibility skills. Good (1992) endorses another strategy by encouraging counseling psychologists to learn the idiosyncratic language and speaking style of medical personnel. Acceptance by medical authorities is enhanced, according to Good, when psychological personnel recognize the "terms, abbreviations, and expressions which are a part of medical care" (p. 71). The ability to communicate across disciplines enhances relationships and supplants professional distance with collaboration and an atmosphere of understanding.

Develop Rapport with Medical Staff

Disharmony between medical and psychological personnel is often the by-product of unfamiliar and insensitive relations. These conditions prompt Good (1992) to recommend that a "way for new psychologists to increase their effectiveness in this setting is to develop working relationships with physicians" (p. 69). Good adds that professional acquaintances create a disposition in which referrals and requests for consultation have more to do with familiarity and less to do with the specific discipline of the consultant. Liese (1986) adds: "Finally, we would probably benefit from continuing our dialogue with primary care medical professionals, because such activity will facilitate our entry into the medical system" (p. 277).

Rapport emerges, also, when novice consultants bridge the gap separating them from the presiding medical hierarchy. When psychological specialists pursue a strict, discipline-driven approach to patient treatment, they risk alienating physicians and other biomedical model proponents. This split prompts Gabinet and Friedson (1980) to admonish psychological consultants to incorporate into their thinking the etiological contributions of "psyche or soma, or both" (p. 944).

Develop Realistic Expectations

The entry of psychological consultants into medical environments should be planned with deliberation and reason. Little advantage results when psychological specialists, in an attempt to gain quick acceptance and recognition, enter the medical setting armed with sensationalized or unfounded promises. Thus, conservative and achievable expectations should underscore the fundamental roles that psychological professionals expect to fulfill (Tucker, 1991). As Tucker (1991) contends, consultants should also enter the medical setting with realistic expectations:

> A counseling psychologist might function very well as a consultant in a health care setting. However, a vision of counseling psychologists that includes their full participation as scientist-practitioners and equal partners in research and theory development in the health field without a health-related subspecialty or some equivalent training is simply not a realistic one. (p. 390)

Real and Potential Consultation Roles

Despite—or because of—the barriers that impede the entrance of psychological consultants in medical settings, some writers urge them to seek health care opportunities with greater determination (Altmaier, 1991; Blancarte, Murphy, & Reilley, 1991; George & Christani, 1995; Lucignano & Lee, 1991; VandenBos, 1993). Miller and Wilson (1979), in support of social workers as integral agents in health care settings, declare that "the growing body of knowledge about the impact of the social environment on man's physical and emotional condition wins reluctant acceptance" (p. 129). Although counselors have been slow to enter health and medical settings, several authors contend that the connection between disease and emotion calls on them to assume more assertive and meaningful roles (Ballou et al., 1992; Nicholas et al., 1988). Indeed, psychological consultants have much to offer the medical establishment, including the potential contributions described in the following paragraphs.

Clinical Consultation

In medical settings, medical professionals frequently treat patients who have complicated syndromes that combine organic and psychological factors. According to Gabinet and Friedson (1980), "In a general hospital, primary physicians often request a consultation because they do not know the source of the patient's mental disturbance" (p. 940). The consequences of misunderstanding or overlooking psychological dynamics are considerable, as Hansen et al. (1990) point out: "In an era in which cost and accountability are becoming paramount, misdiagnosing psychological problems as physical illnesses rates as an expensive mistake" (p. 148). Thus, psychological consultants in medical settings often handle consultation assignments that resemble the clinical consultation model (Altmaier, 1991; Nicholas et al., 1988). Gallessich (1985) describes the clinical model as the first "psychological approach to consulting" in which a consultee requests assistance from a knowledgeable consultant (p. 337). Clinical consultants operate within an expert-oriented framework in which they offer expertise with respect to "diagnosis, treatment, and prescription" (Gallessich, 1985, p. 135). Moreover, clinical consultation points to a unique triadic relationship in which a consultant (psychological specialist) and consultee (medical authority) collaborate to improve the care of a third party, the client (patient). Within a medical framework, the clinical model depicts a medical authority who seeks psychological consultation with respect to the psychological dynamics of a particular case. Box 8.1 contains a case example of the clinical consultation model.

Psychological Liaison-Consultation

The traditions of medical treatment include psychiatric consultation as a means of resolving mental health issues in health care settings. For patients in large hospital settings, physicians seek the liaison-support provided by these mental health specialists. Despite the recognition that conventional liaison-consultation in hospitals is somewhat exclusive to psychiatric professionals, some psychiatrists align themselves with psychological specialists (Schenkenberg et al., 1981). The professional literature provides several descriptions that, together, create a picture of psychological liaison-consultation (Gabinet & Friedson, 1980; Schenkenberg et al., 1981). **Psychological liaison-consultation** might be defined as a consultation service in which psychological specialists serve as integral components of medical settings and contribute insights that traditional medical approaches cannot provide. Stotland (1988), writing about

---

Box 8.1
Case example: A clinical consultation approach

A 26-year-old woman was admitted to a general hospital following an assault that occurred while she was walking to her car from work. She had completed her workday at a brokerage firm just before she was assaulted in a busy down-town area. The attack left her with multiple lacerations and bruises, none serious. She was admitted to the hospital for observation. Her emergency room physician was also concerned that the patient was not able to talk about the incident. In fact, she had not spoken about the attack at all since she arrived at the emergency room nor had she explained the incident to the police, who found her lying, in a fetal position, in the alley behind the brokerage company. The physician ruled out physical damage to the pharynx, esophagus, or any other speech-related mechanism. Following the examination and treatment for the patient's physical injuries, the physician sought consultation with a clinical psychologist on the hospital's staff. Though the physician suspected that the terror of the assault resulted in psychological symptoms, she was unsure how to proceed with treatment or referrals or how to interact with the patient. The consultant visited the patient's hospital room, assessed the symptoms, and rendered a diagnostic impression. Subsequently, the consultant and physician collaborated with respect to medical care, including provisions for psychological treatment.

---

psychiatric consultation, identifies various conditions that could indicate the need for psychological liaison-consultation:

1. When the patient's psychosocial status interferes with her ability to cope with her illness or her personal needs
2. When her psychosocial status causes her to present with successive illnesses or complicates her recovery from illness
3. When, because of her psychosocial status, the patient uses and abuses deleterious substances
4. When the patient's ability to comprehend and to comply with a course of management is in doubt
5. When the patient has clinical features of a psychiatric illness and help is needed in establishing a diagnosis
6. When the available skills and time of the referring physician have not succeeded in resolving the patient's psychosocial symptoms (p. 27)

Gabinet and Friedson (1980) present a success story in which the consultation contributions of a "front-line" psychologist have gained acceptance by primary physicians (p. 939). They summarize several functions psychological liaison-consultants serve, including psychological testing, diagnosing, treatment planning, and implementing behavioral science ideologies. Though the success reported by Gabinet and Friedson kindles optimism and encouragement, their case appears more the exception than the rule. Schenkenberg et al. (1981) remain cautiously optimistic, however, as they offer this warning to those who believe medical programs in general fully appreciate the potential of psychological liaison-consultants: "Effective use of psychologists in such settings is still a matter of promise rather than actual fact" (p. 309).

Interdisciplinary Collaboration

Health care exists in diverse settings that employ professionals and paraprofessionals who represent different orientations or backgrounds. Though each practitioner offers unique skills and theoretical wisdom, some fear that the combination of many specialists is often contradictory, creating blurred professional boundaries. Ballou et al. (1992) prefer an optimistic position: "Ultimately, the possibility of multiple and interwoven involvements offers the desirable scenario of interdisciplinary approaches provided by a multiprofessional team" (p. iii). The rationale is simple. To orchestrate the most comprehensive patient care, health care specialists require the wisdom and support of other professionals. Hylbert and Hylbert (1979) agree:

> As spectacular as has been his contribution, the physician cannot provide comprehensive treatment alone. He finds himself, today, a member of an ever growing team of professionals and paraprofessionals whose competencies are utilized in varying combinations as the individual case may warrant. (p. 32)

Although collaboration often occurs in a collegial, person-to-person form, an alternative model is the multidisciplinary team approach. A **multidisciplinary team** is a collection of health care specialists who contribute to patient care by sharing the expertise of their respective disciplines. Multidisciplinary teams are potentially synergistic groups invested in comprehensive health care (Lucignano & Lee, 1991; Nicholas et al., 1988). Conventional teams include physicians, psychiatric nurses, mental health counselors, social service professionals, speech pathologists, dieticians, exercise physiologists, physical or occupational therapists, and psychologists (Lucignano & Lee, 1991; Nicholas et al., 1988). As a "consultant" to the team, the psychological professional contributes expertise about the behavioral or psychological dynamics of patients' illnesses. Issues that reflect the behavioral or psychosocial needs of patients (for example, patient noncompliance, resistance, family dynamics, posttreatment implications), though baffling to medical personnel, are well known to psychological specialists.

Behavioral Programs

Many psychological consultants are human behavioral specialists skilled in the interpretation of environmental influences and the design of behavioral treatments. Their roles are enhanced when physicians acknowledge that patient ailments require interventions that fall outside traditional pharmacological or biomedical treatment (Fox, 1994; Gabinet & Freidson, 1980). Fox (1994) explains that psychologists, for example, have developed behavioral management protocols for patients with various chronic diseases (such as enuresis and encopresis, obesity, bruxism, hypertension, and coronary illness). As consultants skilled in behavioral modification principles, psychological consultants serve a valuable collaborative role in helping physicians design and implement behavioral programs for patients with these organic disorders. Fox (1994) endorses the psychological professional's participation in developing behavioral programs for patients who must follow "needed and complex (and sometimes unpleasant) treatment regimes" (Fox, 1994, p. 205).

Health Education and Wellness

Many citizens exacerbate health risks by indulging in unhealthy behaviors. Unhealthy behaviors create unnecessary risks to health and require repetitive medical treatment. Mindful of the threats that misinformation or bad habits pose to health, Nicholas et al. (1988) advise that the "prevention of illness and health promotion must become a routine part of the health care system" (p. 92). This health care imperative should prompt health psychologists and counselors to serve as trainers or educators who emphasize health and wellness concepts in their work.

Consultants also engage in psychoeducational roles that target patients' coping and adaptation. **Psychoeducation** denotes the cumulative instructional processes that promote psychological resilience and knowledge. Nicholas et al. (1988), addressing an audience of mental health counselors in a behavioral medicine setting, point out that psychoeducation goals incorporate three assumptions:

1. The mental health counselor's role is comparable to that of a teacher.
2. Medical patient problems involve learning deficits rather than symptoms.
3. Patients should be active in directing their own learning.

In a related capacity, psychological consultants, through their prevention focus, help patients and hospitals reduce the cost of medical treatment. Robson, France, and Bland (1984), for example, in an experimental investigation of the effects of psychological consultation as an intervention supplementing medical treatment, found that consultants provide a valuable service that reduces the cost and intensity of the medical treatment. Fox (1994) agrees:

> Psychology has the potential to become a major health service profession with a vital role in resolving some of society's most vexing problems by significantly reducing the enormous drain on the nation's financial resources that has resulted from an illness-driven approach to health care and health care financing. (p. 205)

Medical Treatment Compliance

Psychological factors influence individuals in ways that speed or delay recovery. Medical professionals sometimes discover that prescriptions for health or recovery from illness are sabotaged by patients' noncompliance and irresponsibility. Although the specific causes vary, Altmaier (1991) highlights several common areas of nonadherence.

Many patients, to the frustration of medical authorities, refuse to initiate, continue, or complete their prescribed course of medical treatment. Others violate the goals of treatment through their failure to attend scheduled appointments. Further, some patients demonstrate a pattern of negligence with respect to taking medication at scheduled times, while others resist recommended changes that result in positive health practices.

As consultants, psychological professionals assess and monitor the source of noncompliance and then collaborate with physicians on methods of increasing patient compliance (Altmaier, 1991). Further, consultants have the skills to study the physician-patient relationship for dynamics that generate noncompliance (Altmaier, 1991).

Medical Staff Training

Many responsibilities germane to medical and health interventions require psychological interpretation and application. Interactions with patients, for example, often call on medical authorities (such as physicians or nurses) to relate, empathize, and comfort. The adaptation of patients to their illnesses and, indeed, their recovery is often accelerated by the psychological insights and skills of medical staff. Mindful of the psychological implications of medical staff and patient interactions, some authors propose psychological training roles within medical settings (Altmaier, 1991; Weinman & Medlik, 1985). Altmaier (1991), responding to physicians' confessions that they are often ineffective communicators, espouses a specific training goal: "Training health care providers in interpersonal skills is a key role for counseling psychology, and one in which considerable activity has occurred" (p. 353). A different training role is implied by Liese's (1986) hypothesis that some physicians want to provide psychological interventions to supplement medical treatment and "appear eager to learn effective and reliable strategies from psychologists" (p. 277). A similar training need emerges from the concern that medical professionals are often unable to detect psychological problems or manage patient behavior (Weinman & Medlik, 1985).

Stress and Hospitalization

Hospitalized patients represent a population often wrought with anxiety and fear (Brannon & Feist, 1992). The stress of hospitalization can sidetrack medical treatment, delay recovery, or exacerbate illnesses. The sources of patient stress are indeed vast. Many are anxious, for example, about the high costs of hospitalization and the disruption that hospitalization creates within occupational and personal arenas. Others worry about uncertain or bleak prognostications about their physical health. Patients who face surgery represent a group whose medical treatment conjures extreme stress and worry (Anderson, 1987).

The stress of hospitalization presents numerous opportunities for psychological consultants, as Weisman (1978) points out: "When the limits of medicine and surgery have been reached, psychosocial problems may just be gathering momentum" (p. 266). Consultation in relation to hospitalization is one attempt to make patients feel better before their treatment. Supporting the delivery of consultation interventions to hospitalized patients are several research studies that conclude that patients' recuperation rests heavily on the successful management of psychological factors (Anderson, 1987; Pinto & Hollandworth, 1988). Through consultant-patient dialogue, consultants can assess the gravity of patients' psychological distress and provide an ambience of empathy and support. Consultants also have the potential to carry out a diverse range of patient stress reduction techniques, including relaxation training and cognitive restructuring. Some medical settings extend training and support programs to help patients prepare for treatment (Brannon & Feist, 1992), roles to which psychological consultants are accustomed.

Employee Assistance Programs

The work environment in many medical settings is stressful and hampers employee performance. Saltzberg and Bryant (1990) recognize the unique psychological concerns prevailing in a hospital setting: "Hospital employees are subject to specific stresses caused by the nature of their work; they are at high risk for drug abuse, burnout, and value conflicts brought about by unsatisfactory job conditions and career prospects" (p. 45).

In response to high-pressure work and the reality that overly stressed medical personnel can make disastrous mistakes, some medical settings offer employee assistance programs (EAPs) that provide psychological interventions to staff and consultation to hospital officials (Saltzberg & Bryant, 1990). In the "consultant" role, EAP specialists collaborate with administrators and the medical hierarchy to identify troubled employees, refer them for appropriate treatment, and maintain a liaison between treatment specialists and the work environment. Supervisory training represents an integral consultant role in many EAP programs. Saltzberg and Bryant (1990) make an additional point with respect to EAPs in medical settings. These authors call attention to the high population of female employees in medical settings and the unique problems they often encounter (for example, the stress faced by single working mothers, various forms of victimization, and the burden of caring for elderly relatives).

Referral Issues

The new paradigm that considers the holistic nature of human dysfunction calls attention to both organic and psychosocial issues for virtually every disease. As Taylor (1990) notes, "One need not be clairvoyant to appreciate certain developments that can be expected as a result" (p. 47). Thus, one reality is that medical professionals are, perhaps more than at any other period in history, faced with the psychological implications of the many health conditions or illnesses they treat. The implications for psychological specialists are considerable. As these multifaceted disorders increase in number and complexity, for example, medical authorities will come to rely on the consultation (and other psychological interventions) input of psychological specialists. The range of conditions that present psychological and organic variants is, indeed, exhaustive, and while a discussion of each is beyond the scope of this chapter, the list that follows cites suggested references for readers who desire more detailed discussion.

1. Alcohol abuse (Mitchell, Thompson, & Craig, 1986)
2. Stress disorders (Taylor, 1990)
3. Eating disorders (Connor-Greene, 1987)
4. Cancer (Koocher, Sourkes, & Keane, 1979)
5. Elderly patients (Rabins, Lucas, Teitelbaum, Mark, & Folstein, 1983)
6. AIDS (Wolcott, Fawzy, & Pasnau, 1985)
7. Burn injuries (Ochitill, 1984)
8. Pain (Hickling, Sison, & Holtz, 1985)
9. Obstetrics (Solyom, 1981)
10. Pediatrics (Rivara & Wasserman, 1984)
11. Surgery (Anderson, 1987)
12. Arthritis (Achterberg-Lawlis, 1982)

SUMMARY

This chapter introduced you to a challenging and perhaps growing role for psychological consultants: consultation in health care settings. The chapter highlighted the importance of health care in America and the relationship of psychological principles to disease and wellness. In addition, it outlined the various types of health care settings and their implications for psychological and mental health interventions.

A major portion of the chapter emphasized the consultation roles that psychological specialists might occupy. We caution that consultants in health settings encounter many barriers and must look to ways of gaining acceptance and overcoming obstacles. The assumption that the functions of consultants need to be developed and refined underlay much of the discussion. The chapter concluded with an examination of the various conditions that have strong psychological elements and of the potential involvement of consultants in the treatment of these illnesses.

GLOSSARY

Behavioral medicine A broad field of health care in which psychological professionals apply principles of behaviorism in treating the behavioral elements that contribute to medical disorders. Behavioral medicine is rooted in the belief that physical illness and behavior are intimately connected.

Biomedical model In medical and health care settings, a model that conceptualizes illness as a biological development in which disease is caused by the natural processes of the body or invasive external agents (bacteria, viruses, or microorganisms).

Health psychology The area of psychology that specializes in health maintenance and disease prevention. Health psychologists are professionals who help individuals develop wellness practices, apply behavioral and psychological strategies to health promotion, and treat health disturbances with psychology as a frame of reference.

Holistic interventions Within the context of health and wellness, interventions that perceive the individual as a "whole" person consisting of dynamic divisions or subsystems (including behavioral, psychological, and lifestyle components) capable of exerting significant influences on that organism.

Multidisciplinary team   With respect to medical settings, includes health care professionals and paraprofessionals, all with similar patient treatment goals. Team members make various contributions depending on their background and training.

Psychoeducation   A term that refers to the cumulative processes used to teach individuals psychological skills and knowledge so that they can cope efficiently with existing illnesses or prevent future illnesses.

Psychological consultation in health care settings   Consultation processes and actions, delivered from the perspective of psychology and mental health, that supplement the efforts of medical personnel in rendering comprehensive care to patients.

Psychological liaison-consultation   An underdeveloped form of consultation in which psychological specialists play a key role in medical settings. They provide assistance with medical problems that cannot be resolved by traditional means.

Psychosomatic medicine   A broad field within the health care arena that views physical illness as the product of interactions between psychological and physical processes.

ANNOTATED BIBLIOGRAPHY

Psychological consultants seeking information about consulting in health care settings will find few sources that offer detailed or formal consultation models. Perhaps because of the underdeveloped status of psychological consultation in the medical arena, most major consultation texts have little to say on this subject. An exception is James Hansen, Bonna Sue Himes, and Scott Meier's 1990 book *Consultation: Concepts and Practices*. Chapter 5 of this book provides some general information on consultation in medical settings. These authors also offer a comprehensive discussion of the need for mental health consultation in medical settings and information about the effectiveness of this type of consultation. In addition, Chapter 6 of June Gallessich's *The Profession and Practice of Consultation: A Handbook for Consultants, Trainers of Consultants, and Consumers of Consultation Services* (1982) provides meticulous detail about clinical consultation approaches that have clear implications for work in medical settings.

Much can be learned from a collection of journal articles that discuss consultation on the part of psychologically trained professionals. Of particular value are Glenn Good's "Counseling Psychologists in Hospital/Medical Settings: Dilemmas Facing New Professionals" (1992) and Elizabeth M. Altmaier's "Research and Practice Roles for Counseling Psychologists in Health Care Settings" (1991).

Several articles highlight the consultation contributions of psychological specialists to medical settings. Laille Gabinet and William Friedson's "The Psychologist as Front-Line Mental Health Consultant in a General Hospital" (1980) describes the firsthand experiences of a psychologist functioning as a consultant. A similar purpose is accomplished by T. Schenkenberg, L. Peterson, D. Wood, and R. DaBell in their article "Psychological Consultation/Liaison in a Medical and Neurological Setting: Physicians' Appraisal" (1981). Another excellent source of information on the staff development and skill-building functions of consultants is John Weinman and Lenka Medlik's article "Sharing Psychological Skills in the General Practice Setting" (1985). Further, you may wish to review a special 1991 issue of *Counseling Psychologist* (Stone, 1991) titled "Counseling Psychology and Health Applications." For background information on counseling and health issues, the January 1985 issue of *Counseling Psychologist* (Fretz, 1985) is a valuable reference.

Other readings serve the worthwhile purpose of outlining future trends that merit the attention of psychological personnel in health and medical settings. Ronald Fox's article "Training Professional Psychologists for the Twenty-First Century" (1994) is an excellent example. An alternative source is R. G. Frank's "Health-Care Reform: An Introduction" (1993).

References and Suggested Readings

Achterberg-Lawlis, J. (1982). The psychological dimensions of arthritis. *Journal of Consulting and Clinical Psychology, 50*(6), 984–992.

Adler, N. E., Cohen, F., & Stone, G. C. (1979). Themes and professional prospects in health psychology. In G. C. Stone, F. Cohen, & N. E. Adler (Eds.), *Health psychology* (pp. 573–590). San Francisco: Jossey-Bass.

Albee, G. W., & Ryan-Finn, K. D. (1993). An overview of primary prevention. *Journal of Counseling and Development, 72,* 115–123.

Altmaier, E. M. (1991). Research and practice roles for counseling psychologists in health care settings. *Counseling Psychologist, 19*(3), 342–364.

Anderson, E. A. (1987). Preoperative preparation for cardiac surgery facilitates recovery, reduces psychological distress, and reduces the incidences of acute postoperative hypertension. *Journal of Consulting and Clinical Psychology, 55*(4), 513–520.

Ballou, M. B., Fetter, M. P., Litwack, K. P., & Litwack, L. (1992). *Health counseling.* Kent, OH: American School Health Association.

Blancarte, A. L., Murphy, K. J., & Reilley, R. R. (1991). Health psychology: Status and trends. *Psychological Reports, 69,* 189–190.

Brammer, L. M., Abrego, P. J., & Shostrom, E. L. (1993). *Therapeutic counseling and psychotherapy* (6th ed.). Englewood Cliffs, NJ: Prentice-Hall.

Brannon, L., & Feist, J. (1992). *Health psychology: An introduction to behavior and health* (2nd ed.). Belmont, CA: Wadsworth.

Bronson, W. H., Butler, A. J., Thoresen, R. W., & Wright, G. N. (1967). A factor analytic study of the rehabilitation counselor role: Dimensions of professional concern. *Rehabilitation Counseling Bulletin, 11,* 87–97.

Cole, H. P., & Lacefield, W. E. (1975). *Skill domains for the helping professions, a conceptual and empirical inquiry: Preliminary report.* Unpublished manuscript, University of Kentucky, Department of Educational Psychology and Counseling, Lexington.

Connor-Greene, P. A. (1987). An educational group treatment program for bulimia. *Journal of American College Health, 35,* 229–231.

Fox, R. E. (1982). The need for a reorientation of clinical psychology. *American Psychologist, 37,* 1051–1057.

Fox, R. E. (1994). Training professional psychologists for the twenty-first century. *American Psychologist, 49,* 200–206.

Frank, R. G. (1993). Health-care reform: An introduction. *American Psychologist, 48*(3), 258–260.

Fretz, B. R. (Ed.). (1985). Counseling for health [Special issue]. *Counseling Psychologist, 13*(1).

Gabinet, L., & Friedson, W. (1980). The psychologist as front-line mental health consultant in a general hospital. *Professional Psychology, 11*(6), 939–945.

Gallessich, J. (1982). *The profession and practice of consultation: A handbook for consultants, trainers of consultants, and consumers of consultation services.* San Francisco: Jossey-Bass.

Gallessich, J. (1985). Toward a meta-theory of consultation. *Counseling Psychologist, 13*(3), 336–351.

George, R. L., & Christani, T. S. (1995). *Counseling: Theory and practice* (4th ed.). Boston: Allyn & Bacon.

Good, G. E. (1992). Counseling psychologists in hospital/medical settings: Dilemmas facing new professionals. *Counseling Psychologist, 20*(1), 67–73.

Hansen, J. C., Himes, B. S., & Meier, S. (1990). *Consultation: Concepts and practices.* Englewood Cliffs, NJ: Prentice-Hall.

Hickling, E. J., Sison, G. F., Jr., & Holtz, J. L. (1985). Role of psychologists in multidisciplinary pain clinics: A national survey. *Professional Psychology: Research and Practice, 16*(6), 868–880.

Hylbert, K., & Hylbert, K., Jr. (1979). *Medical information for human service workers* (2nd ed.). Elizabeth, WV: Counselor Education Press.

Issacs, G. (1975). Experimental training and manpower utilization programs (primary care). In E. J. Lieberman (Ed.), *Mental health: The public health challenge* (pp. 180–183). Washington, DC: American Public Health Association.

Jaques, M. E., Kauppi, D. R., Steger, J. M., & Lofaro, G. A. (1979). The education and training of rehabilitation counselors. In J. Hamburg, D. J. Mase, J. W. Perry, & M. Dulmage (Eds.), *Review of allied health education* (Vol. 3, pp. 61–98). Lexington: University of Kentucky Press.

Koocher, G. P., Sourkes, B. M., & Keane, W. M. (1979, August). Pediatric oncology consultations: A generalizable model for medical settings. *Professional Psychology, 10*, 467–474.

Krusen, F. H. (1971). The scope of physical medicine and rehabilitation. In *Handbook of physical medicine and rehabilitation* (2nd ed., pp. 1–13). Philadelphia: Saunders.

Liese, B. S. (1986). Physicians' perceptions of the role of psychology in medicine. *Professional Psychology, 17*(3), 276–277.

Lucignano, G. L., & Lee, S. (1991, April/May/June). Ethical issues involved in the role of psychologists in medical settings. *Journal of Rehabilitation, 57*, 55–57.

Matarazzo, J. D. (1984). Behavioral health: A 1990 challenge for the health sciences professions. In J. D. Matarazzo, S. M. Weiss, J. A. Herd, N. E. Miller, & S. M. Weiss (Eds.), *Behavioral health: A handbook of health enhancement and disease prevention* (pp. 3–40). New York: Wiley.

Miller, D. A., & Wilson, C. P. (1979). Social work practice in the health setting. In J. Hamburg, D. J. Mase, J. W. Perry, & M. Dulmage (Eds.), *Review of allied health education* (Vol. 3, pp. 129–147). Lexington: University of Kentucky Press.

Mitchell, W. D., Thompson, T. L., & Craig, S. R. (1986). Underconsultation and lack of follow-up for alcohol abusers in a university hospital. *Alcohol Abusers, 27*(6), 431–437.

Nicholas, D. R., Gerstein, L. H., & Keller, K. E. (1988). Behavioral medicine and the mental health counselor: Roles and interdisciplinary collaboration. *Journal of Mental Health Counseling, 10*(2), 79–94.

Nicholas, D. R., Gobble, D. C., Crose, R. G., & Frank, B. (1992). A systems view of health, wellness, and gender: Implications for mental health counseling. *Journal of Mental Health Counseling, 14*(1), 8–19.

Ochitill, H. (1984). Psychiatric consultation to the burn unit: The psychiatrists' perspective. *Psychosomatics, 25*(9), 689–701.

Pinto, R. P., & Hollandworth, J. G., Jr. (1988). Using videotape modeling to prepare children psychologically for surgery: Influence of parents and costs versus benefits of providing preparation services. *Health Psychology, 8,* 79–95.

Rabins, P., Lucas, M. J., Teitelbaum, M., Mark, S. R., & Folstein, M. (1983). Utilization of psychiatric consultation for elderly patients. *Journal of the American Geriatrics Society, 31*(10), 581–585.

Rivara, F. P., & Wasserman, A. L. (1984). Teaching psychosocial issues to pediatric house officers. *Journal of Medical Education, 59,* 45–53.

Robinson, L. (1984). *Psychological aspects of the care of hospitalized patients.* Philadelphia: Davis.

Robson, M. H., France, R., & Bland, M. (1984). Clinical psychologist in primary care: Controlled clinical and economic evaluation. *British Medical Journal, 288,* 1805–1808.

Saltzberg, M., & Bryant, C. (1990). Hospital-based EAPs. *EAP Digest, 10*(6), 45–62.

Schenkenberg, T., Peterson, L., Wood, D., & DaBell, R. (1981). Psychological consultation/liaison in a medical and neurological setting: Physicians' appraisal. *Professional Psychology, 12*(3), 309–317.

Schwartz, G. E., & Weiss, S. M. (1978). Behavioral medicine revisited: An amended definition. *Journal of Behavioral Medicine, 1,* 249–251.

Seaward, B. W. (1994). *Managing stress: Principles and strategies for health and wellbeing.* Boston: Jones and Bartlett.

Solyom, A. E. (1981). Mental health consultant in infant day care: A new frontier of prevention. *Infant Mental Health Journal, 2,* 188–197.

Stone, G. L. (Ed.). (1991). Counseling psychology and health psychology [Special issue]. *Counseling Psychologist, 19*(3).

Stotland, N. L. (1988). When to seek psychiatric consultation for your patient. *Female Patient, 13,* 26–28.

Taylor, S. (1990). Health psychology: The science and the field. *American Psychologist, 45*(1), 40–50.

Thoresen, C. E., & Eagleston, J. R. (1985). Counseling for health. *Counseling Psychologist, 12*(1), 15–87.

Thorne, C. A. (1993). Integrating mental health into family practice. *American Family Physician, 47*(6), 1366–1367.

Tucker, C. M. (1991). Counseling psychology and health psychology: Is this a relationship whose time has come? *Counseling Psychologist, 19*(3), 387–391.

VandenBos, G. R. (1993). U.S. mental health policy: Proactive evolution in the midst of health care reform. *American Psychologist, 48*(3), 283–290.

Weinman, J., & Medlik, L. (1985). Sharing psychological skills in the general practice setting. *British Journal of Medical Psychology, 58,* 223–230.

Weisman, A. D. (1978). Coping with illness. In T. P. Hackett & N. H. Cassem (Eds.), *Handbook of general hospital psychiatry* (pp. 264–275). St. Louis, MO: Mosby.

Wolcott, D. L., Fawzy, F. I., & Pasnau, R. O. (1985). Acquired immune deficiency syndrome (AIDS) and consultation-liaison psychiatry. *General Hospital Psychiatry, 7,* 280–292.

Wright, G. N., & Fraser, R. T. (1975). *Task analysis for the evaluation, preparation, classification, and utilization of rehabilitation counselor-track personnel* (Monograph No. 22). Madison: Wisconsin Studies in Vocational Rehabilitation.

CHAPTER NINE

Consultation in Business and Industrial Settings

Glossary

Annotated Bibliography

References and Suggested Readings

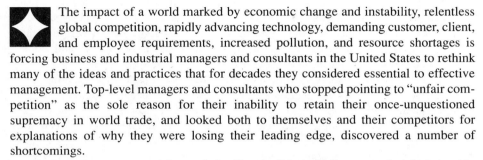 The impact of a world marked by economic change and instability, relentless global competition, rapidly advancing technology, demanding customer, client, and employee requirements, increased pollution, and resource shortages is forcing business and industrial managers and consultants in the United States to rethink many of the ideas and practices that for decades they considered essential to effective management. Top-level managers and consultants who stopped pointing to "unfair competition" as the sole reason for their inability to retain their once-unquestioned supremacy in world trade, and looked both to themselves and their competitors for explanations of why they were losing their leading edge, discovered a number of shortcomings.

Perhaps the most surprising and significant of their findings was that their trust in and expectations of their employees were not nearly as high as those of their more successful competitors in such areas as product and service quality, customer and client satisfaction, and the ability to plan and implement rapid innovation (Boyett & Conn, 1992). A second discovery was that while most high-level executives in this country report that employees are their greatest resource, little support for this belief is evident in such areas as employee selection, training, supervision, performance assessment, compensation, and promotion policies and practices. Indeed, there is less support when management and supervisory practices in relation to employees in lower-level jobs are reviewed (Baird & Meshoulam, 1992; Brill, Herzberg, & Speller, 1985; Clark, 1993; Hersey & Blancard, 1993; Schein, 1987; Waterman, 1992). Once again, they found that their more successful competitors not only view their employees as their most important resource, but also actively encourage personal and professional development. They provide continuous opportunities and rewards for additional education and training, regular reviews of performance assessments, and an appropriate reward system for innovative or increased production and service.

Davidow and Malone (1992), concerned with the revitalization of American business and industry, assert that many of today's businesses and industries are neglecting their most important resource:

> We know that companies that build the highest-quality products in the most efficient factories have relied on techniques such as total quality management and lean manufacturing. These techniques are in turn dependent on worker skills in problem solving and teamwork. (p. 162)

Other managers and consultants agree. As Drucker (1985a) warns, "Business is a human organization, made or broken by the quality of its people. . . . Knowledge is a specific human resource" (p. 3). Schein (1987) points out that "Organizations are becoming more dependent upon people, because they are increasingly involved in complex technologies and are attempting to function in more complex economic, political, and sociocultural environments" (p. 26). More succinctly, Likert (1967) states that "all the activities of any enterprise are initiated and determined by the persons who make up that institution" (p. 1).

Managers in business and industrial settings are beginning to realize that they are far more dependent than ever before on the people who make up their organizations. More and more senior administrators are becoming aware that they depend on the technological skills, the knowledge, and the interest, efforts, and energy of the people in their organizations (Boyett & Conn, 1992; Davidow & Malone, 1992). With this realization, they are looking for better ways to attract, motivate, and keep men and women with specialized knowledge and technical skill.

They are learning, also, that, while they are primarily interested in certain factors— particularly employee recruitment, selection and classification, training, supervision, job assignments, performance evaluation, loyalty, pay, and promotion—employees involved in complex technologies have a different set of personal needs and expectations (Schein, 1987; Conyne & O'Neil, 1992; Clark, 1993; Waterman, 1992). For example, they expect challenging assignments and a reasonable degree of responsibility. They expect fair treatment, acceptance by their immediate supervisor and peers, recognition for their accomplishments, and opportunities for personal and career development. Moreover, they expect to participate in the organization's decision-making process, whether through direct action or consultation. In short, today's skilled technical employees are not simply looking for a job or material gain; they are looking for a career (Drucker, 1985a, 1985b). Their needs and, therefore, the needs of employers who wish to attract and keep them, are related to a work setting in which they feel accepted and worthwhile, and where they believe they will continue to learn and to contribute.

As business and industrial organizations become more complex and require more knowledge in more areas, top-level administrative officers realize they do not have answers to all the problems that may arise, particularly in the area of human development. Many look to psychological consultants for assistance in developing human service systems that are designed specifically for the people in their organizations. In addition to program development, top-level managers in business and industrial settings are contracting with psychological consultants and organization development specialists for key consulting functions. Examples of these functions include forecasting employee needs; assessing difficult-to-measure employee skills (such as leadership, decision-making, and planning skills); and determining suitability and adaptability of employees for transfer to other sites (particularly remote, isolated, or foreign sites). Other examples include developing benefit programs; measuring productivity levels; serving as expert witnesses to testify at employee compensation hearings; and designing, conducting, and evaluating specific training seminars, workshops, and programs.

Because it is impossible to cover all the areas just listed in a single chapter, we focus in this chapter primarily (though not exclusively) on three types of programs:

1. **Employee assistance programs (EAPs):** programs in business and industry designed for the delivery of mental health services to troubled employees whose work performance is impaired and for preventive and health or wellness programs

2. **Organizational development (OD) programs:** programs where the organization itself is the consultant's client and organizational or system enhancement is the primary goal of consultation
3. **Human resource planning and development (HRPD) programs:** programs for recruitment, selection, orientation, training, and retention of employees

Besides exploring these three areas, the chapter also briefly discusses the role of psychological consultants in **collaborative team consultation** in business and industrial settings. (A collaborative team is a consultation team composed of a variety of psychological, technological, and management specialists who work together to resolve complex human resource problems or issues and to facilitate organizational change.)

Be Aware at the Outset

While the primary purpose of this chapter is to discuss the need for psychological and OD consultants in business and industrial settings and to outline their roles and strategies, we should note two assumptions at the outset. The first is that profit remains the "bottom line," and the second is that there are no quick or magic answers.

Profit Is the Bottom Line

Profit is the ultimate mark of success or failure for business and industrial organizations and, therefore, the top priority of their high-level managers and boards of directors. Furthermore, managers and boards of directors guided by profit insist that their employees, including psychological and OD consultants, internalize the profit motive and justify their existence by demonstrating the positive economic results of their work.

Because the majority of psychological consultants in business and industrial settings come from the human service professions, where people are, without question, granted the highest position in the motivational hierarchy, the expectation of consultees that they internalize the profit motive can be difficult to accept. It can be especially difficult for the psychological consultant reporting to a manager of the "old school" who is highly skeptical about the value of human resource planning and development in business or industrial settings. Still, accept they must, for consultants unable to justify the cost-effectiveness of their services will not long remain with the organization (Montana & Charnov, 1987). If external to the organization, they will not be invited to submit future consultation proposals. If internal, they will become victims of **downsizing** (eliminating positions not directly contributing to production or profit), or they will simply be informed that their services are no longer needed.

No Quick or Magic Answers

Action-oriented senior managers may be caught up in the call for radical organizational change after reading numerous success stories in their professional journals of organizations that implemented the most recent recommended organizational innovations.

Eager to share in the success of the corporations cited in these articles, they may need to be reminded by the consultant that failures are seldom reported in journal articles, and that successful organizational change, even when minor, rarely occurs overnight. Baird and Meshoulam (1992) studied 30 corporations ranging from 2,000 to 300,000 employees and varying from financial services to industrial products. They found that, while there is no single or best way to enhance organizational development, most successful programs were implemented over a period of time, usually in seven carefully prepared stages, each built on the foundation of all previous stages (p. 70). They warn their readers that purchasing a state-of-the-art, sophisticated program and trying to implement it before the basics are in place, or adopting a program because it proved successful in another organization, nearly always leads to loss of time and money. In short, Baird and Meshoulam stress that organizational changes only work when they fit an organization's specific needs. Therefore, justification is required before spending time and money to transform an organization. Organizations are distinctive, and managers who want organizational change should first know the basics (the cost, fit, expected outcomes) and the potential contribution of change to their particular organization.

Employee Assistance Programs

While EAPs can be found in most large business and industrial settings today, recognition and acceptance of the need to provide such services were a long time coming. In their review of the history of EAPs, Brill, Herzberg, and Speller (1985) trace the first programs, "initiated at a handful of companies," to the 1920s and report little growth during the next three decades. Indeed, they state, "It was not until the 1970s that American business began once again to pay more attention to the problem of troubled employees" (p. 728).

Early EAPs were designed to assist in the assessment and treatment of alcohol dependency and abuse, usually through referrals to outside counselors in private practice, Alcoholics Anonymous, hospitals, community mental health centers, or rehabilitation programs. Many of today's EAPs are designed to work with employees whose job performance is adversely affected by a much wider range of personal problems.

Factors Determining Number and Types of Services

A number of factors dictate the comprehensiveness of EAPs. These factors include the size of the business or industrial organization, the perceived needs for employee services on the part of the organization's chief administrative officers, and the financial condition of the business or industry. Another determinant is a solid belief that EAPs will be cost-effective (that is, that the cost of treating knowledgeable and technically skilled employees will be less than that of replacing them). A high incidence of absenteeism, tardiness, filed grievances, and reported employee-supervisor conflicts also creates a need for a range of EAP services. While EAPs limited to the assessment and referral of alcohol and substance abusers still exist, an increased number of businesses and industries offer assistance to all their employees (Brown, Pryzwansky, & Schulte,

1995; Gerstein & Sturmer, 1993). The more comprehensive EAPs not only include services for troubled employees whose work performance is negatively affected by problems of alcohol and substance abuse, mental health problems, marriage and family problems, and employee-supervisor conflicts. They also offer both preventive and wellness programs, designed to enhance the health and well-being of their employees. Such programs may help employees find suitable child care facilities, teach methods and techniques for dealing with stress, and provide referrals for employees needing financial or legal advice. They also include exercise and nutrition classes, smoking cessation programs, orientation and mentor programs for new employees, tuition payment programs for job-related courses, career planning programs, and preretirement programs to assist the employee in the transition from full-time employment to retirement. While large corporations are more likely to provide these services in-house, smaller businesses and industries contract specific programs from external consulting agencies or independent consultants. Again, psychological consultants possess the knowledge and skills necessary to plan for and provide these services.

Common Characteristics

The clients of EAPs are either self-referrals or, in some instances, referrals by immediate supervisors who have noticed a severe drop in the level of the employee's work performance. Most directors of EAPs insist that confidentiality is essential to the success of their programs. Troubled employees will often refuse to use EAPs if they believe that there is even a remote chance that their problems, or the information they reveal to an EAP counselor, may become known to others in the organization.

Confidentiality issues also require the records of EAP clients to be kept separate from the organization's personnel records. The EAP client is informed on entry that he or she must sign a release-of-information form before any information in EAP files can be shared with others. Information from clients' files may be shared when the treatment of specific problems requires coordination with the client's supervisor or when the client referred by a supervisor wants that supervisor to receive a general progress report. In most EAPs, initial client contacts are phone inquiries. It is necessary, therefore, that a crisis line be available to callers at all hours of the day and night.

Problems Encountered by Program Directors

Directors of EAPs, whether internal or external, are responsible to both the clients served and the organization that employs them. They must balance their clients' need for confidentiality and the organization's need for the information essential for effective management. This dual, and often-conflicting, client-organization responsibility also creates problems for the directors of EAPs as they consult with the organization's senior managers. On the one hand, they feel responsible to their clients when the organization's culture, personnel policies, and work practices are contributing to the problems of their troubled clients or impeding their treatment. On the other hand, they feel obligated to help the senior managers of the organization find new ways to increase employee productivity and employee job satisfaction and simultaneously keep the costs of EAP services to a minimum.

Internal and External Programs

EAPs are on the increase as upper-level managers of business and industrial organizations recognize that it can be less costly to treat once-effective employees whose problems adversely affect their present work practices than to recruit, hire, orient, and train their replacements. This is particularly true in businesses and industries that require employees with advanced knowledge, training, and technical skills. After a review of the literature, Brill, Herzberg, and Speller (1985) report that, though few and far from conclusive, controlled studies of utilization of medical benefits by troubled employees with access to EAPs have demonstrated cost savings. The types of savings reported in these studies include reduced absenteeism and tardiness, fewer visits to company medical clinics, and decreases in disability and workers' compensation payments. Other forms of savings include decreases in accidents and safety violations and reductions in the numbers of grievances filed and disciplinary actions taken. As consultants, EAP professionals collaborate with organizational leaders and supervisors to train employees in EAP procedures and increase program utilization.

Organizational Development Programs

Today's top-level managers in business and industry are seeking new and innovative ways to cut costs, while simultaneously improving the quality of production and service and meeting the imposed standards and regulations set by the courts and various federal and state agencies. These standards and regulations involve, for example, antitrust laws, tax codes, subsidies, and embargo lists; equal employment opportunity; safety and health hazards; and workplace electronic surveillance. Lacking the necessary expertise in one or more of these areas, they are turning to external business and industrial consultants and OD specialists for assistance (Drucker, 1985b). They realize that, if their business or industry is to survive, they simply cannot afford to continue present management practices and hope things will return to the way they were. The need for change is no longer in question. Rather, the questions they seek answers for are: What present and future changes are necessary for this particular business or industry? Once these changes are determined, how can they be implemented effectively and smoothly? What is the realistic and best time frame for their implementation? And finally the bottom-line question: Will these changes prove cost-effective?

Innovative Changes in Organizational Structure

Structural changes in any organization have consequences. That is, any change, whether major or minor, in an organization's structure has the potential to affect all parts of the organization to some degree, and the more innovative the change, the greater the degree of its impact on the total organization. No matter how critical the need for change or how careful the planning, not all the consequences of change in an organization's structure can be anticipated. Transition from the former to the new structure of an organization will almost certainly present unexpected problems.

Organizations are made up of people, and people are fallible. Perceptions will vary. Events will be misinterpreted. Explanations will be misunderstood. Prejudices will emerge and become manifest. Anxiety can soar. Morale can fall. Suspicions can rise. And the organization's grapevine can sing with false speculations and rumors. Still, there is a time when traditional organizational structures must give way to new and more effective ones. Some of the more creative and risk-taking managers are experimenting with innovative changes in organizational structures. Among their changes are trends in downsizing (a flattening or "delayering" of the management hierarchy), **team systems** (a variety of work teams, project teams, semiautonomous work units), and **nontraditional compensation** (gainsharing, pay-for-knowledge, lump-sum bonus plans, employee stock options).

Downsizing   There is little doubt that attempts to make business and industrial organizations lean, flexible, and competitive will continue well into the next century. One method—downsizing—has already gained wide acceptance by top-level executives and boards of directors. Middle-management positions have been hardest hit. In some instances, entire levels of middle management have been deleted from organizational charts. In others, less certain about how to shift the duties of some middle managers (decision making, supervision, support) to others in the organization, position reductions are less drastic. In the near future, as more intelligent computer programs demonstrate that a computer can not only do most of the work currently performed by middle managers but also can do it with far greater speed and accuracy, more middle managers will become victims of downsizing.

While the economic advantages of downsizing appear immediately evident, executives who jumped too quickly and indiscriminately eliminated middle-management positions quickly discovered that the loss of these positions required numerous other innovations. For example, the decisions formerly made by middle managers now had to be made by lower-level employees who had little or no experience, responsibility, or training for decision making in the past. The same discoveries proved true for the supervisory and support functions once performed by the managers whose positions were eliminated.

Further, executives discovered that by flattening the management hierarchy, they had eliminated the incentive of many employees aspiring to become managers, and along with that, they lost the organization's only management training program. With radical downsizing, there is no organizational ladder to climb, nor are there any managerial promotions as rewards for outstanding performance. New incentive and training programs to motivate and reward employees have to be developed. Realizing their dilemma, top executives may seek the assistance of HRPD and OD experts whose specialties include knowledge of human motivation.

Downsizing is traumatic for all involved. It affects those whose positions are eliminated, the managers who must inform them, the survivors, and the HRPD specialists responsible for offering assistance. While the trauma cannot be avoided, steps can be taken to lessen its intensity. All employees, including the survivors of downsizing, need a full and open explanation of the necessity for downsizing. They need to understand not only *why* the positions were terminated, but also *how* the positions terminated were selected. The survivors need assurance that additional position cuts are not planned, or if they are, when they are likely to occur. Both groups also need to be assured that job performance was not a selection issue. Further, both groups should hear, as soon as possible, what assistance the company offers to those affected by downsizing—for example, severance pay, early retirement options for those eligible, and job search assistance. (Job search assistance can include résumé writing, job interview skills and video practice simulations, training programs for upgrading work skills, partial or full tuition reimbursement for relevant college courses, office space with secretarial assistance for a period of time, networking techniques, and workshops on methods of coping with stress.) Termination and follow-up interviews to determine the success of the assistance offered are recommended.

When involved in planning for downsizing in the early stages, psychological consultants with clinical training in human vulnerabilities and reactions to stress can give valuable assistance to both the employees and the managers. Their clinical knowledge and experience prepares them for dealing with people feeling anger, frustration, shame, embarrassment, worry, and powerlessness. Employees unprepared for downsizing often experience a flood of unexpected and contradictory thoughts and feelings that can lead to a plummeting sense of self-worth, an acute sense of vulnerability and helplessness, and a lack of control. Regardless of the assistance offered, some individuals feel they have been treated unfairly and see litigation as their only recourse.

The needs of survivors must also be attended to. They, too, are likely to experience debilitating feelings, such as anger over seeing their friends lose their jobs; relief, even guilt, at having survived the cut; fear that they may be next; and doubt that they have been fully informed. If their needs go unmet, they may seriously consider looking for work with another company. They may also avoid any contact with those whose positions were eliminated because they do not know what to say or because they fear that their supervisors might frown on their association or their expressed concern. They may begin a review of all stated company policies related to firing, layoffs, relocation, or termination to see if there are any irregularities in this instance. They may also take advantage of their right to review their personnel files to read and, if permitted, to make copies of all past job performance evaluations.

Whether internal or external, psychological consultants working as human resource specialists will almost certainly encounter serious ethical conflicts inherent in downsizing. As consultants, they are employed by the company; yet the employees whose positions were terminated are also their concerns. In their work they may see and hear (overhear?) things that conflict with their personal and professional values. Examples might include promises of managers for excellent letters of reference, regardless of moderate or poor performance evaluations in the past; plans of employees to bring suit against the company; or plans of employees to reveal to the press instances where the company illegally dumped hazardous waste materials or violated safety regulations. Any limitations of confidentiality must be clear to both the consultee and the consultee's clients—in this instance, the employees affected by downsizing.

Team Systems   The traditional bureaucratic management hierarchy has obvious shortcomings: slow and inefficient communication, fixed job roles and responsibilities, a lengthy time frame for decisions, stifling supervisory practices, little or no feedback of ideas from lower-level, on-line employees, and the tendency of upper-level managers to lose touch with the needs of employees, customers, or clients. To avoid these shortcomings, **new-generation managers** began to experiment with a team systems approach as a way to use more fully the knowledge and skills of employees at all levels of the organization to increase production, improve quality, and gain flexibility.

As might be expected, employee adjustment to a team approach is less difficult for those entering a new business or industry than it is for those who have worked in an established business or industry for some time. However, once employees are convinced that the promises of a team approach are "real," their adjustment to a radically different work setting can occur much sooner than either management or employees thought possible. Adjustment time depends on how long it takes the team approach to demonstrate the following to employees:

1. There are no coercive supervisors looking over their shoulders and making demands.
2. Both peers and supervisors are sincerely interested in their ideas.
3. They are recognized and rewarded for ideas adopted by the company.
4. They have input into how their job can best be performed.
5. They are financially rewarded for acquiring the additional knowledge and skills necessary to perform the jobs of other team members when needed.
6. They are rewarded for outstanding team performance.

Work-Unit Teams   Initial attempts of the more traditional businesses and industries to implement a team approach are likely to be limited to the establishment of work-unit teams. **Work-unit teams** require few changes from the traditional organizational structure and no radical changes in the work-flow process. A work-unit team's responsibilities and objectives are clearly defined, and managers of the team are appointed. Team members meet with their managers on a regular basis to discuss the team's performance and to develop action plans to improve the unit's production and quality levels. Members of the work-unit team are invited to participate in an open discussion and to share their ideas and problem-solving abilities with the team manager.

Managers and supervisors may be reduced in number with the establishment of work-unit teams, but their positions are not eliminated, and they are not selected by the work-unit members. Moreover, while work-unit managers and supervisors are encouraged by upper management to facilitate the problem-solving abilities of their team members and to provide the work unit with the information and resources they need to solve problems, the managers and supervisors remain "in charge." They continue to perform traditional management functions, particularly in such areas as budgeting, scheduling, and the hiring, firing, and disciplining of team members. An adversarial relationship between management and workers remains in place, and few of the advantages reported by business and industries that have opted for a self-managed team approach are likely to occur.

Self-Managed Teams   While self-managed teams might evolve from work-unit teams, they represent a radical departure from traditional organizations and management hierarchies (see Chapter 10 for information on the dynamics of teams). In self-managed work teams, no company managers or supervisors are assigned to direct the members' performance. Instead, self-managed teams elect the team leader from their membership to facilitate their meetings and perform administrative functions. The team members assume responsibility for team performance (for example, planning, scheduling, budgeting, hiring, and when necessary, disciplining or firing team members unwilling or unable to contribute to team efforts). In short, self-managed teams operate as semi-independent units with collective responsibility for the unit's performance, and the members' compensation is based on that performance.

In addition to fulfilling the human need for belonging, self-managed groups, like networks, provide members with a horizontal link. Self-managed groups cut across the organization to provide a cross-disciplinary approach to people and issues. When working as a team, all members are peers. The result is greater human interaction, consensual decision making, and willingness to communicate about and attempt to address the concerns and problems that arise during day-to-day task allocations. Members of self-managed teams often report feeling revitalized and more involved in their work. Business and industrial organizations report fewer employee absences and sick days and less employee tardiness on arrival and when returning from scheduled breaks. In addition, managers also note improvement in communication—both vertical and horizontal. Conflicts between supervisors and workers are practically nonexistent. And disciplinary cases are limited to only the most severe, since most are handled by peer pressure. Managers also report smoother production flows. When problems arise they are solved by the team rather than simply shutting down and calling the supervisor to provide the solution.

Semiautonomous Work Units   Occasionally a problem arises that is too complex to be solved by self-managed teams or that requires more time than the teams can give. On such occasions, the coordinating team manager may decide to form a **semiautonomous work unit** to address the problem.

No single set of characteristics exists to describe the work unit. They vary in size. Their members' areas of expertise may be in a single discipline, or they may represent diverse specialties. They may be "insiders" (selected members of different work teams in the organization), or they may include "outsiders" (independent consultants contracted by the organization to serve in the work unit). The work unit may be given an indefinite period or assigned a strict deadline, again depending on the complexity and urgency of the problem. In either case, the leader is usually expected to submit periodic progress reports to a top-level executive, usually the **chief executive officer (CEO)** or the team coordinator, if he or she is a member of the organization's executive board.

Nontraditional Compensation Systems   Traditional systems of compensation, based on position, title, or authority, are no longer applicable in the innovative management systems presently being developed. Downsizing, for example, not only flattens the levels of management hierarchy but also flattens opportunities for promotion and employee incentive. With fewer opportunities for vertical movement, new-generation managers and HRPD specialists are providing opportunities for horizontal movement, along with career-long development programs for all employees. With the exception of pay-for-knowledge programs (see below), most nontraditional incentive programs result in variable compensation systems. That is, employees' salaries will vary from year to year or even more often and are always at risk and subject to change. They are tied to team or company performance and not added to base salary. They are one-time, lump-sum amounts or, as in the case of stock options, they are unavailable to the employee until after a specified vestment period, usually 15 years and/or exit from the company. Examples of some of the incentive programs being experimented with today are gainsharing, pay-for-knowledge, lump-sum bonus plans, and employee stock options. Additional incentive programs (full or partial tuition reimbursements, sabbaticals, repayment for professional meetings, conferences, and workshops, for example) are discussed under the heading "Human Resource Planning and Development."

Gainsharing **Gainsharing** (an incentive for group performance) has been credited with having a positive impact. Gainsharing is based on key indicators, such as cost reductions, value added, profits produced, time saved, sales increased, deadlines met, services delivered, or flexibility to adjust to innovative change. Once the key indicators are selected, they can be compared to current, historical, or base levels. When a team surpasses the base levels, it receives predesignated bonus points in the form of a percentage of base salary or a specified number of dollars. Teams may also lose bonus points when they fall below base levels, though deductions of bonus points will not affect an individual member's base salary. Typical of most incentive plans, gainsharing is not automatic, nor is it based on individual effort. All members of the team, regardless of how hard or how little they work, will receive the same percentage increase or set amount of dollars over their base pay. The age of entitlement (that is, increments for years of service, cost-of-living increases) is over. Individuals gain only when their team contributes to the performance and profit of the organization.

Pay-for-Knowledge One of the more innovative of the nontraditional incentive programs is **pay-for-knowledge** (a series of training programs or knowledge and skill modules to qualify employees for other positions in the organization—team, department, division, company). When organized well, pay-for-knowledge programs benefit both the individual employee and the business or industry.

For the individual employee, pay-for-knowledge programs provide opportunities to learn new job skills and to add increments to his or her base salary. Other benefits reported by those who participate in pay-for-knowledge programs include a sense of personal development and job satisfaction, an increased sense of self-reliance, pride in accomplishment and being viewed by others as multiskilled, wider and more flexible organizational relationships, and a tendency to perceive a brighter future with the business or industry.

Advantages for the business or industry include greater flexibility in the use of human resources—particularly when advanced technical change is introduced in both job tasks and job demarcation—as well as elimination of fixed job attitudes and smoother production flows. Other advantages include greater emphasis on skills and quality, fuller commitment of employees, a training program that can be adjusted as needs change, improved communications at all levels (both vertical and horizontal), and preparation for innovative changes—movement to a team approach, for example. In short, pay-for-knowledge programs prove cost-effective. Production is not interrupted at the loss or illness of a crucial employee; there is a qualified person there to fill the vacancy. When any employee is falling behind, others possessing the necessary knowledge and skills for that position can assist rather than waiting—an automatic action when compensation is based on the work performance of the team or section.

Early experiments revealed that the goal of total flexibility was unrealistic. Employees were unable to retain more than seven skill modules. Retention requires continual experience in the skill modules completed. Providing experience opportunities to perform in all skill modules achieved can be difficult, particularly when team assignments are held to a minimum. One company, reported in Clark's *Human Resource Management and Technical Change* (1993), limited the number of learning modules for an individual to four primary and two secondary. Because employees had been led to believe that the company's original goal was total flexibility and that they had been promised opportunities for unlimited learning modules, the decision to limit them to six was viewed as a broken promise that created problems. Had the managers first turned to psychological consultants, who are aware of the most current research on the retention of learned skills, they would have realized that the goal of total flexibility was impossible to achieve and placed a realistic limit on the number of skill modules an individual could complete. All psychological consultants would be well advised to keep informed of current research on the effectiveness of innovative management strategies and techniques. Informed consultants can help their consultees avoid costly errors such as the one just cited.

Lump-Sum Bonus Plans   As the term implies, **lump-sum bonus plans** are set-figure bonus awards for outstanding performance that benefits the company in some way. They may be awarded to recognize individuals whose ideas have contributed to increased production, improved product quality, or better service delivery to customers or clients. Lump-sum bonuses may also be awarded to all members of teams or work units. Again, these are one-time awards and are not added to the recipients' base salaries. Lump-sum bonus awards motivate workers most effectively when awarded publicly—in view of large numbers of workers and reported in the organization's newsletter.

Consultants or HRPD specialists are often involved in initiating lump-sum bonus programs. They are also often responsible for monitoring them and evaluating outcomes.

Employee Stock Option Plans   Once limited to top executives, **employee stock option (ESO)** plans are being made available to employees at all levels. ESO plans may vary; however, in most instances, the company sets up a trust fund into which it contributes new stock or money to purchase existing shares of stock. Eligible employees receive shares of stock, usually based on a percentage of their annual salary. The employee's right to the stock increases with seniority, and after a set number of years (usually five to seven), he or she is granted ownership of the stock account. When the "vested" employee leaves the firm, the company purchases his or her stock shares at market value. Employees who own stock in the company that employs them are more likely to be interested in seeing the company succeed. As with gainsharing plans, stock option plans serve as incentives to employee performance, for they make the employees financial partners.

Human Resource Planning and Development Programs

Organizations of all types recognize that people are perhaps their greatest resource. With the exception of futurists, top-level managers in high-tech businesses and industries were probably the first to realize that their survival depends on their success at hiring people who not only possess the technical knowledge and skills for present job performance requirements, but are also future-oriented, astute learners who seek opportunities for continual personal and professional development. These same managers were also the first to recognize that the people they need to build a cutting-edge company or industry would (could?) not work at peak performance levels with the rigidities of traditional management practices. A few of the more adventurous set out to create experimental HRPD programs.

Those who reviewed the literature for answers found few reports of hard experimental data they could apply to the development of these programs. Martin (in Dressel, 1971), after reviewing the evaluations of six new, innovative colleges in various stages of development, offers an explanation for the scarcity of empirical research that might also apply to innovative HRPD programs in business and industrial settings: "In swiftly changing times, research instrumentation cannot keep up with innovative activities, samples will not stand still long enough to provide specimen, contexts are not compatible, hypotheses contradict, methodologies break down" (p. 311). Even today, the vast majority of articles in management journals are limited to reports from participant observers, case studies, comparative studies, and experiential reports. Few of these articles report failed attempts; indeed, the majority are success stories. There is a definite lack of longitudinal studies. In short, HRPD evaluation studies require much more explicit reporting than that currently appearing in the journals we have reviewed.

As the economy moves from an industrial to an information base, and as great volumes of complex information must be gathered, classified, and analyzed, managers are required to spend more money, time, and energy on finding, motivating, and training their people. They are also finding HRPD frustrating because the quality of people is more difficult to measure than product quality. Immediate improvement is less evident, and results are difficult to measure in dollars. Further, because traditional managers have little knowledge and experience in the newer human techniques they read about in journals, they are often unable to implement the most recent HRPD innovations.

Baird and Meshoulam (1992) studied 30 corporations and found three major reasons why corporations waste time and money in human resource development: "First, effort is not focused on pressing business problems. . . . Second, the program's information and skills do not interact and support each other, and Third, managers do not manage their resources" (p. 68). In short, they neither expect nor demand cost justification for human resource costs.

Dangers of Prepackaged Programs

Managers who become caught up in the clamor for radical change (for example, quality-control circles, flexible time, and nontraditional compensation) are sometimes tempted to purchase a new sophisticated HRPD program without first attending to the basics that must be in place before it can be implemented. It is not enough for the CEO of a business or industrial firm to recognize the need for innovative change. Before new employees are recruited, corporate goals and objectives must be established, and training and orientation or socialization programs to help new employees adapt to the organization's culture and expectations must be developed. Before formulating an employee appraisal system, the organization must put an employee profile system in place, and critical employee training needs that fit the organization's goals and objectives must have been met. Further, before introducing diversification, decentralization, or off-site product groups or divisions, the company must take steps to prepare employees. They must understand the need, reasons, and advantages. Before flattening the organization (indiscriminately eliminating middle-manager positions, for example), managers need to know that such an action will help them control staffing costs and cut only those areas that are no longer contributing to production, quality, or profit.

Human Resource Planning and Development Central to Managing Technical Change

While there are still fairly large numbers of top-level managers who view technical change in business and industrial settings as solely a technical matter and see no role for the HRPD specialist or consultant in dealing with technical change, new-generation managers and boards of directors are expanding the role of human resource specialists. They are convinced that innovative HRPD is central to managing the processes of technical change. Consequently, they are involving human resource specialists in decisions related to OD, flattening the management hierarchy, team building, knowledge and skill training programs, assessment and evaluation of job performance, qualification of employees to fill additional positions, programs to train line managers and supervisors to work with self-managing and semiautonomous work teams, and innovative communication systems.

Role of Human Resource Planning and Development Specialists

Organizational change can lead to a great deal of frustration for both senior managers and OD consultants. The bureaucratic approach to management and supervision favored by most American business and industrial managers is highly resistant to change, even when the need for change is known and accepted (Davidow & Malone, 1992; Naisbitt & Aburdene, 1990; Peter, 1973; Waterman, 1992). Further, managers often possess little knowledge and experience in the newer human management strategies and techniques, and even less in human development. Many of the innovative changes designed to cut costs, increase production, and improve quality control could be less traumatic for both managers and employees and result in less litigation if HRPD specialists were involved early in the planning. Any change (or even rumors of change) in any part of an organization will to varying degrees affect all other parts of the organization, and the initial reaction of people in the organization is rejection. At the very least, change or innovation creates discomfort. To those not involved in the decision for change, speculation about the reasons for change center on power, politics, and upper-level management, rather than on the rationale for or utility of the change. Curry (1992) asserts: "In the absence of a reasonable explanation, members of an organization attempt to make sense out of what seems to them to be a nonsensical event" (p. 2). Their imaginative reasons, treated as fact, can create a schism between upper and middle management, between employees and management, or between union and management. If involved in the early planning for change, HRPD and OD specialists, with their knowledge and skill of the dynamics of human, group, and organizational behavior, have much to contribute.

Clark (1993) reminds HRPD specialists that one reason they are marginally involved in the processes of technical change is their lack of information technology skill and knowledge. His study of and experience in British businesses and industries lead him to conclude:

> Those people who have responsibility for, or wish to influence, personnel issues under conditions of advanced technical change need to acquire a detailed appreciation of the particular technology and task when considering the choice of the most appropriate organizational arrangements. (p. 214)

While other factors will certainly influence the future role of HRPD specialists, Clark (1993) issues this challenge:

> The question for specialist personnel managers is whether they have the ambition and expertise to play a major role in this endeavor as the wider voice of organizational, work and human resource issues, or whether they wish to follow the recent UK trend of retreating into ever-narrower technical specialisms (employment law, recruitment technology). (p. 222)

Collaborative Team Consultation

There are occasions when consultants in other specialties (engineering, production, marketing, to name only three) wish they could call on a psychological consultant for assistance. For example, an engineer, frequently assigned to conduct on-site consultation with dissatisfied (and often irate) customers of his firm's machinery, informed one of the authors that, in at least 90 percent of his consultations, the problems he encounters are not a matter of technology. They are, rather, problems created by a plant's personnel, usually directly traceable to management, machine operators, maintenance personnel, or supervisors. He then related three instances that he said are typical:

In the first instance, the consultant's firm had installed 5 new machines in the consultee's plant. The salesperson assured the consultee that the 5 new machines would surpass the performance of 20 of the old machines, and that maintenance required for the new machines would be less than a quarter of what they presently spent maintaining the older machines. Otherwise the firm he represented would remove the new machines without charge and return the purchase price, no questions asked. After a trial period, the consultee was convinced that the claims of the consultant's firm were at best unrealistic and at worse dishonest. In his assessment of the situation, the consultant could find nothing wrong with the new machines. Further assessment of the problem revealed that both machine operators and maintenance personnel believed that management's intent in purchasing the new machines was to cut personnel by half. To prove to management that their numbers should not be reduced, the operators intentionally ran the new machines below capacity and shut them down frequently for unnecessary maintenance or repair. Maintenance personnel cooperated with the operators by taking longer to complete the maintenance process and by claiming the company had not stocked necessary replacement parts. The result of their combined efforts was that the production of the new machines was held to the same level as that of the 5 machines they had replaced. When the plant manager assured the machine operators and maintenance crew that there were no plans to cut personnel, that he had purchased the machines to meet a new, long-term contract that required a significant increase in production, the machines suddenly performed as promised by the consultant's company.

In the second instance, a production manager, who had been rewarded with a sizable bonus for a 40 percent increase in production with the new machinery, attempted to keep his record production level by insisting that the machines be operated continuously and that the recommended maintenance schedules for them be ignored. After approximately six months, when the machines began to break down from overuse and neglect, the production manager was confronted by senior management to account for the sudden drop in production. His response was that the new machines were of inferior quality and constantly breaking down, making it impossible for him to continue his former high level of production. The consultant's assessment of the records clearly showed this not to be true. The production manager was replaced, and the consultant's firm received an apology from the consultees.

The consultant traced the third instance to strife between maintenance personnel and the machine operators. During his assessment, each department blamed the other for all production difficulties. Maintenance claimed the operators did not know how to operate the machines properly, and the operators accused maintenance of not following standard maintenance procedures or of taking too long to complete simple repairs. The consultant found some truth in both accusations, and spent most of his time at the site working with the plant manager and the supervisors of both groups to establish more cooperative work relations between the two departments. Once the relations between these two departments improved, production climbed to predicted levels.

These three incidents were resolved because the consultee accepted the consultant's findings and worked to correct on-site employee problems. However, in cases where the consultees refused to believe the consultant or where they could not resolve employee problems, the engineering consultant only had one recourse: pick up the phone and inform his firm that the machines were to be removed and reimbursement was in order. Needless to say, this practice is not cost-effective for either the consultee or the firm that the consultant represents.

Collaborative team consultation requires team ownership of the identified problem and the agreement that accountability for the success or failure of any innovative changes is to be shared. Consensus is both a process and a goal. The process requires all team members to listen to and respect what others on the team have to contribute, to look beyond the boundaries of their own specialty, and to blend their ideas with the ideas of the other specialists. Coordination and cooperation are crucial if consensus is to be reached.

Though the role of psychological consultants is not to act as group leaders, their knowledge and experience in group dynamics, group procedures, learning processes, defense mechanisms, and motivation of human behavior places them in a position to facilitate the cooperative efforts of the group, as well as to contribute to the solution of the problems being addressed. Working in a collaborative team consultation effort with members from diverse specialties can also be a stimulating experience for psychological consultants. It can stretch their perspectives, allowing them to apply their theories beyond their training, to gain new knowledge and skills from experts in a variety of disciplines, to learn about research not usually reported in their journals, and to be confronted with their strengths and weaknesses. In short, working in a collaborative team consultation setting can be an exciting and valuable learning experience.

SUMMARY

Several themes run throughout this chapter:

1. Of all the resources in business and industrial settings (for example, money, time, material, and people), people, or human resources, are the most important.
2. Work in today's business and industrial settings is progressively becoming more information intensive, and consequently, it requires employees possessing a high level of technological knowledge and skill.
3. Present knowledge and skills are likely to be outdated tomorrow; it is therefore necessary that business and industrial organizations provide continual opportunities and incentives for employees at all levels to upgrade their knowledge and skills.
4. Bureaucratic organizational structures and traditional management strategies, though effective in an industrial society, are far too cumbersome and inflexible to deal with the innovative changes necessary in a fast-paced, ever-changing information society.
5. New-generation business and industrial leaders, psychological consultants, and OD specialists are experimenting with innovative changes designed to meet present and anticipated challenges.
6. Unless psychological and OD consultants are willing and able to acquire the high-level technological knowledge and skills necessary to qualify as experts in human resource and organizational development, their future roles

in business and industrial settings will be severely limited. Innovative managers and management consultants, less qualified in human resource development, will quickly step in to fill the need.

Innovative business and industrial changes discussed in this chapter include downsizing or flattening the managerial hierarchy, temporary project or task teams, semi-autonomous work units, nontraditional compensation systems, continuing education and training programs and incentives, EAPs, HRPD programs, and collaborative team consultation.

GLOSSARY

Adhocracy   Defined by Waterman (1992) as "any form of organization that cuts across normal bureaucratic lines to capture opportunities, solve problems, and get results." In an adhocracy, "the boss" is defined as that individual who has the most knowledge and skills *at the moment*. In short, knowledge is granted authority at the time it is needed.

Chief executive officer (CEO)   The top executive officer, responsible to a board of directors or a board of trustees.

Collaborative team consultation   Consultation in which a variety of psychological, technological, and management specialists work together to resolve complex human resource problems or issues in order to facilitate organizational change.

Downsizing   A reduction of an organization's workforce as a method of coping with worsening economic conditions. The impact of downsizing is greatest for employees engaged in staff-oriented work or secondary production processes (staff as opposed to line positions).

Employee assistance programs (EAPs)   Designed originally to provide individual and group counseling to alcohol-abusing employees in business and industrial settings, many EAPs today offer a broad range of remedial and preventive counseling services to troubled employees. Counseling may, for example, pertain to substance abuse, marriage and family problems, career planning and placement, stress, termination, and retirement.

Employee stock options (ESOs)   Based on the premise that employees owning stock in the business or industry in which they are employed take greater interest in its success, some companies and industries have created employee stock option plans as an incentive. Once vested, employees become "financial partners," and the success of the company or industry is in their financial interest.

Gainsharing   An incentive based on key indicators, such as cost reduction, value added, profits produced, time saved, sales increased, services delivered, or receptivity to innovative changes.

Human resource planning and development (HRPD) programs   Any single definition of HRPD programs at this time would have to be so general as to be meaningless (for example, programs to enhance human resource management). First, no one program works in every business or industrial setting. Second, there are successful human resource systems at all stages of development. Third, human resource specialists and psychological consultants in business and industrial settings conceptualize their roles in HRPD programs in terms of an organization's specific needs (see **Organizational development**, below).

Lump-sum bonus plans   Set bonus figure awards for outstanding performance that benefits the company. A lump-sum bonus may be awarded to an individual or a team.

New-generation managers   Managers convinced that traditional hierarchical organizations and management strategies are no longer appropriate for today's conditions, and who are, therefore, breaking with tradition by experimenting with innovative organizational structures, a variety of work units, and continuing education and training programs.

Nontraditional compensation   Examples are gainsharing, pay-for-knowledge, lump-sum bonus plans, and employee stock options. Nontraditional compensation is offered to motivate and reward employees.

Organizational development (OD)   Today's businesses and industries are facing the necessity of radical changes in goals, systems, procedures, structure, strategies, jobs, and roles. These changes require better utilization of human resources, redesign of structures and procedures to facilitate communication flow and decisions, development of reward systems based on performance and motivation, increased involvement of lower-level employees in the decision-making process, and the creation of more humanistically oriented work settings. Psychological consultants who possess interest, knowledge, and competence in OD are in demand, particularly by organizations working toward sociotechnical system changes.

Pay-for-knowledge   A series of knowledge and skill modules to qualify employees for other positions. Completion of a new module adds an increment to the employee's salary base.

Project teams   Adaptive, problem-solving, temporary systems of diverse specialists working as a team to make change happen.

Semiautonomous work units   Often organized to reduce the complexity of managing product diversification in conglomerate organizations, ultimately creating change in both the structure and function of the organization. The establishment of semi-autonomous work units can lead to interunit conflict and confrontation if not handled properly.

Team systems   Systems including a variety of work teams, project teams, quality-control circles, and semiautonomous work units.

Work-unit teams   Teams (appointed by managers) whose responsibilities and objectives are clearly defined. Team members meet regularly with their managers to discuss team performance and develop action plans to improve productivity and raise quality levels.

ANNOTATED BIBLIOGRAPHY

Joseph Boyett's and Henry Conn's *Workplace 2000: The Revolution Reshaping American Business* (1992) is must reading for psychological consultants in business settings making the transition into the next decade. It is particularly critical for those involved in

HRPD. Not only do the writers present evidence of the need for change, they also tell the stories of model companies that have achieved world-class performance in quality, service, and innovation—companies that have demonstrated the way to an "American resurgence." While Boyett and Conn focus primarily on management, their projections and research findings are also highly relevant for the psychological consultant.

Although many writers recognize the importance of dealing with the resistance and reactance behaviors of consultees and staff (see Chapter 5), Fritz Steele is one of the few to study the facilitating and constraining influences of the physical, informational, and emotional properties of the consultant's work setting. In his book *Consulting for Organizational Change* (1975), Steele reports that choice of physical work settings can affect what can be accomplished by creating expectations and attitudes about what should normally be done in these settings. Choice of work locale can also trigger feelings, memories, and other reactions that influence people's moods when they are in the setting (p. 164). For example, there are occasions when holding a meeting with board members *away* from the boardroom can facilitate greater flexibility in the roles board members take. Conversely, when the purpose of the meeting is to gather information, meeting away from the work setting can be counterproductive. Steele warns consultants that, while expediency often dictates a meeting place, consultants must become more aware of how and by whom the choices of work settings are being made. According to him, consultants should consider how the impact of a physical setting may serve or hinder the purposes of the meeting, rather than simply accepting whatever setting is most convenient.

Douglas Bray and associates, in *Working with Organizations and Their People: A Guide to Human Resources Practice* (1991), offer their readers an excellent introduction to the variety and scope of the activities and agendas facing human resource specialists in business and industrial organizations. Not only do they emphasize how psychological consultants can apply the knowledge and skills of their specialty areas in HRPD, they also address the major areas of human resource practices (for example, the evaluation of individuals, their training and development, and OD). In addition, their book provides useful discussions of the key HRPD issues, and of the specialized training they believe necessary for current and future human resource practitioners, if these practitioners are to play a role in planning for changes in business and industrial settings.

Psychology in Organizations: Integrating Science and Practice, a book edited by Keven R. Murphy and Frank Saal (1990), is a good introduction for readers interested in applied psychology. Of particular interest to both current and future psychological consultants preparing for HRPD is Part 3, which deals with applications of psychology in predicting managerial potential, assessment centers, job performance measurement, and productivity measurement and enhancement. Also of interest is the final chapter, "Where Have We Been and Where Are We Going?", by Joseph M. Madden, a veteran psychological consultant with 45 years in the field. Madden makes an attempt "to put our current debate about the scientist practitioner model in I/O psychology into perspective."

Although written for psychiatrists, Peter Brill, Joseph Herzberg, and Jeffrey Lynn Speller's article "Employee Assistance Programs: An Overview and Suggested Roles for Psychiatrists" (1985) should prove both interesting and helpful to readers who wish to know more about EPAs in business and industry. They provide their readers with an overview of the need for, cost-effectiveness of, and current status of these programs.

Then, drawing on their own experiences, they present three broad categories of roles the psychiatrist can assume in such programs: clinician and supervisor, educator and administrator, and organizational consultant. They also discuss problems they have encountered in these roles.

Recognizing the difficulty American businesses and industries have in initiating and coping with change, Robert H. Waterman, Jr., a consultant and author, published *Adhocracy* in 1990 and updated it in 1993. **Adhocracy** focuses on the project team or task force as the ideal system "to cut across normal bureaucratic lines to capture opportunities, solve problems, and get results." Waterman states that he was inspired by and drew lessons from business and industrial organizations that responded quickly and with good affect to the need for change through well-managed adhocracy and the use of **project teams** (adaptive, problem-solving, temporary systems of diverse specialists working as a team to make change happen). Though addressed primarily to company executives, this book will also be a valuable resource for psychological and organizational consultants. You will find the case studies of specific companies both interesting and informative. Although successful project teams are emphasized, Waterman's discussions and comments also cover, in some depth, the risks involved and the problems encountered by both the organizations' executives and team leaders.

REFERENCES AND SUGGESTED READINGS

Alpin, J. C. (1985). Business realities and organizational consultation. *Counseling Psychologist, 13*(3), 396–402.

Andrade, K. M., & Ontiveros, S. R. (Eds.). (1986). *Organizational behavior: Contemporary viewpoints.* Santa Barbara, CA: ABC-Clio.

Axelson, J. A. (1985). *Counseling and development in a multicultural society.* Monterey, CA: Brooks/Cole.

Barcus, S. W., & Wilkinson, J. W. (Eds.). (1986). *Handbook of management consulting services.* New York: McGraw-Hill.

Baird, L., & Meshoulam, I. (1992, January/February). Getting payoff from investment in human resource management. *Business Horizons,* 68–75.

Boyett, J. H., & Conn, H. P. (1992). *Workplace 2000: The revolution reshaping American business.* New York: Plume.

Bradley, S. P., Hausman, J. A., & Nolan, R. L. (Eds.). (1993). *Globalization, technology, and competition: The fusion of computers and telecommunications in the 1990s.* Boston: Harvard Business School Press.

Bray, W. D., & Associates. (1991). *Working with organizations and their people: A guide to human resources practice.* New York: Guilford Press.

Brill, P., Herzberg, J., & Speller, J. L. (1985). Employee assistance programs: An overview and suggested roles for psychiatrists. *Hospital and Community Psychiatry, 36,* 727–732.

Brown, D., Pryzwansky, W. B., & Schulte, A. C. (1995). *Psychological consultation: Introduction to theory and practice* (3rd ed.). Boston: Allyn & Bacon.

Burrus, D., & Gittines, R. (1993). *Technotrends: How to use technology to go beyond your competition.* New York: HarperCollins.

Case, J. (Ed.). (1992). *From the ground up: The resurgence of American entrepreneurship.* New York: Simon & Schuster.

Clark, J. (Ed.). (1993). *Human resource management and technical change.* Newbury Park, CA: Sage.

Cochran, D. J. (1982). Organizational consultation: A planning group approach. *Personnel and Guidance Journal, 60,* 314–318.

Cohen, A. R., & Bradford, D. L. (1989). *Influence without authority.* New York: Wiley.

Conyne, R. K., & O'Neil, J. M. (Eds.). (1992). *Organizational consultation: A casebook.* Newbury Park, CA: Sage.

Curry, B. K. (1992). *Instituting enduring innovations: Achieving continuity of change in higher education* (ASHE-ERIC Higher Education Report No. 7). Washington, DC: George Washington University, School of Education and Human Development.

Davidow, W. H., & Malone, M. S. (1992). *The virtual corporation: Structuring and revitalizing for the 21st century.* New York: HarperCollins.

Davis, R. R. V. (1991, March/April). Using psychotherapy to deal with mental health problems in organizations. *Business Horizons,* 56–66.

Deal, T. E., & Kennedy, A. A. (1982). *Corporate cultures: The rights and rituals of corporate life.* Reading, MA: Addison-Wesley.

Dressel, P. L. (Ed.). (1971). *The new colleges: Toward an appraisal.* Iowa City, IA: American College Testing Program.

Drucker, P. F. (1985a). *Management: Tasks, responsibilities, practices* (2nd ed.). New York: Harper Colophon Books.

Drucker, P. F. (1985b). *Managing for results: Economic tasks and risk-taking decisions.* New York: Harper & Row.

Gerstein, L. H., & Sturmer, L. H. (1993, November/December). A Taoist paradigm of EAP consultation. *Journal of Counseling and Development, 72,* 178–184.

Harrison, M. I. (1987). *Diagnosing organizations: Methods, models, and processes* (Applied Social Research Methods Series No. 8). Newbury Park, CA: Sage.

Hersey, P., & Blancard, K. H. (1993). *Management of organizational behavior: Utilizing human resources* (5th ed.). Englewood Cliffs, NJ: Prentice-Hall.

Hollway, W. (1991). *Work psychology and organizational behavior: Managing the individual at work.* Newbury Park, CA: Sage.

Holman, R., & Zasloff, M. (1983, Winter). Providing consultation to corporate employee assistance programs: The time is right. *Consultation,* 19–24, 26–27.

Holtz, H. (1990). *How to succeed as an independent consultant* (2nd ed.). New York: Wiley.

Huse, E. R. (1982). *Management* (2nd ed.). St. Paul, MN: West.

Kelley, R. E. (1981). *Consulting: The complete guide to a profitable career.* New York: Charles Scribner's Sons.

Kotter, J. P., & Heskett, J. L. (1992). *Corporate cultures and performance.* New York: Free Press.

Landy, F. J. (1985). *Psychology of work behavior* (3rd ed.). Homewood, IL: Dorsey Press.

Likert, R. L. (1962). *The human organization: Its management and value.* New York: McGraw-Hill.

Martin, W. B. (1971). Thoughts on evaluation and imagination. In P. L. Dressel (Ed.), *The new colleges: Toward an appraisal.* Iowa City, IA: American College Testing Program.

Montana, P., & Charnov, B. (1987). *Management.* New York: Barron's Educational Series.

Murphy, K. R., & Saal, F. E. (Eds.). (1990). *Psychology in organizations: Integrating science and practice.* Hillsdale, NJ: Erlbaum.

Naisbitt, J., & Aburdene, P. (1990). *Megatrends 2000: Ten new directions for the 1990s.* New York: Avon Books.

North, D. C. (1990). *Institutions, institutional change, and economic performance.* New York: Cambridge University Press.

Peter, L. J. (1973). *The Peter plan: A proposal for survival.* New York: Morrow.

Pugh, D. S. (Ed.). (1984). *Organization theory: Selected readings* (2nd ed.). Harmondsworth, Middlesex, England: Penguin Books.

Rowan, R. (1986). *The intuitive manager.* Boston: Little, Brown.

Sackman, S. A. (1991). *Cultural knowledge in organizations: Exploring the collective mind.* Newbury Park, CA: Sage.

Schein, E. H. (Ed.). (1987). *The art of managing human resources.* New York: Oxford University Press.

Steele, F. (1975). *Consulting for organizational change.* Amherst: University of Massachusetts Press.

Sweeny, A., & Wisner, J., Jr. (1975). *Budgeting fundamentals for nonfinancial executives and managers.* New York: McGraw-Hill.

Tepper, R. (1985). *Become a top consultant: How the experts do it.* New York: Wiley.

Toomer, J. E. (1982). Counseling psychologists in business and industry. *Counseling Psychologist, 10*(3), 9–18.

Tuller, L. W. (1992). *Cutting edge consultants: Succeeding in today's explosive markets.* Englewood Cliffs, NJ: Prentice-Hall.

Waterman, R. H., Jr. (1992). *Adhocracy.* New York: Norton.

Yeager, J., & Raudsepp, E. (1980, July). Power and organizational politics. *Management Guidelines, 199,* 201, 203–204, 206, 208, 211.

Zare, M. (1990, May/June). The EAP and organizational development: Exploring new territory. *EAP Digest,* 27–30, 50–56.

❖ PART THREE

Issues and Concepts

Like the earlier parts of the book, Part III reflects our commitment to providing practical and useful information. Two chapters—Chapters 10 and 11—comprise Part III. The common theme that bridges these chapters is the emphasis on special issues that consultants often encounter in the diverse settings in which they work. At some point, almost all consultants will confront unique dynamics that force them to respond with more than convenient or routine strategies. Perplexing problems, unforeseen dynamics, and unusual circumstances require consultants to have a comprehensive knowledge base. They must delve deeply into their reservoir of insights and abilities in meeting the demands of consultation assignments. Part III delivers on our promise to discuss several of the issues that consultants most need to understand.

CHAPTER TEN

Special Consultation Applications

Chapter 10 examines special consultation interventions and techniques required by problems across diverse work settings. We have included a chapter on these topics because consultants are often asked to provide interventions directly rather than encouraging consultees to do so. Further, most consultants are aware that they must develop a broad repertoire of intervention skills and behavioral strategies to increase their effectiveness and employability. Therefore, Chapter 10 addresses special applications and related processes with respect to three consultation interventions: training, conflict resolution, and team building. Though the chapter discusses the theory and dynamics of the three interventions, it emphasizes application—clear direction on what the psychological consultant must do to develop and deliver training programs, resolve individual and group conflicts, and organize and lead a team approach to problem solving or task completion.

CHAPTER ELEVEN

Ethical and Legal Dilemmas in Consultation

Like other psychological professionals, consultants face numerous ethical and legal questions as they work with individuals, groups, and organizations. Yet no separate professional organization exists to help psychological consultants with these issues, nor is there a code of ethics written specifically for them. To complicate this deficiency, consultants who are members of professional associations find that their specialty areas often require ethical practices that do not apply to the consultation framework. Confidentiality guidelines for psychological specialists who pursue therapy assignments, for example, appear relatively clear, while the same guidelines offer little information about privacy matters in consultation. Further, ethical codes written specifically for psychologists, counselors, and social workers explain ethical issues as they relate to diadic, rather than triadic, professional relationships. Add the inconsistent laws of the various states and territories, conflicting court interpretations, and different ethical rules across the psychological professions, and it is apparent that psychological consultants often face ethical or legal situations for which they are unprepared. Chapter 11 offers a comprehensive analysis of the ethical and legal dilemmas that psychological consultants must consider in their work. The chapter also introduces the ethical issues of marketing statements, consultee identification, individual versus organizational needs and rights, parameters of confidentiality, role conflicts and dual relationships, assessment and data utilization, research and evaluation, and evaluating and reporting violations. Methods of preventing ethical and legal dilemmas are also discussed.

◆ CHAPTER TEN

Special Consultation Applications

Chapter Overview

Training
  Trainer Roles
  Preparing for Training
    Assessing Training Needs
    The Training Proposal
    Matching Training to Participants' Learning Needs
  Experiential Approaches in Training
  An Orientation to Training Evaluation

Conflict Resolution
  An Emerging View of Conflict
  Causes of Conflict
  Conflict Resolution Methods and Models
    Compromise Versus the "Win-Win" Approach
    Conflict Resolution Processes

Team Building
  Defining the Team-Building Process
  Dimensions of Team Functioning
  Team-Building Processes
    Relationship Building
    Assessment
    Diagnosis
    Feedback/Education
    Implementation

Summary

Glossary

Annotated Bibliography

References and Suggested Readings

 As consultants enter diverse settings to help consultees with organizational or human system problems, they encounter an array of special problems, needs, and characteristics. This reality, and the trend that modern consultants are often asked by consultees to provide specialized interventions they themselves are unable to create, requires consultants to plan and implement a broad spectrum of interventions. The ability to respond positively to such requests, indeed, enhances consultants' effectiveness and employability. Regrettably for many consultants, however, formal training programs rarely expose students and future consultants to an in-depth knowledge base that includes the specialized interventions and techniques they need. As a result, consultants often confront problems that require interventions they are unable to provide.

Chapter 10 introduces readers to three special consultation applications and related processes: training, conflict resolution, and team building. We have included these applications in the chapter because of the widespread interest of consultees in such interventions and because we assume that novice consultants may not have acquired an orientation otherwise. You should be aware, however, that the special applications presented here are not synonymous with consultation in the strictest sense. Rather, each application should be implemented during the intervention stage of consultation and is only one important part of the consultation process. Implicit in the discussion, then, is the assumption that training, conflict resolution, and team building applications address consultation problems as part of the broader framework of consultation. They are preceded and followed by other supportive stages.

Training

The phenomenal push for quality is evident in all sorts of organizations, programs, and human systems as they strive to excel, to satisfy performance standards, and to outproduce organizational rivals. Leaders in human service, corporate, governmental, and even familial settings recognize that the enhancement of organizational members' competencies has a direct bearing on their pursuit of excellence. Thus, the attention paid by modern organizations to training and development activities has accelerated dramatically (Cosier & Dalton, 1993). **Training**, often delivered in a workshop format, involves the application of educational and experientially based interventions that help consultation constituents acquire new information, technologies, or competencies. Whether the purpose is to impart knowledge, alter behaviors and attitudes, or enhance skills, training in its various forms permeates every level of modern organizations. Indeed, some authors have described training as one of the most prevalent consultation roles (Gallessich, 1982). As trainers, consultants provide information, plan or direct participant learning, and implement sequential learning activities designed to achieve training goals.

Trainer Roles

Developing and implementing training programs entails delicate, often complex processes, and to meet the needs of participants, trainers are required to assume multiple roles. These roles fluctuate according to the needs of participants, the objectives of the training program, and the dynamics of the consultation setting. Moreover, though consultants may assume a dominant role in a particular training program, they often assume various subroles as well. A few common trainer roles include:

1. *Information expert*   The trainer is an information expert when vast amounts of technical or specialized information must be conveyed, training content is intricate or confusing, interactive learning is impractical, or training time is insufficient. These roles require the trainer to present information in didactic form as a lecturer or public speaker. A psychiatrist who instructs trainees about the chemical ingredients of a new experimental drug for treating depression serves as an information expert trainer.

2. *Facilitator*   The trainer assumes a facilitator role when trainees are in smaller groups and participants must solve specified problems as the central goal of training exercises (Nilson, 1989). Facilitators "begin with information regarding the situation or the problem and the participants; however, the outcome or resolution is not set when the facilitator begins" (Killion & Simmons, 1992, p. 3). Facilitation therefore focuses less on imparting information and more on experiential learning in which participants acquire skills and make decisions. Killion and Simmons (1992) advise that "asking questions and listening are the primary functions of an effective facilitator. These replace giving answers, assuming the group's needs, or providing solutions" (p. 4). The trainer is a facilitator, for example, in a management group charged with formulating its organizational mission statement.

3. *Group process observer/analyst*   Small-group training programs that emphasize experiential learning and feedback require participants to expose their characteristics, values, and personalities. Trainers must observe such groups, assess group processes, and evaluate the group's progress. When groups are poorly mixed, experience conflict, or become disinterested, the trainer recognizes these dynamics and takes appropriate action. For example, the trainer is a group process observer and analyst when a training program relies on observation and feedback to improve group communication or teamwork skills.

4. *Leadership*   The trainer fulfills a leadership role when members of an instructional group share identical goals and move through the training process together. A group trainer-leader is an authority who sets the pace of learning, establishes the agenda, and monitors the group's progress. The trainer is a leader in a group of parents who move through a parent education class in order to receive certification as child care workers.

5. *Planner/organizer*   Effective training programs depend on conscientious planning and organization. Thoughtful planning allows the trainer to take into account the

dynamics and logistical considerations associated with participant needs and character-istics. Further, matching training programs to participants' needs requires considerable pretraining planning and assessment.

6. *Motivator* Some training programs are designed to motivate and stimulate participants toward improved, and at times, inspired performance. Sustaining or im-proving trainees' motivation demands that trainers stimulate the group's interest and at-tention. Motivational training requires trainers to mix humor, examples, stories, and inspirational illustrations. For example, the trainer serves a motivating role in a training program for sales staff of a large medical supply company with gradually declining sales figures.

Preparing for Training

Successful training programs require proactive planning and organization. Hudson (1973) agrees: "Most of the failures and errors that are made in training can be traced back to action without thought" (p. 33). Too often, trainer-consultants flaw training through haphazard planning, rushed interventions, or unfounded methodologies. Inept or superficial training, however, is the inadvertent by-product of negligence on the part of both consultants and consultees. Consultant-trainers, for instance, often apply re-peated or favored training programs without considering their relevance to participants' needs. Trainers also commit a serious error when they formulate training goals through a noncollaborative or isolated planning process. Consultees contribute to poor training ventures by requesting programs that have little relevance and foundation or allow con-sultants to dictate training content without the benefits of collaboration or dialogue. Trainers, therefore, must adopt a framework that incorporates an ensemble of pretrain-ing responsibilities.

Assessing Training Needs Since training interventions should closely match consultation problems and needs, assessing participants' needs is an integral pretraining task. The basis of this process is a period of pretraining collaboration in which trainers and consultees plan the training intervention. Although assessment methods are often costly and time consuming, valid assessment information prevents wasted or unfounded training interventions. A popular method of assessing participant needs is the partici-pant survey method (see Box 10.1).

Survey methods require consultants to access participants prior to training pro-grams, and when access is limited, survey methods can be impractical. An alternative method, and perhaps a minimal assessment activity, consists of professional dialogue between consultants, consultees, and participants. Trainers should seek the answers to several pretraining questions:

- What needs or problems prompt the interest in training?
- What is the consultee's assessment of training needs?
- How many participants are expected?
- What are the trainees' job responsibilities?

Box 10.1
Sample survey form to assess trainee needs

Training Questionnaire

Name (optional) _____ **Job title** _____

Description of job duties _____
_____
_____
_____
_____

Directions: Your organization is interested in providing a training program, and you can help by completing this form. Your training interests and needs are important to the design and content of the training program. Please rate each skill area below according to your needs for information and skill-building opportunities. Thank you.

Skill Area	No Interest				High Interest
1. Beginning a session	1	2	3	4	5
2. Body language	1	2	3	4	5
3. Eye contact	1	2	3	4	5
4. Empathy	1	2	3	4	5
5. Voice tone	1	2	3	4	5
6. Active listening	1	2	3	4	5
7. Using silence	1	2	3	4	5
8. Questioning	1	2	3	4	5
9. Using humor	1	2	3	4	5
10. Managing resistance	1	2	3	4	5
11. Keeping records	1	2	3	4	5
12. Scheduling	1	2	3	4	5

- What are the present trainee competencies relative to the proposed training information?
- What relevant characteristics (age, gender, training background, learning styles) do trainees bring to the training intervention?
- What are the trainees' views or attitudes about training, particularly about the training topic?
- What training have trainees received early?

Some training needs emerge as needed interventions during the broader process of organizational consultation. Through organizational assessment and diagnosis practices, consultants often discover that knowledge or skill deficits contribute to organizational weaknesses (Harrison, 1987). Though consultants in such cases have not anticipated the need for training, assessment discoveries point to skill or knowledge deficits as organizational problems. Consultants often propose training applications as solutions to organizational deficits. Specific training needs, then, can be determined through the assessment processes that characterize consultation (see Chapter 2).

The Training Proposal   Trainers often devise written proposals that assist consultees in trainer selection and program planning. The **training proposal** serves as a planning document that presents the consultant's credentials and training plans (Holtz, 1993). Although the length and detail of training proposals vary according to the dynamics of each training project (Holtz, 1993), most proposals include the (1) consultant's credentials and experiences, (2) purpose of the training program, (3) design of the training program, (4) training schedules and time frames, and (5) logistical arrangements. A brief training proposal (fictitious example) is included in Exhibit 10.1.

1. *Consultant credentials*   Of necessity, consultees are interested in the consultant-trainer's professional qualifications, formal training background, and consultation experiences. Such data provide a documented and visible record that facilitates a correct match between the consultee's training needs and the consultant's professional characteristics. Psychological consultants must adhere strictly to ethical principles when documenting descriptions of professional competencies and characteristics (see Chapter 11).

2. *Rationale*   Training proposals include a statement of purpose or rationale that elucidates the need for training. The written proposal reflects the consultant's understanding of consultation problems and any assessment data that have been synthesized or categorized. From the rationale statement, the consultee evaluates the trainer's assessment and understanding of training needs.

3. *Training design*   The **training design** is a brief account of how the training intervention is to occur; that is, it identifies the training program's methods and desired results. The training design is a planning draft that ensures that the training intervention is specially tailored to the consultee's setting and problem. Even polished, sophisticated trainers risk unsuccessful training when they fail to design properly matched training content and methodologies.

4. *Schedule*   Training programs occur in a myriad of time frames—hours, days, or weeks. A principal consideration is the expediency with which training programs are delivered; that is, to be cost-effective, training must be delivered efficiently enough that the benefits outweigh the losses associated with the trainees' time away from routine work activities. Further, training programs must be scheduled in convenient time frames that avoid unnecessary intrusions or disruptions.

5. *Logistical arrangements*   Training interventions often entail a range of logistical issues and arrangements. Clarification of such matters prior to training prevents

**Training Proposal
for
XYZ Child Development, Inc.**

Trainer Credentials and Experience: Consultant X is an experienced trainer and consultant. She holds professional licenses in counseling and psychology and has acquired a doctoral degree in the counseling psychology field. X has served as a trainer for organizations, human service agencies, residential programs, and child development programs for 15 years. References are available on request.

Purpose of the Training: XYZ Child Development, Inc. has decided to integrate an affective education component into its educational curriculum serving three- and four-year-old children. Its teaching staff has indicated an interest in learning about affective education and various instructional techniques and exercises. Moreover, the administrative staff reports that annual program reviews cite the lack of affective education curricular components as an area needing more attention and depth in the program.

Design of the Training Program: The proposed training program consists of a one-day training session blending lecture and experiential activities. XYZ staff will have the opportunity to observe demonstrations and role-playing activities designed to illustrate affective education techniques. In addition, participants will view videotapes, rehearse learning, and review written material. Of particular importance is the emphasis on the application of information to the specific needs and questions of XYZ staff.

Schedules and Time Frames: The proposed training program should be scheduled during the late summer months, prior to the beginning of the agency's fall classes. It is recommended that the program be offered as a preservice training activity. The proposed training program should begin at 9:00 A.M. and conclude at 4:00 P.M. with one hour for lunch. The days available are August 25, 27, and 30 of this year.

Logistical Arrangements: A meeting room to accommodate 20 participants is required. The training setting should be comfortable, with seating arranged in a conference style, although individual chairs should be portable. The workshop will require an overhead projector, screen, flip chart, videocassette recorder, and monitor to be supplied by the XYZ Agency. Handouts will be included and supplied by the trainer. A fee of $300 includes all materials, travel costs, meals, and other expenses.

Exhibit 10.1
Sample training proposal (fictitious)

confusion or inappropriate arrangements. Consultants should include logistical information that appears essential to training planning and implementation (for example, information about fees, required media equipment or materials, copying, and training space).

Matching Training to Participants' Learning Needs   A training program accomplishes little when trainees are unable to comprehend and relate to its content. Too often, trainers plan training programs so impulsively that they overlook participants' needs. The **learning styles** (a unique blend of receiving, processing, and responding to information) of participants represents one factor that should receive careful analysis. As they structure the training curriculum or outline, for example, trainers should consider the pace, sequence, and communication characteristics of training.

The *pace* of training refers to the rate and progression that characterize the training session's content and activities. Training programs that move too quickly can exhaust participants' attention and energy, and those paced too slowly can be exhausting and unstimulating. Anticipating the training pace points to the importance of pretraining planning and the consultant's familiarity with participants. Although deciding the correct pace is a subjective process, the trainer, through theoretical and intuitive reasoning, should prepare for participants' special learning needs. Tailoring the pace of training programs, for instance, to participants' educational or occupational status, previous training experiences, backgrounds, learning styles, and individual characteristics, is essential to successful training.

Sequence refers to the ordering of training information according to complexity. For example, consider the training program that instructs mental health technicians on the dynamics and processes of empathic understanding. The sequence is ill-planned should the trainer begin a section on the complex skills of advanced empathy before teaching the concept of basic empathy. Silberman (1990) advises trainers to adhere to several basic sequencing principles:

1. Build interest and introduce new content before you delve more deeply.
2. Have demanding activities follow easy activities.
3. Maintain a good mix of activities.
4. Teach easier concepts before teaching more difficult ones.
5. Provide sub-skills before practicing complex skills.
6. Close training sequences with a discussion of "so what." (p. 141)

Since each individual possesses a unique way of receiving, processing, and responding to information, trainers must be alert to how they communicate information. Experts in business, communication, and the behavioral sciences have increasingly recognized that when individuals pay attention to information external to them, they perceive through visual, auditory, or kinesthetic mechanisms. The effective transference of information from trainer to learner occurs when training material is presented in ways that match an individual learner's preferred modality for perceiving information (Eicher, 1987). The trainee who prefers learning through auditory, step-by-step instructions, for example, will have difficulty relating to training exercises that rely on visual modalities.

Experiential Approaches in Training

An **experiential** training program emphasizes a "learning-by-doing" format in which participants have opportunities for interaction, rehearsal, and participation. Experiential approaches emphasize the intrinsic sense of accomplishment and involvement participants feel, and indeed, add to their stimulation and involvement. Johnson and Johnson (1991), alluding to the work of Kurt Lewin, point out that "people will believe more in knowledge they have discovered themselves than in knowledge presented by others" (p. 42). Although experiential approaches are useful tools, their implementation must be viewed with caution; that is, some methods can be intimidating for participants who prefer passive or listening roles. Some experiential methods (such as role playing and demonstration) require risk-taking behaviors that exceed participants' readiness for participation. Nevertheless, with careful planning, experiential methods promote success in training, and for the trainer's benefit, several methods are available:

1. *Processing*   **Processing** is a practice that allows participants to clarify, interpret, and analyze their experience. Following training demonstrations or exercises, the trainer's attention is turned to participant questions and dialogue. Through critical reasoning, participants express their reactions, clarify confusing issues, or volunteer information.

2. *Role playing*   **Role playing** is a common experiential training activity where participants, in groups of two or more, "can experience concretely the type of interaction under examination" in training (Johnson & Johnson, 1991, p. 47). Role-playing exercises can address real or hypothetical situations, can utilize spontaneous interactions or prepared scripts, and can be completed in groups in which two participants perform their roles for neutral observers.

3. *Rehearsal*   **Rehearsal** can be a practical and powerful experiential exercise in training programs targeting specific relational or behavioral skills (for instance, assertiveness, interpersonal conflict resolution, active listening, and empathy training). Rehearsal activities can be observed by trainers and participants with opportunities for processing and feedback. When the setting, format, and technology allow, rehearsal exercises can be videotaped and feedback provided during playback.

4. *Simulation*   The purpose of **simulation** is to involve trainees in realistic situations matched to actual job situations (Spitzer, 1986). The provision of work samples—real examples of trainees' job tasks—is a simulation activity where trainees perform with supervision and feedback. Simulated experiences have alternative purposes. They can be useful as icebreaking exercises to ease tension and increase participant comfort. Games or exercises include fun and entertaining qualities that add to group cohesion. In addition, simulated experiences at the close of training programs are useful to assess instructional gains (Silberman, 1990).

5. *Demonstration*   Trainers can teach skills, processes, and concepts through overt **demonstration** or modeling of desired behaviors (for example, assertiveness training, empathy training). Especially useful in training programs that emphasize behavioral goals, the experiential benefits of demonstration are strengthened when participants themselves model existing or newly acquired competencies and time is provided for processing and feedback.

6. *Subgroups* **Subgroups** are helpful when the training audience is large or fore-boding and the trainer wishes to add an experiential element. Smaller groups give participants opportunities for interaction, disclosure, and input as they address specific tasks that require group decision making and problem solving.

An Orientation to Training Evaluation

Evaluation as it relates to training entails systematic processes that determine the worth of training. Davidove and Schroeder (1992) point out that "tracking the return on a training investment can be time-consuming, but it's more important now than ever" (p. 70). Regrettably, too many trainers ignore this imperative. Many perceive training programs as brief, time-limited interventions that have few far-reaching effects. Others have insufficient time to implement training evaluation procedures. Still others are unclear about valid and reliable evaluation methods or are intimidated by the technical implications of evaluation processes.

Hartley (1973) proposes that training evaluation should consider two primary purposes. First, trainers and consultees must consider the impact a training program has on participants' organizational environment. Has the training resulted in increased skill or knowledge? Are new skills applicable? Has the training intervention resulted in increased performance? What is the status of the organization's efficiency relative to the training intervention? Second, evaluating the effects of training provides data and feedback that allow the trainer to assess the training process, its techniques, and the trainer's role.

Trainers should design training interventions with close consideration of the importance of evaluation. Keeping the following points in mind can be helpful:

1. *Ongoing evaluation* A training evaluation plan should be integrated into the overall training design, rather than attached to the termination point of training as a peripheral activity. Evaluation built into the training plan should be "undertaken before, during, and after a training program" (Phillips, 1991, p. 62). Such integrated evaluation tactics guide the training content and methods, include training objectives and content that match evaluation methods, and occur, as needed, during various phases (for example, pre- and posttest evaluation designs).
2. *Results-oriented training* A training program is likely to have an impact on participants when it is fine-tuned to produce desirable and recognizable outcomes (Robinson & Robinson, 1989). Indeed, the training design is a direct product of the trainer's anticipation of desired results.
3. *Evaluation from multiple sources* Since individuals, groups, and organizations can feel the impact of a training program, evaluation practices should target feedback from multiple sources. Participants provide immediate feedback about the relevance and usefulness of the training process, consultees evaluate training programs by comparing outcomes with work-related needs and goals, and trainers reflect introspectively on their performance and training design to assess their methods and decisions.
4. *More than a "one-shot" activity* Training programs are wasteful, at least partially, when they are conducted as separate or isolated activities that have little

connection to the expected job performance of training participants (Robinson & Robinson, 1989). In contrast, training interventions should reflect a futuristic, problem-solving purpose. Indeed, a valid measure of the success of a training program is its impact on trainees' future behavior and problem-solving efficacy.

In summary, training programs are popular consultation interventions. As consultants, psychological specialists must address organizational problems that will likely continue unless skill and knowledge deficits are corrected. Upgrading the competencies of organizational members becomes the central task of the overall consultation process. We have demonstrated in this section that successful training requires assessment and preparation rather than hasty implementation.

Conflict Resolution

As consultants apply their skills within a diverse range of work settings and organizations, they discover that individuality and interpersonal differences often contribute to the problems they have been asked to address. Indeed, some consultation problems stem directly from the unsuccessful blending of human values and traits, and for many individuals, interpersonal conflict is the inevitable result (Jandt & Gillette, 1985). Human **conflicts** occur anywhere disagreement exists between or among people. Although occasional conflicts are common, they become disturbing when they escalate into frightening confrontations, harsh dialogue, and weakened work and personal performance.

When conflicts escalate beyond the competencies of managers or administrators, third-party consultants are often asked to help. **Third-party consultation** requires experienced and knowledgeable consultants who help consultees resolve significant, lingering conflicts. Consultants engage in a process of **conflict resolution**—the application of planned and organized principles that constructively manage or end conflicts and enrich interpersonal relationships. Gordon (1991) describes the role of the conflict resolution consultant:

> Third parties must demonstrate professional expertise and control of the social processes used, control over the situation at hand, moderate knowledge of the principles, issues, and background factors, and neutrality or imbalance with respect to substantive outcomes, personal relationships, and conflict resolution methodology. (p. 486)

An Emerging View of Conflict

Although to many individuals conflict "signals contention, dissatisfaction, and potential disruption" (Kolb, 1992, p. 66), modern conflict resolution models reflect a positive, accepting view. That is, while conflicts challenge the relational strength of those in families, social groups, and organizations, they also present opportunities for growth, creativity, and interpersonal problem solving (Fisher, Ury, & Patton, 1991; Jandt & Gillette, 1985; McFarland, 1992; Tjosvold, 1991). Indeed, the consequences of conflict are often "double-edged," depending on how conflict is addressed and resolved (Tjosvold, 1991, p. 1). Box 10.2 illustrates the two-sided character of human conflict.

Box 10.2
Two-sided character of human conflict

Positive Potential	Negative Potential
Establishes trust	Creates mistrust
Resolves problems	Magnifies problems
Heightens morale	Leads to demoralization
Leads to identification of problems	Obscures problems
Improves quality of relationships	Impairs quality of relationships
Mediates differences	Causes differences to escalate
Improves communication	Stifles communication
Enhances creativity	Produces stagnation

Causes of Conflict

Conflicts can range from simple differences of opinion to major confrontations. Although conflicts come in many forms, show varying intensities, and appear to have multiple contributing factors, their etiologies can usually be traced to a few broad sources:

1. *Conflict caused by psychological factors*   Psychological factors that cause conflicts include the personal and relational qualities (feelings, self-esteem, perceptions, values, and needs) that, in turn, lead to differences in thinking and understanding (Lederach, 1987). Indeed, it is difficult to conceive of any conflict situation where psychological factors do not contribute in an integral way.
2. *Conflict caused by miscommunication*   Ineffective interpersonal communication can lead to vague interactions, misperceptions, unintended messages, and eventually, conflict. Miscommunication can contribute to the imbalance in relationships that results when one party perceives the other party inaccurately. Any reasonable attempt to understand conflict should consider the messages that reflect the differences between or among those involved (Fahs, 1982).
3. *Conflict caused by arbitrary decisions or solutions*   Decisions and solutions often set work standards, establish policies, and result in advantages for some and disadvantages for others. When one party feels that personal needs or interests have been ignored, or that the decision-making process has been hasty, unclear, or exclusive, conflict is the likely consequence (Kraybill, 1987). Further, highly authoritarian decisions and solutions that coerce others into compliance lay the groundwork for significant conflict.
4. *Conflict caused by competitive interests*   In conflict situations, vested interests and values are often at stake. Writing about the structural elements of social conflict, Himes (1980) emphasizes that "in conflict the contending parties struggle for status, power, scarce resources, and other values. Structurally inherent

potential for conflict is heightened when one party believes that access to such values is blocked by the other party" (p. 39).

5. *Conflict caused by a power imbalance*   The misuse of power in interpersonal relationships and organizations can be a continual source of conflict. As people seek to be heard and to have an influence on their surroundings, others often oppose or block their interests altogether. When individuals sense that their ability or opportunity to influence their environment is threatened, conflict results (Kraybill, 1987). Power in relationships represents an interesting paradox: The more power one strives to exert, the greater the resistance by others.

Conflict Resolution Methods and Models

Consultants rely on a mix of processes and strategies as they approach conflict resolution assignments. They recognize that situations vary from setting to setting and that a range of competencies and tactics can be helpful. Numerous conflict resolution processes and models are available to guide the consultant's actions.

Compromise Versus the "Win-Win" Approach   Compromise has long been acclaimed as an effective way to resolve conflicts. While **compromises** often provide quick solutions, their efficacy is perhaps overstated. As Cohen (1980) points out, "By its very definition, compromise results in an agreement in which each side gives up something it really wanted. It is an outcome where no one fully meets his or her needs" (p. 197). Compromise requires opposing parties to agree to terms somewhere in the middle of their two positions. As an illustration, consider how compromise is used to resolve the conflict presented in Box 10.3.

Following a long period of heated debate, harsh accusations, and complaining, Worker X and Worker Y in the example featured in Box 10.3 eventually decide on a compromise. They agree to purchase a partition seven feet high to allow more privacy to Worker X and some openness to Worker Y. With this compromise, the conflict appears resolved. However, a closer examination of the compromise reveals several restrictive features. For example, the solution requires a partition that provides only minimal privacy for Worker X and diminished openness for Worker Y. Neither is fully content with the new height of the partition, and it is likely that the damage incurred by their superficial compromise will continue, making future conflict highly probable.

Conflicts can be resolved so that both parties achieve everything they want (Fisher, Ury, & Patton, 1991; Jandt & Gillette, 1985). Mutual satisfaction of both parties and a focus on the maintenance of harmonious relationships are integral by-products of collaborative "win-win" conflict resolution strategies. **Win-win solutions** reflect the belief that a creative settlement exists for each conflict, that conflict outcomes meet the needs of each party, and that all parties benefit.

Once again, consider the example of the two feuding workers in Box 10.3. An alternative to a settlement where both parties remain dissatisfied or their needs are not fully met is the win-win solution. If they think creatively and collaboratively, Worker X and Worker Y could agree to focus more on the problem and less on personal differences. If they integrated win-win thinking into the problem-solving process, they could

Box 10.3
Case example: Feuding workers

Two coworkers, Worker X and Worker Y, are involved in an ongoing conflict about the height of a partition separating their workstations in the clerical office of a small company. Their workstations are side by side, and they share a common partition. Worker X desires the partition to extend from floor to ceiling for greater privacy, while Worker Y prefers the openness of a five-foot-high partition. The conflict has evolved into significant performance problems for both workers, and their more frequent outbursts are disturbing to the morale of other employees. The owner of the company has requested that the two feuding workers resolve their dispute soon or face serious job action.

generate various creative solutions. For example, it is feasible for one of the workers to exchange office space with another worker who has compatible privacy interests. Or perhaps the two workers could request a specially constructed acoustical partition that gives Worker X greater privacy and Worker Y the desired openness. A third win-win alternative may be the installation of a translucent partition that allows privacy as well as openness. Whatever the final arrangement, the critical feature of win-win solutions is that the parties reach a settlement in which each wins while sacrificing little or nothing.

Models   Because conflict resolution can be a tedious, emotionally laden process, consultants should rely on established intervention processes rather than highly reactant or purely intuitive methods. To their advantage, the conflict resolution field is replete with alternative methods and models, and the consultant's assessment of conflict situations should determine the best approach. Conflicts may be widespread throughout organizations or occur as ongoing differences between various work units or groups within an organization. Some conflicts may be small in scale, limited to a few individuals. Regardless of the setting and scope of conflicts, consultants should be experts at conflict resolution.

Widespread *organizational conflict* occurs when conflict exists at multiple organizational levels, among large numbers of people, or cannot be isolated to small groups or a few individuals. Ignored or tolerated, such conflicts are potentially costly to the organization at several levels. As Tjosvold (1991) observes, "Uncontrolled conflict rips apart relationships, sabotages collective work, and devastates people" (p. 3). Ironically, avoiding open discussions of conflict often accentuates the problem.

Organizational leaders must acknowledge the presence of disturbing or uncontrolled conflict rather than disavow its presence. Tjosvold (1991) proposes a model of conflict resolution that encourages organizations to invite and appreciate conflicts. The "conflict-positive" organization cultivates an open, inviting climate in which managers, supervisors, and employees view conflict situations as opportunities for positive and creative outcomes (p. 8). Through experience and leadership, the organization molds its policies and procedures to the inevitable truth that human conflict is a persistent and common aspect of organizational life. The conflict-positive organization encourages freedom of expression, airing of differences, and win-win solutions. Through a mixture of "tough" policies that require confrontation and problem settlement, and "soft" policies that entail sensitivity and trust, positive organizational leaders display their determination to deal with conflict (Tjosvold, 1991, p. 13).

Tjosvold (1991) describes four measures organizations can take to become conflict-positive. First, the culture of the organization should adopt the view that conflict is a positive experience. Managers and employees should perceive the experience of conflict as healthy and productive. Second, managers and employees, through purposeful study and experience, should increase their knowledge and understanding of conflict and resolution processes. The third step requires a collaborative approach to conflict resolution. That is, managers and employees should appreciate their differences, develop mutual goals, empower one another, and assess their progress. Fourth, organizational managers and employees should seek affirmation of conflict-positive views throughout the organization. If conflict-positive strategies are to work, they should be reflected throughout the organization and at each level.

As groups vie for attention, pride, resources, or recognition, rivalries naturally emerge. Maintaining a "competitive edge" is not only acceptable in organizations, it is a prerequisite to successful futures (Blake & Mouton, 1984, p. ix). As organizations compete, so too do groups or work units within organizations. Specialization and the need to arrange people into functional, separate units are dynamics common to modern organization structures. Such units often evolve into high-achieving teams capable of phenomenal performance. Unfortunately, as members identify more with their team than with the surrounding organization, competition and rivalry emerge. Occasionally, team competition evolves into major conflicts. The potential consequences include divided loyalties, poor decision making, mistrust, and weakened performance (Blake & Mouton, 1984). Such conflicts can be classified as *intergroup conflicts,* and their handling requires special conflict resolution approaches.

Blake and Mouton (1984) propose an Interface Conflict-Solving Model that provides a framework for addressing intergroup conflicts. Separate work groups, despite their loyalties and team characteristics, must occasionally cross group or unit boundaries, share portions of work projects, or "interface" with other groups in some way to satisfy organizational goals (p. ix). An **interface** is a point of connection, overlap, or interchange where competitive groups cross boundaries to accomplish their desired result. The reunion of earlier separated work groups creates the probability of conflict between the groups. For example, consider two groups that must complete separate portions of the same overall project. An interface exists as the performance of one group significantly affects the work of the other. When one of these groups works at a slower pace than the other or conforms to a different work standard, the interface is likely to be conflictual.

The Interface Conflict-Solving Model, implemented within a framework of managerial support and participant cooperation, requires several conflict-solving sessions that representatives from each conflict faction attend. Blake and Mouton (1984) outline six general steps. The initial step requires each group to propose its model or ideal solution to the conflict situation. Thus, each group, independent of the other groups, submits its proposal to resolution specialists or leaders for comparison. A second step requires interface groups, in a climate of cooperation and mutual purpose, to work to consolidate separate proposals into a single ideal settlement. Third, each group, independent of the other groups, describes the actual situation or interface conflict. At this point, the groups rely on their own understanding to realistically describe the conflict situation. The next step requires consolidation of the actual relationship. In this conflict-solving phase, the groups combine their separate descriptions to form a joint, unifying description. Collectively, they decide on necessary changes and future plans. They achieve agreement about what is necessary for them to work together. A final step is a progress review and re-planning stage. That is, groups reconvene at a designated time to review their progress or to reassess interface status. Additional planning continues as needed.

Individual conflicts involve interpersonal conflicts between individuals rather than groups or divisions. Although limited to small numbers of people, unresolved or ignored interpersonal conflicts can become deeply embedded in relationships and significantly influence the future interactions between or among the individuals involved (Kolb & Putnam, 1992). Seemingly permanent interpersonal differences and future conflict episodes are the likely consequences. Moreover, long-standing relational conflicts often continue as covert conflicts that future interpersonal events or situations can easily trigger. Such conflicts take on a cyclical quality, continually fluctuating between covert and overt states (Hansen, Himes, & Meier, 1990). As Walton (1987) points out, "Two persons who are opposed are only periodically engaged in manifest conflict" (p. 65). As a result, any conflict, though erupting with seemingly new issues and etiologies, can actually be an alternative form of the lingering conflict.

While the traditional goals of third-party consultants are to resolve highly visible conflict situations, they often fail to address the covert conflict associated with hidden relationship problems. Walton (1987) presents the Interpersonal Dialogue Model, which focuses on human relational issues. Interpersonal dialogue methods are founded on the principle that successful individual conflict resolution practices should address underlying relational issues that remain suppressed and hence are avoided as topics of overt discussion. Through the dialogue approach, conflict parties "engage each other and focus on the conflict between them, including aspects of the relationship itself" (Walton, 1987, p. 5).

Walton's interpersonal dialogue methods rely on an array of functional techniques that can be implemented by third-party consultants. Their goals are to help conflict factions better manage their conflict (either through conflict resolution or control), reduce the costs of conflict, and improve the quality of the working relationship (Walton, 1987). An ultimate objective is the adeptness of the opposing parties in utilizing communication and collaboration skills when future interpersonal differences emerge.

Conflict Resolution Processes   Consultants should not begin the conflict resolution process arbitrarily or without assessing the conflict situation. Although they may observe disturbing conflicts within organizations, perhaps as the primary consultation issue, or as peripheral characteristics of other consultation issues, the decision to pursue active conflict resolution rests with the consultees and parties to the conflict. Forcing or enticing unwilling parties into active conflict resolution, or prematurely addressing conflict situations, can be inappropriate and harmful. Further, the consultant must anticipate that some intraorganizational conflicts, although somewhat uncomfortable or disconcerting to the parties involved, can indeed serve important functional purposes that move the organization forward.

When conflict is disturbing or unproductive and the parties in conflict seek active resolution, the consultant adds an objective, informed, third-party element to the conflict situation. The immediate aim is to bring the conflicting parties together to agree to work toward solutions. At this point, the cooperation of both parties is essential to the conflict resolution venture and in itself represents a major agreement.

An Atmosphere for Conflict Resolution   Establishing an atmosphere of trust is critical to beginning the conflict resolution process (Tjosvold, 1991). Trust implies a reciprocal dependence by each party on the other party to adhere to conflict resolution principles. As McFarland (1992) states, "Conflict parties must speak and behave in ways that demonstrate trust, thereby encouraging the other conflict party to respond in a trusting and cooperative manner" (p. 19).

At this early stage, an important function is **synchronizing** of each party's readiness for conflict resolution. Synchronizing requires that one party's initiative to enter a conflict meeting matches the other party's readiness (Hansen, Himes, & Meier, 1990). Conflict parties' mutual readiness facilitates collaborative approaches that require each party to engage in a joint, two-way process that extends throughout the resolution effort. Once an atmosphere of cooperative problem solving exists, the consultant can begin to actively address the conflict, determine its cause, and pursue workable solutions.

Regardless of the models or methods consultants utilize, conflict resolution is more likely when each party is confident that a successful outcome is within reach. Filley (1975) identifies a number of beliefs that foster successful outcomes. First, the parties to a conflict should believe that a mutually agreeable solution exists and that each party can achieve its mission. Second, the parties must believe that cooperation is preferable to competition and rivalry. Third, the opposing factions should acknowledge that they are equal in status; the conflict situation is devoid of any hierarchical imbalance or coercion. Fourth, each party should accept the other's position statement as authentic and fair. Fifth, differences of opinion are viewed as helpful and positive; creative solutions emerge from differences. Sixth, each faction should trust the intentions and actions of the other party. The final point Filley makes is that, though other parties could compete, they have chosen cooperation as the best course of action. Consultants may wish to check the views of the opposing parties against these principles before proceeding with the resolution process.

Consultant Roles   Although the third-party consultant's role entails a range of activities and responsibilities, resolving conflicts and enhancing interpersonal relationships are the primary aims. The consultant must possess a repertoire of conflict management skills, applied situationally across organizational, group, and individual conflict situations. Several techniques and practices merit special definition.

Consultants are often asked to assess the severity of organizational conflicts and their causes. Diagnosing conflict not only provides a general understanding of the conflict situation, it answers many questions about how to proceed with the resolution process. To begin their investigation, they may want to know how severe and how pervasive a conflict situation has become within the consultee's setting. Several practical issues should be addressed during the formative stage of conflict resolution:

- Does unproductive conflict exist, and if so at what intensity?
- What is the conflict history, its contributing factors, and its consequences?
- How do the opposing parties view conflict?

- What methods or strategies are commonly applied to conflict situations?
- What relationship dynamics exist between the parties?
- To what extent is conflict embedded in relationships?
- Are the parties ready to assume responsibility for resolving conflicts?

Consultants may set in motion a more elaborate diagnostic approach. Greenhalgh (1991), for example, proposes a model in which conflict specialists predict the severity of conflicts and the potential for successful resolution by analyzing various conflict dimensions. Greenhalgh lists seven critical dimensions:

1. *The conflict issue in question* If the conflict issue represents a matter of principle rather than a practical process or action, conflict resolution is more difficult.
2. *The size of the investment that may be lost.* Conflicts are easier to resolve when each party makes a relatively small investment. Larger investments translate into more difficult conflict resolution.
3. *The relationship of the parties* The interdependence of the parties to a conflict means that one party may gain or lose as the opposing party gains or loses. If one party gains at the expense of the other, conflicts are more difficult to resolve.
4. *The continuity of the interaction* The parties involved in a conflict are almost always engaged in interactions over a period of time. Long-standing relationships lead to easier conflict resolution because the existing disagreement may be a minor element in the overall relationship.
5. *The structural features of the parties* Parties that are cohesive and have strong leadership make conflict resolution easier. Weaker groups are often fragmented and unresponsive to the leader's authority and thus create barriers to the conflict resolution process.
6. *The role of third parties* When trusted and respected third parties participate in the resolution process, positive outcomes are more likely. The absence of neutral third parties makes conflict resolution difficult.
7. *Perceptions of the progress or escalation of conflict* Conflict resolution is easier when the parties believe that the conflict situation is improving. Conflict worsens, however, when either faction perceives that the conflict is escalating or becoming more divisive.

Applying Greenhalgh's (1991) model requires consultants to review each dimension and the alternative perceptions of the opposing parties. Ultimately, through their diagnostic review, consultants can heighten their understanding of the conflict situation.

Negotiation is a bargaining process that appears useful in conflict situations in which parties wish to come to an agreement but cannot decide on the nature and terms of the agreement (Johnson & Johnson, 1975). Johnson and Johnson (1975) describe the negotiation process: "It is aimed at achieving an agreement that determines what each party gives and receives in a transaction between them" (p. 176). Operationally, negotiation procedures require parties to bring their demands and expectations to a central forum for discussion. Third-party consultants, who fulfill neutral roles during negotiations, can be helpful in clarifying issues or positions, facilitating discussions, and motivating parties when negotiations are stagnant. Further, consultants can strongly influence the relational variables that accompany negotiated settlements; that is, they can facilitate a psychologically healthy climate as they monitor each party's reaction to the settlement process.

As individuals become personally entangled or preoccupied with conflict situations, emotionally charged and volatile behaviors often emerge. These actions may impede resolution, generate mistrust, and ultimately exacerbate conflicts. Third-party consultants often find themselves in the midst of such tension-filled arenas. In such cases, they should adopt a peacemaking role.

Consultants have the potential to restore calm and encourage an atmosphere of cooperation. Several principles characterize their peacekeeping function. First, the consultant's mere presence can have an immediate calming effect. The consultant's impartial or nonevaluative status implies that all sides of a dispute will be recognized, considered, and respected (Kolb, 1992). Moreover, since the consultant signals hope that conflicts will end in positive settlements, cautious optimism emerges and leads ultimately to deescalation (Gordon, 1991). Indeed, it is through the consultant's watchful presence that open discussions begin and calm-restoring ground rules established. Peacekeeping roles are enhanced, also, through the empathy and support skills that psychological consultants bring to the process. When the parties air tensions in a supportive atmosphere, their confidence is heightened and antagonism diminishes.

When direct exchanges or dialogue between disputing factions are impossible or it is evident that a neutral party is needed, consultants assume **mediation** roles. As mediators, consultants are impartial, trusted agents who represent all parties. Consultant-mediators convey information, including oral or written statements or positions, present points of debate, and foster communication. The mediator role, however, is much broader and more complex than may appear at first glance. That is, consultants should help create mediation processes that allow people to vent feelings and tensions in an empathic setting (Kolb, 1992). Further, consultant-mediators must objectively and accurately represent each party's position to the other, encourage constructive dialogue, and work to restore calm.

Groups often reach an impasse when debating important decisions. When poorly managed or ignored, an impasse can evolve into disturbing conflict. **Consensus** is a helpful consultant strategy for maintaining group cohesion while groups work through deadlocked decision making. Consensus emphasizes the importance of all group members giving input and consenting to the final decision (Avery, Auvine, Streibel, & Weiss, 1981). Although consensus processes do not require all members to agree completely with the final outcome, they do agree to support it.

Team Building

Teams, or at least potential teams, are everywhere. They form in virtually every human setting in which people come together for a common purpose. Families, organizations, work units, educational institutions or programs, and community groups are examples of groups that have the potential to develop into functioning teams. Larson and LaFasto (1989), describing the emergence of team philosophies in society, provide a succinct definition of a **team**: "A team has two or more people; it has a specific performance objective or recognizable goal to be attained; and coordination of activity among members of the team is required for the attainment of the team goal or objective" (p. 19).

Teamwork provides the blueprint for working together and solving problems. The benefits of teamwork (the process or state of working as a team) are well chronicled in group and organizational literature (Alexander, 1985; Blake & Mouton, 1964; Likert, 1961; Mayo, 1933; McGregor, 1960; McKee, 1992; Pfeiffer, 1981). Clearly, there is little doubt that teams function more effectively than nonteams.

Regrettably, effective teams are conspicuously rare. Zimbardo and Ebbeson (1969) describe an emerging trend in our society where we possess the capacity to resolve vast social problems, yet because of our inability to work together, little is accomplished. Ineffectual groups create an unfortunate paradox in organizations in which, despite specialized technology and a desire to succeed, inefficiency, dissatisfaction, and wasted opportunity are the norm.

Defining the Team-Building Process

Organizational leaders often rely on skilled consultants to help them blend existing work groups into cohesive teams. Molding groups into motivated and **synergistic teams** (teams propelled by a collective, unidirectional, and motivating energy) is no easy task, however, since team building requires more than hopeful thinking. According to Johnson and Johnson (1975), **team building** involves an experiential process: "Team building refers to a method under which groups experientially learn to increase their skills for effective teamwork by examining their structures, purpose, setting, procedures, and interpersonal dynamics" (p. 300).

According to Blake, Mouton, and Allen (1987), team-building consultants must identify and seek to abolish processes or actions that impede effective teamwork. Their work is complete when team obstacles are replaced with team-oriented behaviors or conditions. To these ends, consultants must observe groups in action, assess team functioning, and isolate obstacles to effective team functioning.

Dimensions of Team Functioning

Effective teams maintain a structure that transcends the splintered actions that characterize a mere collection of individuals. Moreover, effective teams do not emerge haphazardly or randomly (Alexander, 1985). For consultants, knowing the characteristics of effective teams and nonteams is essential to their team-building work. The professional literature describes a range of team characteristics:

1. *Individualism versus team synergy* Excessive individualism characterized by the idiosyncratic interests and actions of individual group members impedes the group's teamwork. When members seek personal agendas or individual rather than team goals, group momentum diminishes. When members' individual energies are collected into a team-building synergy, the team's potential for accomplishments is unlimited. In syner-

gistic teams: "The whole is greater than the sum of its parts. The team result has exceeded the sum of individual contribution" (Blake, Mouton, & Allen, 1987, p. 6).

2. *Misused authority versus team leadership*   Highly authoritarian leaders abuse their **power** (the ability of one group member to influence others to behave in ways that satisfy the individual exerting the power) when they undermine member participation and creativity, and ultimately, teamwork. When group relationships are patterned according to a rigid or hierarchical order, individual autonomy and egalitarian principles are sacrificed. In effective teams, leadership is not a coercive, unidirectional process. According to Kouzes and Posner (1990), "Leadership is a reciprocal process that occurs between people. It is not done by one person to another" (p. 29). Both internal and external leaders must acquire and maintain a team philosophy. Teamwork should be evident at the highest level of the organization as group members recognize that working together is an expected norm of organizational behavior. Further, within effective teams: "The development and cohesion of a team occurs only when there is a feeling of shared leadership among all team members" (Alexander, 1985, p. 102).

3. *Interpersonal conflict versus collaboration*   Misperception and ineffective communication often lead to conflict in groups. Poorly managed conflicts are destructive and create excessive tension. Moreover, conflict contributes to stressed relations and the inability to mediate differences. Larson and LaFasto (1989) point out that "the potential for collective problem-solving is . . . often unrealized and the promise of collective achievement . . . often unfulfilled" (p. 13). Effective teams expect and invite conflict. The health of the team is strong and can promote divergent ideas or actions. Conflicts represent opportunities for problem solving and collaboration. The collaborative process requires that each team member have a joint responsibility for negotiating and resolving interpersonal differences.

4. *Mistrust versus trust*   Trust refers to group members' confidence that each member is sincere, truthful, and reliable in working toward the best interests of the group. Mistrust threatens the very heart of the team. Dishonesty and deception encourage mistrust among members, who, in turn, feel unsupported and betrayed. Effective teams promote an atmosphere of trust and loyalty. One team member can expect other team members to behave in ways that nurture the team and support its goals. Risk taking and experimentation are encouraged because members trust that it is safe to express novel ideas or attitudes. The sense of trust throughout the team enhances collaboration among team members (Larson & LaFasto, 1989), allowing the healthy management of differences (Alexander, 1985).

5. *Incompatible goals versus team spirit*   Unmatched, oppositional objectives and unconstrained rivalry among team members impede effective teamwork and create resistance. According to Johnson and Johnson (1975), "When group members have incompatible goals, however, or are in competition with one another, then their power assertions will conflict and there will be resistance to accepting another's influence" (p. 204).

Effective teams proclaim a shared purpose with supported goals or objectives. Central to the team's commitment is the concept of **team spirit**, an intangible, collective sense of unity and commitment to the team. Team spirit is evident in teams that express loyalty and dedication, an unrestrained sense of excitement, a willingness to help the team, an intense identification with the team, and a loss of individualism within the team (Larson & LaFasto, 1989).

Team-Building Processes

Each consultant approaches team-building consultation differently (Johnson & Johnson, 1975). Since all groups and their team obstacles are unique, it is difficult to devise a precise list of actions and processes that address the needs of all groups. Nevertheless, we describe a generic, step-by-step team-building model that outlines the consultant's procedures: relationship building, assessment, diagnosis, feedback/education, and implementation. Each step requires the consultant's attention to various tasks that, collectively, make up the team-building process (see Figure 10.1).

Relationship Building   Consultants enter the team-building process in the same way they enter other consultation activities and roles. A few points are noteworthy, however. For example, relations with consultees and other consultation participants are particularly critical to successful team building. The consultant must encourage an atmosphere of trust and rapport, in which observation, feedback, and evaluation can take place without intimidation. Participants should recognize that the consultant's role is supportive and objective and does not involve the type of performance evaluation that highlights performance weaknesses. Further, the consultant should serve as a model who is prepared to engage the consultee's needs as a team-oriented consultant.

Assessment   The goal of assessment activities is to evaluate group weaknesses, strengths, and the potential for team behavior. Assessment processes begin with important questions about the group and the organization it comprises. Wigtil and Kelsey (1978) provide fundamental questions that should begin the assessment process:

1. Is there organizational support for teaming?
2. Were the participants provided organized preparation for teaming?
3. Is there a positive management system operating that is willing to examine climate related to leadership style, decision making, planning, organization, and monitoring?
4. Are individual and organizational needs being met? and,
5. Do members of the team have opportunities to participate in different functional team roles? (p. 416)

Whether the group is small and spatially contained or large and scattered, data are collected through various processes. Particularly helpful are observational methods, the use of standardized instruments, and individual or group interviews. Data can be gathered in either qualitative or quantitative forms (Phillips & Elledge, 1989). **Qualitative data** include estimates of team functioning that result from group or individual observations, supervisory accounts, or interviews. Alternative qualitative variables include the presence of intangible employee apathy or morale problems, strained worker relations, and incomplete or inaccurate communication (Dyer, 1987).

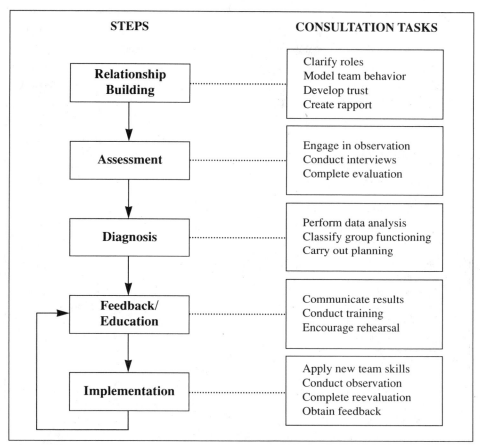

STEPS   **CONSULTATION TASKS**

Relationship Building
- Clarify roles
- Model team behavior
- Develop trust
- Create rapport

Assessment
- Engage in observation
- Conduct interviews
- Complete evaluation

Diagnosis
- Perform data analysis
- Classify group functioning
- Carry out planning

Feedback/ Education
- Communicate results
- Conduct training
- Encourage rehearsal

Implementation
- Apply new team skills
- Conduct observation
- Complete reevaluation
- Obtain feedback

FIGURE 10.1
Steps and tasks of team-building consultation

Quantitative data require more formal measurements and perhaps standardized instruments. Global measures (for example, declining productivity or sales, number of employee grievances, turnover rates) provide additional sources of quantitative information used to assess team variables. Standardized instruments can be a valid and reliable source of team information. Alexander's (1985) Team Effectiveness Critique is an example of a brief team rating instrument (see Exhibit 10.2).

When groups are small and contained, the consultant may observe the target group as it conducts its business, record notes or ratings of important group dynamics and processes, and make notes on the group's potential for teamwork. Although assessment activities are ongoing, the formal assessment period concludes when the consultant synthesizes data into hypotheses about the characteristics and needs of the team.

Diagnosis When sufficient data are collected, the consultant pursues the highly specialized task of diagnosing team functioning. The chief diagnostic objective is to provide a valid impression on which team-building training and education are planned.

THE TEAM EFFECTIVENESS CRITIQUE
Mark Alexander

Instructions: Indicate on the scales that follow your assessment of your team and the way it functions by circling the number on each scale that you feel is most descriptive of your team.

1. Goals and Objectives

There is a lack of commonly understood goals and objectives.

Team members understand and agree on goals and objectives.

1	2	3	4	5	6	7

2. Utilization of Resources

All member resources are not recognized and/or utilized.

Member resources are fully recognized and utilized.

1	2	3	4	5	6	7

3. Trust and Conflict

There is little trust among members, and conflict is evident.

There is a high degree of trust among members, and conflict is dealt with openly and worked through.

1	2	3	4	5	6	7

4. Leadership

One person dominates, and leadership roles are not carried out or shared.

There is full participation in leadership; leadership roles are shared by members.

1	2	3	4	5	6	7

5. Control and Procedures

There is little control, and there is a lack of procedures to guide team functioning.

There are effective procedures to guide team functioning; team members support these procedures and regulate themselves.

1	2	3	4	5	6	7

6. Interpersonal Communications

Communications between members are closed and guarded.

Communications between members are open and participative.

1	2	3	4	5	6	7

EXHIBIT 10.2

Team effectiveness critique

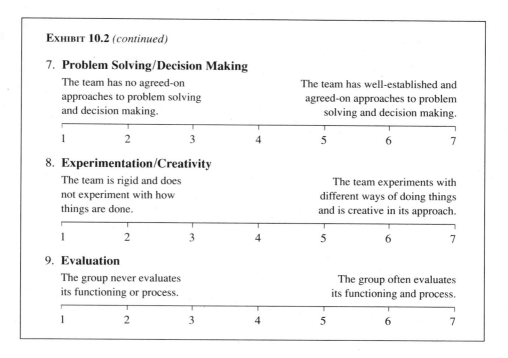

Exhibit 10.2 *(continued)*

7. **Problem Solving/Decision Making**

The team has no agreed-on approaches to problem solving and decision making.

The team has well-established and agreed-on approaches to problem solving and decision making.

1   2   3   4   5   6   7

8. **Experimentation/Creativity**

The team is rigid and does not experiment with how things are done.

The team experiments with different ways of doing things and is creative in its approach.

1   2   3   4   5   6   7

9. **Evaluation**

The group never evaluates its functioning or process.

The group often evaluates its functioning and process.

1   2   3   4   5   6   7

Relying heavily on group process and analysis theory, the consultant studies the group's actions, its strengths and weaknesses, and members' behavior. Diagnostic thinking, within the context of team building, embodies two main calculations: current level of team functioning, and possible strategies to enhance team functioning.

Feedback/Education   When data have been gathered, analyzed, and synthesized into a diagnostic impression and agreed-on course of action, the consultant distributes the results of observations, rating forms, and interviews to group members. Feedback can be provided orally or through a written report (Phillips & Elledge, 1989). According to Phillips and Elledge (1989), a feedback meeting includes collaborative discussions among all constituents. It accomplishes three purposes: sharing assessment and diagnostic information, encouraging the group's ownership of feedback information, and agreeing on the next step in team building.

Although the consultant's feedback often enlightens group members, a range of more direct interventions, closely matched to assessment and diagnostic information, are available. Training sessions, for example, can be effective ways of instructing participants in team concepts and skills. Moreover, training opportunities have the potential for experiential learning in which group members participate in a broad range of planned exercises, role playing, and simulations.

Implementation   If team-building efforts are to be worthwhile, they must be integrated into the organization or group. At this point, group members are alert to their group's teamwork barriers and have experienced opportunities to learn and apply new team-building skills. Team members, newly committed to a team philosophy, should work diligently to avoid or eliminate team barriers. As teams demonstrate their competencies, "they are given increasing responsibility for decisions that affect their work" (Jessup, 1990, p. 79). When team-building interventions are effective, the consultant gradually withdraws, allowing the team to mature in its new team approach. Until this point, however, team-building interventions should continue with observation, feedback/education, and implementation activities.

SUMMARY

Consultation problems create the demand for specialized interventions that address a range of problems or needs. Although none of the applications described in this chapter are strictly synonymous with consultation, they do represent interventions that consultants may implement to resolve consultation problems. The chapter detailed three popular consultation interventions: training, conflict resolution, and team building. For each intervention, we gave close attention to the importance of application and process. In addition, we discussed some novel approaches that may guide the consultant's actions. The chapter's primary purpose was to increase your knowledge and facilitate your readiness to conduct specialized applications.

GLOSSARY

Compromise   A conflict resolution strategy that requires parties in conflict to agree to terms somewhere in the middle of their two positions.

Conflict   A clash in values, attitudes, or behaviors resulting from natural and expected human differences.

Conflict resolution   Planned and organized consultation applications aimed at the mediation, resolution, or management of conflicts and the enrichment of interpersonal relationships.

Consensus   A decision-making technique particularly useful when groups experience conflict over a course of action or a decision. Consensus requires all members to consent to the final disposition of the decision.

Demonstration   An experiential training method in which trainers or participants model desired interactions, skills, and other behaviors.

Experiential   A term that describes a style of learning emphasizing a "learning-by-doing" format. Participants are active in the training process as they realize opportunities for interaction, rehearsal, participation, and performance evaluation.

Interface   A point of connection, overlap, or interchange where competitive groups cross boundaries to accomplish their desired result.

Learning style   A unique blend of receiving, processing, and responding to information.

Mediation   A process of conflict resolution in which a third party serves as an agent in conveying information or communication between parties.

Negotiation   A practice that entails bargaining where parties that wish to come to an agreement dispute the nature and terms of the agreement.

Power   The ability of one party to influence others to behave in ways that satisfy the individual exerting the power.

Processing   In training, an experiential method that allows participants to clarify, interpret, and analyze their participation in training activities.

Qualitative data   A type of subjective data that provides important generalizations or estimates of quality. Qualitative data are often informal estimates expressed in non-numerical form.

Quantitative data   Observable, objective, and measurable information that can be synthesized and expressed numerically. Quantitative results often yield important factual information about a hypothesis or variable.

Rehearsal   A practical and powerful experiential exercise in training programs in which participants practice targeted relational or behavioral skills.

Role playing   A common experiential training method in which participants, in groups of two or more, practice or rehearse interactions pertinent to training goals.

Simulation   An experiential training method that involves the application of games, exercises, or situations that mimic real circumstances or project participants into contrived roles.

Subgroups   An experiential training method in which larger groups are divided into smaller groups to increase participants' interactions and involvement.

Synchronizing   Implies that one party's initiative to enter a conflict meeting matches the other party's readiness.

Synergistic teams   Teams propelled by a collective, unidirectional, and motivating energy.

Team   A group that shares a common purpose and employs cooperative problem-solving techniques.

Team building   A collection of diverse methods that encourage groups to function as teams. Team building encourages groups to learn the fundamental skills of effective teamwork.

Team spirit   An intangible, collective sense of unity and commitment to the group among team members.

Teamwork   The process or state of working as a team.

Third-party consultation   An approach to conflict resolution that requires the active participation of an objective consultant, skilled in conflict resolution practices.

Training   The application of educational and experientially based interventions that help learners acquire new information, technologies, or competencies.

Training design   An account of how a proposed training intervention is to occur; the design includes the training program's purpose, method, and format.

Training proposal   Usually a written document that presents the consultant's credentials and training ideas. A training proposal outlines relevant information about a proposed training program.

Win-win solutions   In conflict resolution, an approach founded on the philosophy that each faction has a vested interest and that a creative solution can be achieved where both parties benefit.

ANNOTATED BIBLIOGRAPHY

The applications discussed in Chapter 10 describe three broad consultation interventions. Because the professional literature on each intervention is expansive, only a few key sources are mentioned in this bibliography.

An excellent resource that emphasizes a practical, handbook approach to training is Mel Silberman's *Active Training: A Handbook of Techniques, Designs, Case Examples, and Tips* (1990). Throughout this comprehensive guide, Silberman gives detailed instructions for each phase of training. Chapters 1 and 2 in particular provide worthwhile reading for beginning and advanced trainers alike. These chapters address the design and implementation of training programs. An alternative source is Carolyn D. Nilson's *Training Program Workbook and Kit* (1989). Dana G. Robinson and James C. Robinson's 1989 book, *Training for Impact: How to Link Training to Business Needs and Measure the Results,* is an excellent resource for the consultant trainer who wants to study the process of training evaluation. To remain abreast of contemporary approaches to training, consultant-trainers should subscribe to *Training and Development Journal,* the professional journal of the American Society for Training and Development.

Popular models of conflict resolution are discussed separately in Dean Tjosvold's *The Conflict-Positive Organization: Stimulate Diversity and Create Unity* (1991), Robert Blake and Jane Mouton's *Solving Costly Organizational Conflicts* (1984), Fred Jandt and Paul Gillette's *Win-Win Negotiating: Turning Conflict into Agreement* (1985), and Richard E. Walton's *Managing Conflict: Interpersonal Dialogue and Third-Party Roles* (2nd ed., 1987). Collectively, these sources examine conflict across interpersonal, group, and organizational variables. Further, Roger Fisher, William Ury, and Bruce Patton provide enlightening information relative to the art of negotiating in their mass market book *Getting to Yes: Negotiating Agreement Without Giving In* (1991). This work highlights the importance of managing minor disagreements and major conflicts without jeopardizing interpersonal relationships. One additional source that teaches practical negotiation skills and strategies is Herb Cohen's *You Can Negotiate Anything* (1980). In this helpful book, Cohen adds a user-friendly touch by citing numerous personal examples of negotiation.

For those who wish to continue the study of team-building consultation, we recommend a few cogent and well-rounded selections. Robert Blake, Jane Mouton, and Robert Allen's 1987 book, *Spectacular Teamwork,* is an excellent practical source of information. Additional information can be found in Carl E. Larson and Frank K. LaFasto's *Teamwork: What Must Go Right, What Can Go Wrong* (1989). Mark Alexander's brief article, "The Team Effectiveness Critique" (1985), provides a basic discussion of the characteristics of effective teams and describes the construction of a team assessment instrument.

REFERENCES AND SUGGESTED READINGS

Alexander, M. (1985). "The team effectiveness critique." In J. Pfeiffer and L. Goodstein (Eds.), *The 1985 annual: Developing human resources* (pp. 101–104). San Diego, CA: Pfieffer.

Avery, M., Auvine, B., Streibel, B., & Weiss, L. (1981). *Building united judgment: A handbook for consensus decision making.* Madison, WI: Center for Conflict Resolution.

Blake, R. R., & Mouton, J. S. (1964). *The managerial grid.* Houston, TX: Gulf.

Blake, R. R., & Mouton, J. S. (1984). *Solving costly organizational conflicts.* San Francisco: Jossey-Bass.

Blake, R. R., Mouton, J. S., & Allen, R. (1987). *Spectacular teamwork.* New York: Wiley

Cohen, H. (1980). *You can negotiate anything.* New York: Bantam Books.

Cosier, R., & Dalton, D. (1993). Management consultant: Planning, entry, performance. *Journal of Counseling and Development, 72*(2), 191–198.

Dastoor, B. (1993). Speaking their language. *Training and Development, 47*(7), 17–20.

Davidove, E., & Schroeder, P. (1992). Demonstrating ROI of training. *Training and Development, 46*(8), 70–78.

Dyer, W. (1987). *Team building* (2nd ed.). Reading, MA: Addison-Wesley.

Eicher, J. (1987). *Making the message clear: Communicating for business.* Santa Cruz, CA: Grinder, Delozier, and Associates.

Fahs, M. (1982, October). Communication strategies for anticipating and managing conflict. *Personnel Administrator,* 28–34.

Filley, A. C. (1975). *Interpersonal conflict resolution.* Glenview, IL: Scott, Foresman.

Fisher, R., Ury, W., & Patton, B. (1991). *Getting to yes: Negotiating agreement without giving in.* New York: Penguin Books.

Gallessich, J. (1982). *The profession and practice of consultation: A handbook for consultants, trainers of consultants, and consumers of consultation services.* San Francisco: Jossey-Bass.

Gordon, J. (1991). *Organizational behavior* (3rd ed.). Boston: Allyn & Bacon.

Greenhalgh, L. (1991). Managing conflict. In J. Gordon (Ed.), *Organizational behavior* (3rd ed., pp. 491–496). Boston: Allyn & Bacon.

Hansen, J., Himes, B., & Meier, S. (1990). *Consultation: Concepts and practices.* Englewood Cliffs, NJ: Prentice-Hall.

Harrison, M. (1987). *Diagnosing organizations: Methods, models, and processes.* Newbury Park, CA: Sage.

Hartley, J. (1973). The role of training evaluation. In I. Davies (Ed.), *The organization of training* (pp. 83–89). London: McGraw-Hill.

Himes, J. (1980). *Conflict and conflict management.* Athens: University of Georgia Press.

Hudson, E. (1973). A practical approach to the planning of training. In I. Davies (Ed.), *The organization of training* (pp. 33–42). London: McGraw-Hill.

Jandt, F., & Gillette, P. (1985). *Win-win negotiating: Turning conflict into agreement.* New York: Wiley.

Jessup, H. (1990). New roles in team leadership. *Training and Development Journal, 44*(11), 79–83.

Johnson, D., & Johnson, F. (1975). *Joining together: Group theory and group skills.* Englewood Cliffs, NJ: Prentice-Hall.

Johnson, D., & Johnson, F. (1991). *Joining together: Group theory and group skills* (4th ed.). Englewood Cliffs, NJ: Prentice-Hall.

Killion, J., & Simmons, L. (1992). The Zen of facilitation. *Journal of Staff Development, 13*(3), 2–5.

Kolb, D. (1992). Women's work. In D. Kolb & J. Bartunek (Eds.), *Hidden conflict in organizations* (pp. 63–91). Newbury Park, CA: Sage.

Kolb, D., & Putnam, L. (1992). Introduction: The dialectics of disputing. In D. Kolb & J. Bartunek (Eds.), *Hidden conflict in organizations* (pp. 1–31). Newbury Park, CA: Sage.

Kouzes, J., & Posner, B. (1990, January). The credibility factor: What followers expect from their leaders. *Management Review,* 29–33.

Kraybill, R. (1987, Summer). Directors' circle. *MCS* [Mennonite Conciliation Service] *Conciliation Quarterly,* 10–12.

Larson, C., & LaFasto, F. (1989). *Teamwork: What must go right, what can go wrong.* Newbury Park, CA: Sage.

Lederach, P. (1987, Summer). Understanding conflict: The experience, structure, and dynamics of conflict. *MCS* [Mennonite Conciliation Service] *Conciliation Quarterly,* 2–12.

Likert, R. (1961). *New patterns of management.* New York: McGraw-Hill.

Mayo, E. (1933). *The human problems of an industrial civilization.* Boston: Harvard University, Graduate School of Business Administration, Division of Research.

McFarland, W. (1992). Counselors teaching peaceful conflict resolution. *Journal of Counseling and Development, 71,* 18–21.

McGregor, D. (1960). *The human side of enterprise.* New York: McGraw-Hill.

McKee, B. (1992, July). Turn your workers into a team. *Nation's Business,* 36–38.

Nilson, C. (1989). *Training program workbook and kit.* Englewood Cliffs, NJ: Prentice-Hall.

Pfeiffer, S. (1981). The problems facing multidisciplinary teams: As perceived by team members. *Psychology in the Schools, 18,* 388–394.

Phillips, J. (1991). *Handbook of training evaluation and measurement methods* (2nd ed.). Houston, TX: Gulf.

Phillips, S., & Elledge, R. (1989). *The team-building source book.* San Diego, CA: University Associates.

Robinson, D., & Robinson, J. (1989). *Training for impact: How to link training to business needs and measure the results.* San Francisco: Jossey-Bass.

Silberman, M. (1990). *Active training: A handbook of techniques, designs, case examples, and tips.* San Diego, CA: University Associates.

Spitzer, D. (1986). *Improving individual performance.* Englewood Cliffs, NJ: Educational Technology Publications.

Tjosvold, D. (1991). *The conflict-positive organization: Stimulate diversity and create unity.* Reading, MA: Addison-Wesley.

Walton, R. (1987). *Managing conflict: Interpersonal dialogue and third-party roles* (2nd ed.). Reading, MA: Addison-Wesley.

Wigtil, J., & Kelsey, R. (1978). Team building as a consulting intervention for influencing learning environments. *Personnel and Guidance Journal, 56*(7), 412–416.

Zimbardo, P., & Ebbeson, E. (1969). *Influencing attitudes and changing behavior.* Reading, MA: Addison-Wesley.

◆ CHAPTER ELEVEN

Ethical and Legal Dilemmas in Consultation

This chapter should be approached with certain assumptions in mind:

1. No profession can afford to ignore ethics and values. Indeed, a sense of ethics may be the single most distinguishing characteristic of the true professional.
2. Without the support and enforcement of a strong professional group (professional organization, association, or society), no code of ethical standards for the behavior of psychological consultants will be developed or, if developed, will exert significant long-term influence.
3. Without a separate professional organization and a clear code of ethics developed by and written specifically for psychological consultants, both consultants and consultees engage in a high-risk endeavor.
4. No separate professional association organized specifically for psychological consultants currently exists. In fact, psychological consultation lacks many of the essential characteristics that distinguish professions from other occupations.
5. An ethical code, with all its values and virtues, is useless unless it is functional, shared, and enforced by other members of the profession.
6. Finally, no single chapter, regardless of how carefully written or how comprehensive, can possibly acquaint the reader with all the ethical and legal issues facing today's psychological consultants.

While this chapter, and the articles and books cited in it, may prove helpful, a cursory reference to a code of ethics is insufficient. You are encouraged, therefore, to carefully review the ethical codes of your professional associations. You should also attempt to gain a thorough understanding of the laws and legal decisions, both federal and state, related to the practice of psychological consultation. Further, while it is recommended that all who practice psychological consultation carry adequate liability insurance to protect them against malpractice and negligence suits, psychological consultants, like other mental health professionals, are far more likely to be absolved from guilt in such suits when it can be established that they have been functioning ethically (Van Hoose & Kottler, 1985).

The primary goal of this chapter is to increase psychological consultants' awareness of and concern for the ethical and legal dilemmas they will encounter in their daily practice. Awareness alone is not enough; there is much at stake in the resolution of every ethical dilemma. Ethical actions have consequences. We believe that psychological consultants will not only improve the quality of their consulting efforts but also make themselves less vulnerable to external regulation by being alert to both ethical and legal questions they may be forced to confront. A secondary goal is to encourage psychological consultants to develop a personal code of professional conduct to which they can look for direction.

Differences in the ethical codes of the psychological consultant's primary or related professional affiliations, the consultant's personal value system and moral empathy, inconsistent laws of the states and territories, and conflicting court interpretations and decisions force the psychological consultant to "function in a legal no-man's land" (Van Hoose & Kottler, 1985, p. 16). For this reason alone it is worthwhile to begin this chapter by looking at some of the reasons psychological consultation has fallen so short of the predicted movement toward true professionalization (also see Chapter 1).

Profession or Occupation?

Unlike many of the business and industrial consultation specialties (marketing, management, finance, tax planning, and public relations, among others) that have established professional associations or societies and published codes of ethical conduct for their members, psychological consultation lacks this mark of professionalism. Indeed, psychological consultation currently lacks many of the essential characteristics that distinguish professions from other occupations. For example:

- There is no commonly accepted knowledge base that can be identified and communicated through present graduate programs.
- There is no corporate group (professional organization, association, or society) to ensure minimum competency for entry into the profession of psychological consultation.
- There is no effort to ensure that psychological consultants continually take positive steps to update their competency. "A profession is never mastered" (Duke, 1993, p. 702).
- Finally, there is no standard for professional conduct made explicit by a functional code of ethics developed specifically for psychological consultants.

Lowman (1985) echoes Duke's (1993) concerns about the lack of movement towards professionalization, when he states that "there are virtually no commonly accepted principles or procedures" for the practice of psychological consultation in organizations (p. 468).

Some attempts are being made to address these problems. The **Council for Accreditation of Counseling and Related Education Programs** (**CACREP**) is working to strengthen the training of consultants through the accreditation of graduate programs. Although continuing education is not required of psychological consultants, as members of professional associations in related specialty areas of human services, practitioners are required to meet standard levels of competence and continuing education for certification and licensure. Gallessich (1982) called for professional autonomy for consultants apart from other human service disciplines.

Part-Time Practitioners

Although the number of human-service specialists interested in psychological consultation has increased recently (see Chapter 1), the majority of today's psychological consultants are enterprising, part-time, sole practitioners in related professions with no (or at best limited) formal education and training in consultation. Some view their part-time work in consultation as a transition to a new profession. They actively seek new approaches and methodologies to improve their technical skills. They read the professional literature and attend workshops, seminars, and national, regional, and state conferences. Others, recognizing the increased demand for psychological consultants, view their part-time consultation engagements as an opportunity for additional income. Both groups appear to enjoy their status as "free agents." Further, since most part-time consultants also hold a full-time position in their specialization (for example, academic positions in colleges and universities, administrative positions in institutions and agencies, managerial positions in business and industry), they have neither the time nor the energy to engage in organizational efforts necessary for professionalization of psychological consultation.

Complacency and Inertia

Because most professional specialists drawn to psychological consultation have already undergone a lengthy period of specialized training in their disciplines and are already members of and identified with their own professional associations, they may not be highly motivated to become involved in the difficult task of establishing a new profession. Indeed, because they are already viewed as professionals in their specialty areas, many see little reason to change their professional identities. Why leave an established profession in which they are recognized as experts to become amateurs in consultation? Underrating the power of complacency and inertia resulting from interest in and loyalty to specialty and attachment to profession may be the primary reason psychological consultants have failed to move toward professionalization at the pace anticipated.

Professionals by Proclamation

Writers in the field (including the authors of this book) are guilty of speaking of psychological consultation as if it were already a profession in the true sense. In doing so, they add to the complacency of their readers—another impediment to true professionalization. Professionalization of psychological consultation will *not* occur through proclamation, regardless of the number of times such a proclamation is repeated.

The Role of a Code of Ethics

Mabe and Rollin (1986) address the role of a code of ethical standards in counseling that seems equally applicable to psychological consultation. In addition to focusing on the *ACA Ethical Standards* (formally *AACD Ethical Standards*), they also "provide some of the lessons learned in other professions," medicine in particular, as they view both the problems and limitations involved in the construction and use of a code of ethics (p. 294). They conclude that the items essential to a code of ethics are:

a. the specific duties or rights that differ from ordinary ethical requirements;
b. the specific duties or rights that may simply be the application of general ethical principles in a particular professional area;
c. a reiteration of certain ordinary ethical requirements that need emphasis for some reason;
d. aims or general goals that the profession should aspire to realize;
e. requirements that relate to coordinating or protecting the interest of members of the profession; and

  f. a statement of the responsibility of members of the profession for reporting code violations or other violations. (Mabe and Rollin, 1986, p. 294)

Even when the code meets all the above requirements, Mabe and Rollin (1986) stress that a professional code, though necessary, is not sufficient. There will be many occasions when the code provides only the most general guidelines for deciding a position on an ethical issue, compared to the few when it offers the clear answer the consultant seeks. The ultimate responsibility for deciding an ethical issue is left to the individual consultant. Individual decisions, however, are often subjective and intuitive. They are influenced by personal values, beliefs, attitudes, and interpretations. A code of ethics, Van Hoose and Kottler (1985) point out, is normative rather than factual: "It is concerned with principles that *ought* to govern human conduct rather than with those that do govern it" (p. 3; emphasis added). There is, then, an inherent ambiguity in the application of ethical standards to the practical situations consultants encounter. In addition to feelings and intuition, rational reasoning and critical analyses are required before acting on an ethical dilemma. Psychological consultants can increase the rationality of their decisions by following certain steps for ethical decision making (see Box 11.1).

Advocates of Professional Autonomy

As pointed out earlier, most human service specialists drawn to psychological consultation are already members of the professional association in their individual discipline or specialty area. However, while they may employ their association's ethical guidelines with some degree of confidence for activities generic to their professional roles, they soon learn that their association's code is not only inadequate, but often creates numerous ethical dilemmas when applied to large numbers of people with conflicting interests in the consultation process (Crego, 1985; Gross & Robinson, 1985; Lowman, 1985; Tannenbaum, Greene, & Glickman, 1989).

  Three sharply delineated positions appear to exist among psychological consultants regarding the establishment of a separate professional group and the development of a code of ethics. There are those who would move immediately toward true professionalism (for example, Gallessich, 1982), others who would prefer to wait for a greater knowledge base and further testing of theories (see Robinson & Gross, 1985; Lowman, 1985), and still others who would like to see the ethical codes of the professional organizations in which they hold memberships expanded to include psychological consultation (for instance, Brown, Pryzwansky, & Schulte, 1991; Huey & Remley, 1988).

  A powerful advocate for the establishment of a separate professional organization for psychological consultants, Gallessich (1982) warns her readers that until psychological consultants develop separate and enforceable ethical standards, consultees, their clients and staff, and the consultants themselves remain at risk. Further, she warns, "viable ethical codes can come into existence *only* when professional groups are able to agree on their principles—and when these principles are sanctioned by the larger society" (p. 396). While it is true that all human service professionals encounter ethical and legal dilemmas in their work, the nature of the tripartite relationship of the consultant (see Chapter 1) is especially sensitive and constantly vulnerable to exploitation and

---

Box 11.1
Steps in making ethical decisions

Psychological consultants uncertain what to do when faced with an ethical dilemma may find the following steps for ethical decision making helpful:

1. Check personal values and motives carefully.
2. Review relevant sections of related professional associations' ethical codes.
3. Search the literature for reports of similar and related cases, noting decisions and recommended actions.
4. Seek the advice of colleagues, particularly those who work in the same settings and may have encountered the same or a similar ethical dilemma.
5. Contact the chairperson of the professional association's committee on ethical standards.
6. Project possible outcomes and consequences for alternative decisions on the issue.
7. Make a decision and act on it.
8. Document reasons for all choices and actions.

---

abuse. Indeed, each stage of the consultation process (see Chapter 2) seems to present its own set of ethical and legal dilemmas.

A smaller, though influential group (those considering or currently pursuing consultation as a career, conducting research in the field, publishing the results of their research in their professional journals, writing textbooks, and developing formal courses and programs at the graduate level for psychology, counseling, and social work programs) realize that establishing a new profession is an arduous, costly task attended by numerous obstacles. They realize, also, that unless they move quickly to develop a common knowledge base, graduate programs of specialized training, credential or license requirements, and a minimum competency level for entrants, psychological consultation will soon face the inhibiting controls and mandates of the government and the courts. The lack of a functional code of ethics and too little emphasis on personal responsibility for judgments made and acts performed will have the same result.

Not only does a profession's code of ethics lay the foundation for the professional's competency, behavior, and responsibility to clients served and to the profession itself, the code also functions as an expression of a professional identity and a symbol of a profession's maturity and autonomy. Autonomy is impossible for any group of professionals without a clear and enforceable statement of standards and ethics. Indeed, if the profession does not establish and regulate standards of behavior and responsibilities for its members, history clearly shows that federal and state legislators and the courts will do it for them.

Though ethical standards and codes of conduct are necessary to protect society, consumers of professional services, and members of the profession, codes are not without problems and conflicts. By their nature, codes of professional conduct are finite; they do not offer ultimate answers. Neither do they respond to every ethical question that may arise in the daily practice of psychological consultation. Furthermore, codes are subject to various and conflicting interpretations. They are often ambiguous when applied to specific cases. Consequently, they are difficult to enforce, for ethics cannot be guaranteed by decree.

Until psychological consultants form a separate professional group of their own, they must continue to rely on the codes developed by their professional specialties. Indeed, Brown, Pryzwansky, and Schulte (1991) point out that consultants are *"bound* to abide by the ethical standards of the organizations to which they belong" (p. 373, emphasis added). Multiple codes present serious ethical dilemmas, for individuals who hold memberships in more than one professional organization discover that they are bound to the conflicting standards and sanctions of the different organizational codes.

Levy's (1976) summary of the ethical dilemma involving professional codes of conduct faced by consultants is most descriptive:

> Codes of ethics are at once the highest and the lowest standards of conduct expected of practitioners; the awesome statement of rigid requirements and the pro forma blurb issued primarily for public relation purposes; the gradually evolved essence of moral expectations and the arbitrarily concocted shortcut to professional prestige and status; the handy guide for the legal enforcement of ethical conduct and for punishment for infringements thereof, or the unrealistic, unimpressive, and generally unknown or ignored guide to wishful thinking. (pp. 209–210)

Advocates of Expanding Existing Professional Codes

At present, Lowman (1985) disagrees with the appeals for professional autonomy. Rather than a new code at this stage of professional development, he recommends "a more detailed application of the existing codes" (p. 648). Most psychological consultants' primary identifications and loyalties remain with the professional associations in their individual specialty areas. Examples include the **American Psychological Association (APA)**, which has formulated the *Ethical Principles of Psychologists* (1991); the **American Counseling Association (ACA)** and its *Ethical Standards* (1995); and the **American School Counselor Association (ASCA)** and its *Ethical Standards for School Counselors* (1984).

Believing that organization of such a diverse group of specialists is highly unlikely at the present time, Brown, Pryzwansky, and Schulte (1991) provide their readers with "a number of ethical principles keyed to the codes of ethics of APA and ACA," which they believe "can serve as the basis for ethical behavior in psychological consultation" (p. 373). They also identify and discuss a number of potential legal pitfalls for psychological consultants (for instance, negligence, defamation, sexual misconduct, misrepresentation, confidentiality, invasion of privacy, and breach of contract) (pp. 367–373). Though focused on counseling in the schools, a similar stance is found in Huey and

Remley's *Ethical and Legal Issues in School Counseling* (1988). Both sources draw on the ethical codes of counseling (ACA) and psychology (APA) to frame a separate code for psychological consultants.

Consultant's Knowledge of Personal Competence

The question of personal competence, reflecting the consultant's professional training and preparation, is a continual ethical concern. Indeed, issues of ethics and competence often overlap. Each psychological consultant must consider whether the demands of a particular consulting engagement are within his or her personal and professional limitations. In a very real sense, psychological consultants are expected to determine their own assets—measure their own deeper character, their knowledge, skills, experience, and techniques.

Consultants who lack the knowledge, technical skills, or experience to do the job are in no position to make informed ethical choices concerning the manner in which they will do it, whether to fulfill the contract responsibly, to avoid infringement of the rights of the consultee or the consultees' employees and clients, or to evaluate moral consequences encountered in the consultation process. Though addressing therapists, Lakin (1988) offers good advice to consultants when he informs his readers that "competence must be defined in terms of ethical actions as well as the requisite knowledge and skills" (p. 143).

Existing ethical codes recognize the tendency of some consultants to overestimate their knowledge and abilities and the temptation of others to succumb to an enticing fee for consultation engagements calling for knowledge and skills beyond their present training and experience. Indeed, a consultant's narcissism may prevent the consultant from perceiving or acknowledging personal weaknesses and limitations. Practically all existing codes of the human service associations state that psychological consultants must limit their services to areas in which they have acquired adequate knowledge and skills and to employ only those methods and techniques in which they are qualified by both training and experience. We are reminded of a graduate student in counseling who, after taking a course titled "Consultation Roles in Counseling," accepted a paid request to help an organization resolve personnel conflicts. The class was the student's only consultation preparation.

Should the consultant determine that his or her services are not beneficial to the consultee, the consultant is obligated to make this known. To do otherwise is unethical and subject to sanction. Consultants are also responsible for informing their consultees of any personal values or impairments that might limit their effectiveness (such as strong beliefs, emotional problems, and addictions). Further, consultants are obligated to correct any faulty expectations of the consultee. Van Hoose and Kottler (1985) warn that to ignore doing so is both an ethical and a legal issue: "The understanding that develops during the first contacts becomes, in effect, an unwritten contract. Each party has a responsibility to abide by the contract. If the contract is breached, the remedy may be legal action" (p. 47). The consultant assumes the legal duty to communicate clearly and honestly to the consultee his or her skills and methods, the conditions of consultation, fees, appointment schedules, and any special obligations of both the consultant and the consultee. Consultants are ethically and legally responsible not only for what they do and the way they do it, but also for what they should reasonably have been expected to do, based on the knowledge available and currently accepted practice guidelines.

Because psychological consultation is a young and growing field, it is characterized by change. The practicing consultant must continually take advantage of learning opportunities—professional workshops and seminars, graduate coursework, professional meetings, current articles reporting relevant research studies, theoretical approaches, and new strategies and interventions.

Consultants must individually determine whether the demands of a particular consulting engagement are within their personal level of expertise. To do this, they must be aware of their personal and professional limitations. In short, consultants must be able to fulfill their responsibilities to the consultee. Not only are psychological consultants bound to adhere to the ethical codes of the professional associations in their related specialties, they also run the risk of having to defend their consulting practices in court. Where knowledge and expertise are the major products and services contracted, full commitment to continuous learning, training, and retraining is a necessity. The psychological consultant is ethically obligated to stay current—that is, to be aware of training alternatives, recent research, and newly developed and tested consulting strategies, methods, instruments, interventions, and techniques.

An exception to the issue of competency is possible only when certain conditions are present:

1. If it can be clearly established that there is no other consultant in the area who is better qualified
2. If the consultant possesses parallel training and experience for the consulting task
3. If the consultant has adequate time to prepare for the consulting task
4. If the consultant makes all these limitations clear to the employing agency
5. If it is a crisis situation that requires immediate intervention

For example, a mental health therapist working in substance abuse at a rural outreach clinic is approached by an administrator of a federal program to conduct a brief smoking cessation workshop with heavy smokers in the organization. Though the therapist has stopped smoking personally, he has neither the experience nor training necessary to conduct smoking cessation workshops. The administrator informs the therapist that there is no other mental health professional in the area. Before accepting the invitation, the therapist may first wish to verify that there are no other mental health professionals better qualified than he to conduct the workshop. He may, for example, call the nearest offices of the American Cancer Society and the American Lung Association, since the directors of these organization are most likely to know if there are smoking cessation specialists in the area. If, indeed, there are none, the therapist may want to request the teaching aids and informational materials these organizations provide for their smoking cessation workshops. Even though he may choose to use a different approach from the one these groups use, their materials may prove helpful as he prepares for the workshop. The therapist is aware that he will be able to draw on his graduate training and work experiences in group therapy and substance abuse counseling. After informing the administrator who contacted him of these conditions, he may ethically accept the invitation.

Ethical Issues of Marketing Statements

Only in recent years have the codes of the human service professions permitted their members to advertise their services. Even today, the term *announcements* is preferred over the term *advertising*, and the information permitted in the announcement is limited to name, highest degree earned, certification and/or licensure, office address, hours, telephone number, and a brief description of the services performed (Section F.2, *Ethical Standards*, 1988, ACA). Further, the description of services is not to emphasize the uniqueness or skill level unless determined so by accepted methods of research. Any misuse of institutional affiliation to recruit clients/consultees for private practice is to be avoided. An announcement should also not include endorsements of former consultees. For example, a consultant advertising consulting services risks professional sanction if the advertisement includes favorable quotations regarding performance obtained from the evaluation forms of past consultees. Fortunately, advertising is only a part of a total marketing effort.

Current attitudes toward advertising and marketing the professional services of psychological consultation are mixed. However, a number of writers support appropriate advertising. Hall and Barker (1988), for example, encourage the consultant in private practice to consider certain marketing strategies and offer seven "guidelines" the consultant may wish to follow. Though addressing counselors, Gilchrist and Stringer (1992) conclude that ethical and effective marketing practices can benefit the counseling professional. Further, they assert, counselor educators and supervisors should ensure "that marketing concepts, practices, and ethics are addressed in counselor preparation programs . . . by incorporating marketing education and training into existing core courses," as well as in continuing (postdegree) education seminars and workshops (pp. 160–161).

Kelley (1981) agrees that most consultants lack the training and experience necessary to market their services effectively. He contends that most psychological consultants dislike "selling" themselves and their services. However, he points out that effective marketing is as essential for success in consultation as it is in any business. According to Kelley, **marketing** "is the total effort directed at convincing your clients [consultees] to satisfy their needs and wants through your services" (p. 105). "Marketing is not an isolated activity"; rather, it is a total, continuous, and integrated process that yields four distinct benefits (Kelley, 1981):

- *"Marketing focuses your business and your efforts"* (p. 105). Attention is on the consultees' needs rather than on the consultant's services or products.
- *"Marketing makes you do today what is required to secure next year's business"* (p. 105). Psychological consultants, particularly part-time consultants, frequently neglect planning for the future. They are too occupied with present consulting engagements to be concerned with the identification of new consultees, the analysis of future trends, or the development of new skills and techniques.
- *"Marketing makes you visible to your clients and your community"* (p. 105). Marketing is an opportunity to educate potential consultees—to communicate who you are and what you can do for them. Visibility can come from referrals,

brochures, membership and active participation in professional associations and societies, published articles and books, speeches, and newsletters.
- *"Marketing improves your organization"* (p. 105). A good reputation, established through marketing and successful performance, often leads to growth.

As a total effort, effective marketing practices may occur through luncheon meetings, phone calls to prospective clients, advertisements in trade or professional publications, referrals from friends or present and former consultees, and donated services or special financial arrangements to worthy causes or community service.

Consultee Identification

Consultee identification would be a simple matter *if consultants defined consultees as the institutions, organizations, agencies, businesses, or industries employing them.* Fortunately, few focus exclusively on organizations or groups at the expense of individuals. Not only are psychological consultants faced with numerous, complex, diverse, and often conflicting issues and relationships that may call their loyalties into question, their personal and professional ethical codes extend their loyalties beyond their employer. For example, psychological consultants may have to decide between conflicting standards:

- Between personal values and the values of the consultee
- Between the needs of the consultee and the rights and well-being of the consultee's clients and staff members
- Between the goals of the consultee and the ethical code of the consultant's professional association

Because the consultee pays for the consultant's services, the consultation relationship is a fiduciary arrangement. In today's litigious environment it may be tested in a court of law. Although employed by an agency, institution, organization, business, or industry, the psychological consultant will almost certainly be obligated on occasion to serve individuals (clients or employees, for example), to act for the good of society, or to adhere to the standards set by his or her professional affiliation. Psychological consultants must spell out their personal values explicitly for themselves, and, when appropriate, present these values to their consultees to avoid conflicting allegiances.

Parameters of Confidentiality

In psychological consultation few ethical issues are more sensitive than the issue of confidentiality. There are numerous occasions in the consultation process when confidentiality is essential (data gathering and reporting are but two examples). However, while the ethical codes of all the related professions stress confidentiality in the one-to-one therapeutic relationship, none directly address the issue of confidentiality in the multiple, complex relationships of the psychological consultant. How, for example, do psychological consultants establish an ethical balance between the needs and goals of the agencies that hire them and the needs and aspirations of the professionals employed by those agencies, or the needs and rights of the clients those agencies serve? What does the psychological consultant do when faced with the agency's "need to know" and the agency's employees' or clients' rights to privacy, to refuse to participate in any of the stages of the consultation, or to withdraw from participation at any time? What should be the consultant's reaction to a consultee's/manager's coercion of a study's participants? What can consultants do when they learn that data gathered for their study of an agency are to be used for purposes other than that for which they were originally intended (for instance, by the personnel manager to reduce the number of professional staff)? What stance should the consultant take when the agency demands control over all data collected during the consultation process, insists on reviewing all reports with full veto power, or holds permission rights on all interventions to be employed?

As we pointed out in Chapter 2, psychological consultants must address the issues of confidentiality at the entry stage. There must be explicit agreements about the types of data needed, how these data will be gathered and used, and how the consultant's findings will be reported.

Individual Versus Organization

The individual's right to informed consent, confidentiality, and competent treatment is a basic ethical concern addressed in the ethical codes of all the human services professions. It is imperative, then, that consultants investigate the goals of an organization or agency before initiating a contract to provide consultation services so that they may determine whether or not they can ethically provide them. Just as in marital therapy where the goal of one client may not be the goal of the other, in consulting, what is good for the agency or organization may not be good for the agency's or organization's clients or employees. Early reservations or skepticism about organizational goals can prevent future ethical dilemmas regarding the parameters of confidentiality, as well as the dilemmas that might arise from inappropriate or premature implementation of consultation interventions. For example, during the entry stage an agency director asks a consultant for assistance in restructuring the organization of the agency. It becomes evident as the meeting progresses that the director wants the consultant to recommend specific organizational changes (already determined by the director) to "take the heat off" the administration when the changes are announced. Had the consultant simply accepted the consultation engagement, the director's hidden agenda would have remained hidden, and the consultant would have unknowingly participated in an unethical activity. Certainly not all unethical consultee goals can be anticipated at the entry stage. Opportunities for using data in ways other than those intended may not occur to the consultee until late in the consultation engagement. For example, following a stress management workshop with agency employees, the executive director who hired the consultant asks for a list of job-related complaints. The director also wants to know which departments were most vocal. To comply with the request would be a breach of confidentiality. The only announced purpose of the workshop was to assist participants by introducing them to stress-reducing techniques. For the consultant to report the information requested, workshop participants must have been informed beforehand that the information would be gathered and reported to the director of the agency. The consultant, therefore, must refuse the director's request.

Individual rights, especially the rights of those in the organization who did not voluntarily seek the consultant's help, yet who are expected to be involved in the consultation process and who will be affected by the consultant's actions, must be considered. Robinson and Gross (1985) refer to these individuals as the consultant's **hidden clients** and warn that when the consultee is viewed as an agency or organization, the welfare of "hidden clients" is often sacrificed. Lakin (1988) asserts: "The ethical challenge for practitioners is in finding a balance between the needs and aims of the organization and the legitimate needs and aspirations of the individuals in the work setting" (p. 119). He is quick to point out, however, that the ideal balance is difficult to attain and maintain. Ethical problems take on a unique complexity for the psychological consultant working in an organizational setting. The positions held by employees are hierarchical, and relationships often create overlapping and conflicting interests (see Chapter 5). The consultant's concern for protecting "hidden clients" from coercion and manipulation may not be shared by an organization's consultees—administrators, managers, or supervisors. Indeed, the values of consultees may be antithetical to the consultant's values. It is possible, too, that consultants may in the course of the consultation process discover that their consultees are involved in unethical or illegal practices (for example, funding irregularities, exploitative or coercive practices, distortion of data contained in the consultant's reports to the press or to the chief executive officer or board of directors). Again, many of these difficulties can be avoided by the consultant's insistence on a clear understanding of the parameters of the consultation process with the agency's or organization's chief executive officer.

Role Conflicts and Dual Relationships

Academic part-time consultants are assailed by conflict-of-interest issues and dual relationships, particularly if, in addition to their personal codes of ethics, they are subject to their universities' written policies about faculty consulting (for instance, these policies may specify a set limit on the number of hours permitted each month or financial penalties—a set percentage of gross fees). Constantly pressed for time, academic part-time consultants must make decisions almost daily regarding ethical issues created by their dual roles. Should they operate out of their offices (use their office computers to prepare consultation proposals and reports, the office telephone to make contacts and receive calls from consultees, and in some cases, the office receptionist or secretary to make or confirm appointments when they are unavailable to take calls)?

Although some part-time academic consultants would not consider conducting their consulting business from their university offices or using office equipment or personnel for personal business, they may choose not to inform the university administration or their colleagues of their part-time consulting engagements. Their justification, if discovered, is often based on the conviction that "what I do on my own time is a private matter." As the major employer, does the university have the right to know of the part-time academic consultant's outside employment, even when there is no written policy governing outside activity?

Whether part-time or full-time, consultants may make errors of omission and commission (Metzger, 1993). Errors of omission may include the following: not requesting all available data relevant to the consulting effort; not doing a thorough analysis at the entry stage; and not including some executives or managers in early planning or progress meetings, because the consultant was unaware of them, finds them difficult, or simply does not like them. Ethical dilemmas may arise in instances where the consultant uncovers information that can negatively affect the organization or when someone in the organization shares sensitive information that could, if shared with the consultee, result in that person's dismissal. Perhaps the most difficult ethical issue in omission, according to Metzger (1993), occurs when the consultant discovers that the major cause of the organization's problems is the consultee or the chief executive (p. 132). Is the consultant ethically obligated to report his or her findings to the board of directors or the executive committee?

Errors in commission "would include blatant favoritism to one manager or another, sharing sensitive data with people who ought to know, colluding with senior management to lend your name to a report supporting precluded decisions and evaluations, excessively socializing with client executives of either sex, and accepting favors in exchange for sensitive data or preliminary observations" (Metzger, 1993, p. 132). What is the consultant's ethical obligation if he or she learns that the company employing him or her is a major polluter? What is he or she to do if the consultee is untruthful or deliberately withholds vital information? How is he or she to respond if it becomes obvious that the organization employs discriminatory employment or promotion policies?

Is it unethical for the consultant to make copies of internal company research reports or the reports of another consulting firm? Suppose a consultee or internal research report reveals the weaknesses of a competing company, agency, or business; is it unethical for the consultant to use this information to prepare a proposal to the competitor to correct these weaknesses? What is the ethical stance for a consultant questioned about the competency of a colleague? Is the consultant obligated to confront and, if necessary, report a colleague who he or she believes to be guilty of unethical practices?

Ethical Issues in Research and Evaluation

Psychological consultants today are certainly aware of the need for and the value of research to both their practice and their profession (Dixon & Dixon, 1993; Froehle & Rominger, 1993; Schein, 1993). Indeed, few would deny that the future of psychological consultation depends on the development of an adequate research and knowledge base. Many practicing psychological consultants are already experiencing a growing pressure for accountability, and they are witnessing an increase in litigation (both threatened and actual) toward themselves and their colleagues in the field. In short, they are being asked to justify their work—to demonstrate *through accepted methods of research* the efficacy of their theories and the effectiveness of their intervention strategies (Lakin, 1988). After reviewing the research literature, Froehle and Rominger (1993) assert that psychological consultation is still in an early stage and then conclude that a more basic concern than the quantity and quality of research at this time should be "the readiness of psychoeducational consultation to advance research" (p. 693).

Practicing consultants may see numerous potential research studies in their work settings, but their motivation to design and conduct those studies often vanishes when they discover that each setting also presents a unique and difficult set of formal and informal constraints on research. Further, they learn that adding the dual role of the consultant-researcher to the already difficult triadic roles of consultant–consultee–consultee's clients presents a great many ethical dilemmas, some apparently impossible to resolve. Unlike the laboratory where it is possible to set boundaries, the work settings of the psychological consultant (agencies, institutions, businesses, and industries) are administered by others who are primarily interested in immediacy of impact and budgetary constraints—the quickest possible, most cost-effective answers to problems or resolutions to crises. Seldom do consultees view research as meeting either of these criteria.

Certainly, blame for the lack of significant research in psychological consultation does not rest entirely with consultees or their work settings. Concerned over some consultants' tendency to inappropriately separate research and practice, Witt (1987) writes:

> Research in consultation seems to occur more in response to convenient questions than important questions and to be born more out of a desire to add notches to a vita than out of a systematic and methodological pursuit of questions which impede organizational development. (p. 274)

If the psychological consultant and the consultee agree that research is necessary, the consultant-researcher must answer a number of questions. For example:

- Do I have the necessary research skills, experience, and resources to design and conduct this study properly?
- How can I set the parameters for confidentiality and privacy with any degree of confidence, even if I am able to delineate the parameters clearly in the contract? Will assurances of confidentiality place me at too great a risk?
- Who has access to and, at the termination of the consulting engagement, owns the data gathered for the study—will I, as the researcher, own the data or will the data belong to the consultee who employed me and paid for the research study?
- Can I be assured that the data gathered for research will not be used for purposes other than those intended by the study?
- How do I protect the research participants' rights to choose not to be studied if that is what they wish?
- Closely allied with the issue of informed consent, how do I ensure that coercion and deception play no part in this study?
- Who has the final word on whether the results of the research study can be submitted for professional publication?

Informed Consent

Psychological consultants are responsible for informing all research participants of their rights, including their right *not* to be involved in the study and their right to withdraw as a research participant at any point they choose, without prejudice or fear of retaliation by their instructors, supervisors, or administrators. Research participants should receive a full explanation of the study, its purposes, and the procedures to be followed—including any instruments to be employed (for example, tests, questionnaires, individual or group interviews). All experimental procedures must be identified. Research participants should be made aware of any attendant discomforts or risks, as well as any expected benefits or advantages. They also must be offered the opportunity to ask for and receive answers to any questions they may have about study procedures. Finally, participants should be debriefed at the conclusion of the study.

Coercion and Deception

Addressing the issue of coercion, Robinson and Gross (1986) assert: "Organizations are, by nature, systems of coercion, compliance, and accountability, and because of these characteristics employees are at risk if they refuse to participate" (p. 332). It is important to note, also, that coercion is possible even when the research study may benefit the participants and the organization by helping both to become more efficient and effective.

Deception, even when well-intentioned, is not only unethical behavior on the part of the consultant and therefore to be avoided; it is also an invitation to legal redress when the research participants learn they have been deceived at the termination of the study. Although certain studies cannot be conducted without withholding information (for example, the true purpose of the study, the use of placebos), psychological consultants should look for alternative methods to deception.

Reporting and Publishing Research Results

The primary purpose of preparing a consultation report—whether an interim report of progress or an exit report of outcome—is to inform and to show, through documentation whenever possible, that the consulting services are on schedule and worthwhile.

Reports of Assessment or Termination Experienced psychological consultants are aware that their reports to the consultee can have negative, as well as positive, consequences. In addition to the ethical dilemmas already discussed, there is also the question of how (or if) to report unexpected or incidental findings to consultees. For example, what does a consultant do when, in the assessment stage of the presenting problem, the consultant uncovers other more serious problems that may cause the consultee embarrassment or may lead the consultee to become uncooperative? An even greater dilemma would be when the assessment data gathered by the consultant clearly indicate the problem is caused by the consultee who sought the consultant's assistance. For example, the consultant could learn that the consultee who seeks assistance for improving staff morale is employing covert methods of supervision by reading the files and "private messages" on the hard disks of the linked computer terminals of the department staff and clerical personnel and then uses this information in evaluation reports.

There undoubtedly will be instances when the psychological consultant will want to confer privately with the consultee before submitting a report, to redefine the consulting service, to confront the consultee with the assessment data, or to terminate consultation if the differences cannot be resolved. Should the consultant decide to terminate services and there is the possibility of litigation from a defensive consultee, one course of action is to prepare a letter or report stating the reasons for termination and then to send the original to the consultee and a self-addressed copy through certified mail. The sealed copy and delivery receipt can be kept on file for as long as the consultant deems necessary.

Publication of Research   There is, without question, a paucity of well-formulated, empirically supported research studies in the psychological consultation literature. Moreover, some reviewers criticize the majority of the published studies severely as being marginally significant, suffering from definition problems, lacking a strong theoretical base, failing to include comparison or control groups, avoiding cultural concerns, and overusing surveys as the major data collection procedure. Numerous reasons are suggested for the scarcity of published research in psychological consultation:

1. Shore and Mannino (1983) assert that it is time for psychological consultation to cut its links with other human services and to "set its own priorities, assess its own values, and operate as a separate entity" (p. 121)—in short, to fix the boundaries of its definition. Clear and explicit operational definitions are necessary if both practice and research in consultation are to move forward. Bardon (1985) suggests that consultant-researchers should start by "finding out what consultants do, in an atheoretical way" (p. 359).
2. The myopia of critics that leads them "to dismiss the research of others as irrelevant inhibits development of a unified body of research" (Froehle & Rominger, 1993, p. 694). Related to this, strong criticism, even censure and ridicule, of research attempting to study the qualitative experiences of the tripartite relationships of consultation discourages the practitioner-consultant-researcher.
3. The publication policies of some professional journals (for instance, behavioral and social science journals) "tend to discourage replication studies and the reporting of contrary evidence" (Froehle & Rominger, 1993, p. 694).
4. The desire for rigorous empirical studies discourages rather than nurtures the scientific work of creative, subjective speculation (Coulson & Rogers, 1968).
5. The emphasis on statistical methodology can lead to tailoring research to fit methodology and, unfortunately, to the avoidance of significant and consequential research studies.

Evaluating and Reporting Ethical Violations

When psychological consultants learn of ethical misconduct by a colleague, they are bound to intervene through active and appropriate evaluation and reporting by the code of their professional association or society and, in certain instances, by the laws of the states in which they practice. Determining the appropriateness of evaluating and reporting an ethical violation adds to the stress of the consultant's natural reluctance to report a colleague. Not only are reporting procedures complex and potentially costly in terms of time, energy, and money, there may also be competing ethical principles when a client or consultee is involved (for example, confidentiality or autonomy versus client or public welfare). Not only do the ethical guidelines of different professional associations vary in specificity and mandate, but the procedures for processing reports of ethical violations also vary between the interrelated professions and within a particular profession from state to state. In addition, when reporting a colleague for ethical misconduct, there is the risk of ostracism and the loss of referrals from one's colleagues, particularly those who believe that professionals have an obligation to protect each other. Still another risk of reporting a colleague is that he or she may respond by filing a libel suit. Finally, in those professions with poor enforcement histories of ethical violations, the consultant may decide that the risks outweigh the effort, time, costs, and consequences of reporting and take no action.

Preventing Ethical and Legal Dilemmas

Experienced consultants prevent many of the ethical and legal dilemmas that can arise during a consultation engagement by working with the consultee and others integral to the consultation process to agree to the contractual responsibilities of all parties. Thorough and carefully devised contracts consider the idiosyncratic qualities of each consultation situation. Not only is it important that the consultant extend contract negotiations beyond the consultee to organizational leaders or directors for administrative approval and consensus on the ground rules from all *consultation participants* (administrators, consultees, and policymakers, for example), but it is important also that anticipated ethical and legal issues be addressed and included in the contract. Examples of such issues might be the consultant's authorization or limitations in reference to reviewing confidential materials, assessment instruments and methods; permission to write and publish the results of research; periodic progress meetings; and fees.

Exhibit 11.1 presents an example of a formal consultation contract. This illustration is only a *sample contract*, not to be copied or considered a standard for all consultation situations. Each consultation engagement is unique; therefore, contracts will differ (at times significantly) from one situation to another.

An alternative to a formal, written contract is the consultant's letter of understanding, which summarizes and confirms the consultant's understanding of the consultation request. A letter of understanding, similar to the formal contract, includes the consultant's description of consultant and consultee responsibilities, along with the pertinent logistical information agreed to during the entry stage of the consultation process. It serves as a source of reference for both the consultant and consultee should misunderstandings or disagreements emerge at a later stage in the consultation process.

Box 11.2 contains an example of such a letter. Again, this sample of a consultant's letter of understanding is not to be considered as a model or standard to be generalized from one consultation situation to another. It is offered only as an example of one such letter written specifically for a particular consultation project.

When consultation requests involve short-term applications (such as a training workshop or a conference on a specific case), some consultants rely on an informal, oral

CONSULTANT EMPLOYMENT CONTRACT

This agreement, made this first day of September 1993, is between Dr. John H. Doe, hereafter referred to as the "CONSULTANT," whose office is located at 1423 Rear 5th St., Anywhere, USA, and XYZ Child Development Program, hereafter referred to as the "PROGRAM," whose office is located at 827 Highlawn Road, Anywhere, USA.

Whereas, the purpose of this agreement is to promote mental health among preschool children and their families enrolled in the Program. And, whereas the Consultant possesses the skills, training, and experience to provide important services related to this goal, this agreement is therefore drawn.

TERM: The term of this agreement shall commence on the first day of September 1993 and continue through the 31st day of August 1994. Should either party decide that early termination is necessary, it may be arranged with 30 days written notice, and the terms of early termination should be acceptable to both parties.

CONSULTATION ELEMENTS: The Consultant shall provide the following elements of services:

1. Extend 20 days of on-site consultation during the contractual period. A day is defined as a normal workday, 9:30 A.M. to 3:30 P.M.
2. Activities of consultation include: observing children in the classroom, accepting and following up on referred children, staff consultation, writing evaluative reports on referred children, and referring children and families to community agencies.
3. The Consultant will serve on the Program's advisory board to assist the board with mental health planning.
4. Participate in two progress status meetings during the contract year, one during each six-month period.
5. The Consultant will complete the necessary forms of documentation regarding referral, billing, and travel reimbursement. A summary report of services for each six-month period is to be completed by the Consultant.

PROGRAM ELEMENTS: The Program will provide these elements:

1. Assist the Consultant with scheduling and classroom visits and observation.
2. Make accessible necessary records, documents, and referral forms and seek parental authorization prior to each consultation referral.
3. Provide office space in each of the program locations for the consultant to conduct private interviews with children and parents.
4. Reimburse the consultant $0.23 for each mile of travel, and an annual fee of $2000 for documented consultation services.

APPROVED BY:

_____ (date)	_____ (date)
Dr. John H. Doe	Ms. Jane Q. Public
Consultant	Director, XYZ Child
	Development Program

Exhibit 11.1
Formal consultation contract (fictitious)

November 29, 1994

Ms. Jane Q. Public, Director
XYZ Child Development Program
5942 Highway Road
Mahood, WV 40766

Dear Ms. Public,

I am pleased that you have asked me to provide an inservice, "Communicating Child Mental Health Needs to Parents," for your Head Start social services staff. The purposes of this correspondence are to confirm my availability and outline the details of the training program.

Pursuant to our telephone conversation on November 24, I have examined my schedule and confirmed that Friday, December 9, 1994, is a convenient date. I understand the program will begin at 9:00 a.m. and conclude at 11:30 a.m. As you indicated, the program will be conducted in Room 343 D of your central administrative building. I will arrive 15 minutes before the program begins to set up my equipment and to check the arrangements.

I expect approximately 20 participants and a room arranged in a conference-style format. As we agreed, I will be responsible for providing handouts and other materials. As we discussed, there will be no fee for the inservice.

Again, I wish to thank you for your interest in my training and development services. Please contact me at your convenience should you require additional information about the inservice program.

Sincerely,

John H. Doe, Ed.D.
L.P.C.
Licensed Psychologist

Box 11.2
Sample letter of understanding (fictitious)

consultant-consultee agreement. Consultants who follow this practice, however, should be aware that the courts view oral agreements as a form of contractual agreement. We prefer written agreements over the less-formal and too-often-hurried oral agreements.

Experienced consultants are well aware that contracts and letters of understanding, regardless of how carefully and thoughtfully written, cannot always prevent ethical and legal dilemmas. Consultants may find themselves faced with unexpected issues, conditions, or obstacles that eluded earlier discussions and existing contracts. Anticipating unexpected problems—particularly in long-term consultation engagements—the consultant may insist that the contract provide for a specific series of progress meetings with the consultation participants. Conventionally, contracts indicate the termination of consultation by including dates and deadlines. Although consultation participants may desire that contracts conclude at the conventional time (that is, at the conclusion of consultation), it should be noted that consultees' participation in consultation is voluntary, and prematurely calling an end to the consultation process is usually an option. Consultants who want to terminate a contract prematurely must be guided by sound ethical and legal reasoning, provide legitimate explanations, and avoid abandoning needy clients and consultees.

SUMMARY

In summary, the ethical and legal dilemmas that psychological consultants in the human services encounter can be especially serious and difficult to resolve. The triadic nature of consultation (see Chapter 1) only adds to the seriousness and complexities of the psychological consultant's ethical dilemmas in the human services, for the consultant's ethical decisions can affect large numbers of people (consultants, consultees, and the consultees' clients and staff members).

Practically all psychological consultants publishing in the field today agree that a consultants' code of ethics is urgently needed (Brown, Pryzwansky, & Schulte, 1991; Brown, Kurpius, & Morris, 1988; Gallessich, 1982; Robinson & Gross, 1985). Indeed, psychological consultation is fraught with ethical and legal dilemmas. Current leaders in the field point out the inability of the present ethical codes of the various professional organizations to offer clear directions for consultants. These codes also fail to reflect the complexity of ethical issues confronting practitioners of psychological consultation. Regrettably, today's leaders cannot agree on whether this is the appropriate time to develop a code of ethics specifically for consultants or to move toward making consultation a true profession.

GLOSSARY

American Counseling Association (ACA)   The major organization of counseling professionals who work in educational, health care, residential, private practice, community agency, government, and business and industry settings. The ACA's mission is to enhance human development throughout the life span and to promote the counseling profession.

American Psychological Association (APA)   The major professional association for psychologists in the United States.

American School Counselors Association (ASCA)   One of the divisions of the ACA. The ASCA publishes two journals, one for elementary and another for secondary school counselors.

Council for Accreditation of Counseling and Related Educational Programs (CACREP)   An accrediting body for graduate counselor education programs. Graduate counselor education programs seeking professional program accreditation are required to perform a lengthy self-study, submit a report of the study for review, and arrange for an on-site visit of an accreditation team.

Hidden Clients   The employees and clients of an organization who were not involved in the decision to seek consultation services, who may be expected to participate in a study of the organization, and who may be affected by the outcome of the consultation process.

Marketing   The total effort of consultants to convince consultees that their needs and wants can be satisfied through the consultant's services (Kelley, 1981). Emphasis in marketing is on needs rather than on services or products.

ANNOTATED BIBLIOGRAPHY

As indicated by the title of their book, *The Counselor and the Law,* B. R. Hopkins and B. S. Anderson (1990) have written primarily for counselors; however, we believe that all psychological consultants in the human services would benefit greatly from reading it. Indeed, it should be required reading in consultation training programs and on the shelves of every consultant's professional library. Litigation today (and possibly even more so in the years immediately ahead) is a pervasive part of American society, and psychological consultants must become aware of the broad legal pitfalls that can trap the unwary and uninformed. In the preface to their book, Hopkins and Anderson state that their intent is "to establish, as clearly as possible, the permissible bounds of conduct within which the counselor can perform his or her job effectively and legally" (p. vii). They have done this and much more.

In *Ethical and Legal Issues in Counseling and Psychotherapy* (2nd ed., 1985), W. H. Van Hoose and J. A. Kottler identify and discuss the major ethical and legal issues helping professionals encounter. Although they focus on the ethical and legal issues that most directly affect counselors and psychotherapists, there is much of value in this book for students interested in consultation as a career option as well as for the experienced professional. They address in depth such topics as ethical versus legal approaches, privacy and confidentiality, truth in marketing and consumer protection, licensure and certification, unethical and incompetent practice, and diagnosis and assessment. In addition, readers will find the authors' 48 brief synopses in the Annotated Bibliography both interesting and helpful if they wish to pursue further reading. The appendixes also contain ethical codes for APA, ACA, AAMF, and NASW.

Written for both graduate and undergraduate students and for practitioners seeking to upgrade their knowledge of ethical and legal issues, Gerald Corey, Marianne Schneider Corey, and Patrick Callanan's 1993 book, *Issues and Ethics in the Helping Professions,* is recognized by practitioners and educators as a popular textbook or supplementary reading for courses in professional ethics, counseling and clinical practica, internships, seminars, and workshops. It emphasizes the basic issues counselors and psychologists will face as practitioners. Citations of the ethical codes of various professional organizations appear throughout the text. The authors give readers the opportunity to respond to their discussions of ethical and legal issues and to draw on their personal experiences. Every chapter "begins with a self-inventory designed to help readers focus on the key topic to be discussed in the chapter" (p. xii). The latest edition includes 50 percent new material. Not only have Corey, Corey, and Callanan updated coverage of ethical and legal issues, but they have also added three new chapters—on ethical decision making, multicultural counseling, and ethical issues specific to marriage and family therapy.

Student service specialists in higher education considering consultation as a possible full- or part-time career may want to read *Applied Ethics in Student Services,* edited by H. J. Canon and R. D. Brown (1985). Concerned because the few convention programs of the past several years that dealt with ethics were poorly attended and because major student service journals received few articles dealing with ethical issues, the authors attempted to fill that void. The introductory chapter is written in case-study format and introduces a variety of ethical issues that student service professionals encounter. Later chapters cover such topics as the construction of ethical codes, their biases, strengths, and deficiencies when applied to actual ethical dilemmas, and five key ethical principles that can be applied to defining core issues of an ethics case. Here, too, the reader will find the codes of the American College Personnel Association and the National Association of Student Personnel Administrators.

Ethical and Legal Issues in School Counseling, edited by W. C. Huey and T. P. Remley (1988), is a collection of articles, primarily from AACD (formerly APGA, now ACA) publications on legal and ethical issues that the editors believe merit the attention of all school counselors. We would add all school consultants. In addition to addressing the ethical concerns covered by most books on the subject, the book contains articles/chapters on such topics as child rights, avoiding ethical violations, reporting unethical practices, counselor liability and duty to warn, statutory trends, child abuse, ethical considerations in using group techniques, computer-assisted counseling, microcomputers, and a survey of state laws and practices. Again, many of the articles are relevant to consultation in the school setting.

Although published specifically for counseling psychologists seriously considering engagements in the justice system, the special issue of the *Counseling Psychologist,* edited by J. M. Whiteley (1983), presents major ethical and legal dilemmas encountered in a very difficult environment for consultees in great need of help. We strongly recommend it to interested readers. Examples of dilemmas that the contributors to this special issue discuss are the distinctions of confidentiality, informed consent, the dichotomized relationships between class-caste stratifications of staff and inmates, problems of coping versus growth, crossing staff and inmate cultural boundaries, overcrowding and overwhelming caseloads, the obligation of staff conformity and allegiance, and the assessment dilemma. Again, though the focus is on counseling in the justice system, much of the material may apply to other consultation settings.

REFERENCES AND SUGGESTED READINGS

American Counseling Association. (1995). *Ethical standards*. Washington, DC: Author.
American Psychological Association. (1978). Report of the task force on the role of psychology in the criminal justice system. *American Psychologist, 33,* 1099–1133.

American Psychological Association. (1991). *Ethical principles of psychologists.* Washington, DC: Author.

American School Counselor Association. (1984). *Ethical standards for school counselors.* Alexandria, VA: Author.

Bardon, J. L. (1985, July/August). On the verge of a breakthrough. *Counseling Psychologist, 13*(3), 335–362.

Binder, V. L. (1993). Ethical and legal issues in criminal justice counseling. In J. M. Whiteley (Ed.), *Counseling Psychologist, 11*(2), 85–89.

Brown, D., Kurpius, D. J., & Morris, J. R. (1988). *Handbook of consultation with individuals and small groups.* Alexandria, VA: Association for Counselor Education and Supervision.

Brown, D., Pryzwansky, W. B., & Schulte, A. C. (1991). *Psychological consultation: Introduction to theory and practice* (2nd ed.). Boston: Allyn & Bacon.

Canon, H. J., & Brown, R. D. (Eds.). (1985). *Applied ethics in student services.* San Francisco: Jossey-Bass.

Conoley, C. W., Conoley, J. C., Ivey, D. C., & Scheel, M. J. (1991, July/August). Enhancing consultation by matching the consultee's perspectives. *Journal of Counseling and Development, 69,* 546–548.

Conyne, R. K., & O'Neil, J. M. (Eds.). (1992). *Organizational consultation: A casebook.* Newbury Park, CA: Sage.

Corey, G., Corey, M. S., & Callanan, P. (1993). *Issues and ethics in the helping professions* (4th ed.). Pacific Grove, CA: Brooks/Cole.

Coulson, W. B., & Rogers, C. R. (Eds.). (1968). *Man and the science of man.* Columbus, OH: Merrill.

Crego, C. A. (1985). Ethics: The need for improved consultation training. *Counseling Psychologist, 13*(3), 473–476.

Dixon, D. N., & Dixon, D. E. (1993, July/August). Research in consultation: Toward better analogues and outcome measures. *Journal of Counseling and Development, 71*(6), 700–702.

Dougherty, A. M. (1992, February). Ethical issues in consultation. *Elementary School Guidance and Counseling, 26,* 215–220.

Downing, J., & Downing, S. (1991, April). Consultation with resistant parents. *Elementary School Guidance and Counseling, 25,* 296–301.

Drucker, P. (1974). *Management: Tasks, responsibilities, practices.* New York: Harper & Row.

Duke, D. L. (1993). Removing barriers to professional growth. *Phi Delta Kappan, 74*(9), 702–704, 710–712.

Erchul, W. P., & Conoley, C. W. (1991, February). Helpful theories to guide counselors' practice of school-based consultation. *Elementary School Guidance and Counseling, 25,* 204–211.

Ethical Code for the International Association of Marriage and Family Counseling. (1993, January). *Family Journal: Counseling and Therapy for Couples and Families* (American Counseling Association, Alexandria, VA), *1*(1), 73–77.

Fisher, L., & Sorenson, G. P. (1985). *School law for counselors, psychologists, and social workers.* New York: Longman.

Froehle, T. C., & Rominger, R. L. III. (1993). Directions in consultation research: Bridging the gap between science and practice. *Journal of Counseling and Development, 17,* 693–699.

Fuqua, D. R., & Newman, J. L. (1989, December). Research issues in the study of professional ethics. *Counselor Education and Supervision, 29*(2), 84–93.

Gallessich, J. (1982). *The profession and practice of consultation: A handbook for consultants, trainers of consultants, and consumers of consultants' services.* San Francisco: Jossey-Bass.

Garn, K. F., Gelwick, B. P., Lamb, D. H., McKinley, D. L., Schoenberg, B. M., Simono, R. B., Smith, J. E., Wierson, P. W., & Wrenn, R. L. (1982). Accreditation guidelines for university and college counseling services. *Personnel and Guidance Journal, 61,* 116–121.

Gibson, W. T., & Pope, K. S. (1992, January/February). The ethics of counseling: A national survey of certified counselors. *Journal of Counseling and Development, 71,* 330–336.

Gilchrist, L. A., & Stringer, M. (1992, February). Marketing counseling: Guidelines for training and practice. *Counselor Education and Supervision, 31,* 154–162.

Gross, D. R., & Robinson, S. E. (1985, September). Ethics: The neglected issue in consultation. *Journal of Counseling and Development, 64,* 38–41.

Gross, D. R., & Robinson, S. E. (1987, March). Ethics, violence, and counseling: Hear no evil, see no evil, speak no evil. *Journal of Counseling and Development, 65,* 340–344.

Hall, D., & Barker, L. W. (1988, Spring). Pursuing private practice in consultation. *Association for Counselor Education and Supervision Consultation Network Newsletter, 1*(2), 1–3.

Hopkins, B. R., & Anderson, B. S. (1990). *The counselor and the law* (3rd ed.). Alexandria, VA: American Association for Counseling and Development.

Huey, W. C., & Remley, T. P., Jr. (1988). *Ethical and legal issues in school counseling.* Alexandria, VA: American Association for Counseling and Development.

Hummel, D. L., Talbutt, L. C., & Alexander, M. D. (1985). *Law and ethics in counseling.* New York: Van Nostrand Reinhold.

Jennings, C. L. (1992). The growing importance of multiculturalism for independent consulting. In A. Vaux, M. S. Stockdale, & M. J. Schwein (Eds.), *Independent consulting for evaluators.* Newbury Park, CA: Sage.

Kelley, R. E. (1981). *Consulting: The complete guide to a profitable career.* New York: Charles Scribner's Sons.

Kurpius, D. (1985, July). Consultation interventions: Successes, failures, and proposals. *Counseling Psychologist, 13*(3), 368–387.

Kurpius, D. J., & Fuqua, D. R. (Eds.). (1993a, July/August). Consultation I: Conceptual, structural, and operational dimensions [Special issue, vol.1] *Journal of Counseling and Development, 71*(6).

Kurpius, D., & Fuqua, D. R. (Eds.). (1993b, November/December). Consultation II: Prevention, preparation, and key issues [Special issue, vol. 2]. *Journal of Counseling and Development, 71*(7).

Lakin, M. (1988). *Ethical issues in the psychotherapies.* New York: Oxford University Press.

Lenning, W. (1992, December). Ethical codes and responsible decision-making. *Guidepost* (ACA Newsletter), p. 21.

Levenson, J. L. (1986, January). When a colleague practices unethically: Guidelines for intervention. *Journal of Counseling and Development, 64,* 315–317.

Levy, C. S. (1976). *Social work ethics.* New York: Human Sciences Press.

Lippitt, R. L. (1983). Ethical issues and criteria in intervention decisions. In S. Cooper & W. F. Hodges (Eds.), *The mental health consultation field* (pp. 139–151). New York: Human Services Press.

Lowman, R. L. (1985, July). Ethical practice of psychological consultation: Not an impossible dream. *Counseling Psychologist, 13*(3), 466–472.

Mabe, A. R., & Rollin, S. A. (1986, January). The role of a code of ethical standards in counseling. *Journal of Counseling and Development, 6,* 294–297.

Martin, R. P. (1983). Consultant, consultee, and client explanations of each other's behavior in consultation. *School Psychology Review, 12,* 35–41.

Metzger, R. O. (1993). *Developing a consulting practice.* Newbury Park, CA: Sage.

Robinson, S. E., & Gross, D. R. (1985, July). Ethics of consultation: The Canterville ghost. *Counseling Psychologist, 13*(3), 444–463.

Robinson, S. E., & Gross, D. R. (1986, January). Counseling research: Ethics and issues. *Journal of Counseling and Development, 64*(5), 331–333.

Rubin, S. E., & Rice, J. M. (1986). Quality and relevance of rehabilitation research: A critique and recommendations. *Rehabilitation Counseling Bulletin, 30,* 33–42.

Schein, E. H. (1993, July/August). Legitimating clinical research in the study of organization culture. *Journal of Counseling and Development, 71*(6), 703–708.

Shore, M. F., & Mannino, F. V. (1983). Accountability and economics in consultation. In S. Cooper & W. F. Hodges (Eds.), *The mental health consultation field* (pp. 119–138). New York: Human Services Press.

Smith, D. K., & Lyon, M. A. (1986). School psychologists' attributions for success and failure in consultations with parents and teachers. *Professional Psychology: Research and Practice, 17*(3), 205–209.

Tannenbaum, S. I., Greene, V. J., & Glickman, A. S. (1989). The ethical reasoning process in an organizational consulting situation. *Professional Psychology: Research and Practice, 20*(4), 229–235.

Thompson, A. (1983). *Ethical concerns in psychotherapy and their legal ramifications.* New York: University Press of America.

Tuller, L. W. (1992). *Cutting edge consultants: Succeeding in today's explosive markets.* Englewood Cliffs, NJ: Prentice-Hall.

Van Hoose, W. H., & Kottler, J. A. (1985). *Ethical and legal issues in counseling and psychotherapy: A comprehensive guide* (2nd ed.). San Francisco: Jossey-Bass.

Welfel, E. R., & Lipsitz, N. E. (1983). Wanted: A comprehensive approach to ethics research and education. *Counselor Education and Supervision, 22,* 320–332.

Whiteley, J. M. (Ed.). (1983). Counseling in prisons [Special issue]. *Counseling Psychologist, 11*(2), 27–34.

Witt, J. C. (1987). Linking research and practice: Issues in research methodology and the utilization of knowledge. *School Psychology Review, 3,* 274–275.

Witt, J. C., & Elliott, S. N. (1983). Assessment in behavioral consultation: The initial interview. *School Psychology Review, 12,* 42–49.

PART FOUR

Looking Ahead

The future is the central theme of Part IV. Whether preparing for a career, currently practicing, or providing education and training, psychological consultants are, in a very real sense, agents of change. The future must be introduced into their preparation, since technological advances and social changes are rushing far ahead of existing graduate education and training programs.

Regardless of the settings in which psychological consultants work, their consultees (individuals, families, groups, organizations, institutions) are already being overwhelmed by the rapid pace of change; therefore, they are seeking the assistance of psychological consultants to help them prepare for that change. Part IV is directed both to those who wish to become psychological consultants and to those currently practicing, whether they practice full- or part-time.

CHAPTER TWELVE
Becoming a Consultant

Although already widely practiced, psychological consultation is still an emerging profession. Most psychological consultants today began as full-time practitioners in their professional specialties and were drawn to psychological consultation by consulting opportunities that emerged during their careers. Many, though originally having no intention of becoming full-time consultants, found the challenge invigorating and decided to make a career change. Chapter 12 provides information that either full- or part-time practitioners will find helpful. The topics covered range from the personal characteristics and skills of successful consultants, to preparation, markets and marketing, advantages and disadvantages of incorporation, liability, tax planning, charging and collecting fees, and establishing an independent practice or partnership or joining or creating a consulting firm.

CHAPTER THIRTEEN

Trends in Psychological Consultation

We are convinced that psychological consultants must be aware of current decisions and trends likely to shape the future of the field. Chapter 13 discusses seven trends that futurists and consultants in the field identified as most likely to exert an impact on the next generation: information technology, computer technology, globalization, demographics, educational reform, biotechnology, and industrial modernization and robotics. As John Naisbitt noted more than two decades ago, high-tech calls for high-touch. With their knowledge, skills, and experience in human development and organizational behavior, psychological consultants are in position to play a vital, high-touch role in the years ahead.

◆ CHAPTER TWELVE

Becoming a Consultant

Even a cursory review of the literature reveals that the paths taken to a career in psychological consultation are both numerous and varied. Few, if any, of today's psychological consultants entered college with the specific goal of becoming a consultant. Weinberg (1985), who asked a number of consultants why they decided on a career in consultation, believed the choices of many could be classified as "accidental." That is, the subjects of Weinberg's informal survey of practicing consultants did not consider their entry into consultation a matter of careful decision making, but rather something that just seemed to happen to them. "Evolved" might be a more descriptive term, since those interviewed spoke of a series of accidents rather than a single event.

While Bandura (1986), a social-cognitive personality theorist, would undoubtedly disagree with such a simplistic explanation, he, too, recognized that **chance encounters** (unintended meetings with previously unknown persons) could exert a tremendous impact on the paths one takes in life. For example:

> Assigned to teach the introductory course in a graduate counselor education program, Jim Simpson (a fictitious name) decided to introduce the course with a mini-workshop that addressed the skills necessary to effective listening. To encourage student participation and involvement early in the course, he prepared a number of experiential exercises that would demonstrate how effective listening requires the listener to *hear* more than words. He also invited an experienced counselor to model empathic listening with volunteers from the class.
>
> Two weeks after the workshop, Jim received a letter from an A. J. Marshall (fictitious name), vice president of national sales for a large insurance company. He informed Jim that he had occasion to overhear a group of students talking about their experiences in their first class session. Not only was he impressed with their enthusiasm, but as he listened, he was also convinced that his company's sales people could benefit from similar experiences. He invited Jim by letter to contact him if he was interested in contracting, as a training consultant, for a series of 10 regional workshops, designed specifically to improve the listening skills of the company's regional sales staffs.
>
> In brief, Jim's decision to begin his course with a workshop on empathic listening and his later chance encounter with Mr. Marshall led to his first experience as a training consultant. The fact that this experience augmented his salary as an assistant professor by $5,000, plus expenses, for conducting 10 Saturday workshops only added to his interest in finding other marketing opportunities for his professional specialty. Within two years, Jim founded a successful part-time practice and left teaching to become an independent psychological consultant.

University professors often work as part-time consultants. While they have no intention of leaving their academic careers, they enjoy their consulting endeavors and only select consulting engagements compatible with their academic responsibilities. A colleague of one of the authors is a fairly typical example. Like the example given earlier of the full-time consultant, the career of the author's colleague is also marked by unexpected circumstances and chance encounters and opportunities:

> Unable to find an opening for a counseling psychologist position in the location he preferred, he accepted the only position available—consultation and education (C&E) specialist in a mental health agency. Disappointed and viewing the position as temporary,

he planned to remain with the agency only as long as it took to find an opening in his field. His doctorate program had not prepared him for consultive and preventive roles.

To his surprise, he found that the C&E position offered exciting potential—mental health work that focused on psychological education, positive growth, and mastery over stressful life situations. He began to modify his original priorities and values. He visited other C&E practitioners, assisted in community planning, joined advisory groups, and participated in governing boards for human service agencies. In addition, he volunteered for speaking engagements, seminars, and even radio talk programs. Within a year he became a technical assistant for Head Start programs in West Virginia, Kentucky, and Maryland. During his fourth year with the agency, he was awarded a major contract to coordinate an employee assistance program with a large federal program. In his fifth year, he was asked by the local school board to coordinate testing and diagnostic services for the system's special education department. Subsequently, he has served in various capacities associated with organizational consultation, training and development, and mental health consultation. After six years with the mental health agency, he accepted a tenure-track position as assistant professor in a university counselor education department. One of his academic responsibilities was to develop a graduate course in psychological consultation. Many of his former consultees, including civic, education, business, and family leaders, continue to contact him for training and consultation projects. While he presently has no plans to enter the field of consultation full time and must work around a heavy teaching schedule, neither does he plan to give up his work as a psychological consultant or to discontinue his effort to improve his knowledge and skills in this area.

A fairly common path to becoming a psychological consultant, particularly for university-affiliated consultants, is an invitation to join an established consultant or consulting team. Independent consultants or consulting firms often contract academicians when a consulting project requires a team approach, when they lack competency in a particular specialty area (such as when upgrading the technology of a business or industry creates personnel or managerial problems), or when the appearance and fact of objectivity are necessary.

While entry into psychological consultation may, at times, be accidental, long-term success in the consulting business is not. Those who have achieved continued success all agree that psychological consulting is a highly demanding and competitive profession. Their paths are more likely to be successful if they possess certain personality characteristics and professional competencies, knowledge, and skills that are "not commonly available" (Holtz, 1990). It is evident, also, that from their perspective, consulting is to be "performed as a regular activity and managed as a business" (Metzger, 1993, p. 2).

Holtz (1990), Kahn (1987), Kelley (1981), Metzger (1993), and Tuller (1992) recommend that every individual entertaining the idea of becoming a psychological consultant should first conduct a serious, objective, and comprehensive self-assessment before proceeding further in the decision-making process. They are convinced that aspiring consultants can benefit from being aware of their personal values, motives, attitudes, feelings, strengths, weaknesses, and current level of personal and professional functioning.

The same writers then address, in some depth, the personal characteristics and professional skills they believe most successful consultants possess, and they suggest that the aspiring consultant compare the results of his or her self-study with their findings. While their lists of the personal characteristics of successful consultants are based on limited research, simple surveys, and personal observations, there is surprisingly little disagreement among them.

Although certain personality characteristics are identified as desirable for consultants, no exclusive, single set of personality characteristics defines a model or ideal personality type toward which aspiring consultants should strive. Indeed, such a model would eliminate spontaneity, genuineness, and authenticity, all listed below as positive personality characteristics of successful consultants.

Personality Characteristics of Successful Consultants

As one might expect, successful people in other professions share the positive personality characteristics of successful psychological consultants. Whether by intention or coincidence, successful psychological consultants also share many of the characteristics of Rogers's (1980) fully-functioning person, Maslow's (1970) self-actualizing person, and Allport's (1955) mature person. Viewed as a group, successful consultants appear to have a rare growth-motivated personality. They constantly seek opportunities to explore their boundaries and to expand their present knowledge, skills, and experience. Two additional advantages of growth-oriented consultants, according to Dougherty (1990), are the following: "By experiencing growth in their own lives, consultants are better able to empathize with consultees about the barriers to growth that consultees normally experience and to be authentic 'role models' for those with whom they work" (p. 18).

Efficient and Objective Perceptions of Reality

Successful psychological consultants appear to have a firm grasp of reality; their perceptions are both efficient and objective: "Because they perceive their world and the people in it accurately, they are excellent judges of character and value. The false and the dishonest are easily detected and their true motives uncovered" (Wallace, 1993, p. 325). Conversely, accurate perception also leads to greater acceptance and tolerance of reality, for perfection is neither expected nor demanded. There is no need to deny reality, nor to insist that it be different. Reality for the successful consultant is neither fair nor unfair; it simply is. It should be noted at this point that "acceptance and tolerance" are not to be mistaken for uncaring passivity. Successful consultants are deeply involved in their work and are strong advocates for healthy change, both in themselves and in their consultees.

Acceptance of Self, Others, and the World

Acceptance and tolerance of self, others, and the world are significant personality traits of successful psychological consultants. Not only do they accept their own weaknesses and strengths without shame, guilt, or pride, they also accept the faults they find in others without anger, complaint, or blame. Prejudices and stereotypes are neither useful nor rational from the standpoint of successful consultants. They seek an **empathic understanding** of their consultees' problems (an understanding of their consultees' inner subjective perceptions and interpretations, without the loss of either their own sense of self or their objectivity).

Authentic and Enthusiastic Involvement in Their Work

Successful consultants find it comfortable to be themselves, to be spontaneous and genuine. While they do not permit convention to keep them from doing what they believe is ethically right and just, they do not make great issues of trivial matters. They will generally conform to rules and customs (manners and dress, for example) when they think their nonconformity might make their consultees uncomfortable.

Problem-Oriented

Successful consultants focus strongly on problems or issues. They are fully committed to their consultation tasks. They have a strong sense of responsibility and obligation to their consultees and their consultees' problems. While they rely on their own potentials and resources, they encourage and facilitate the same self-reliance in their consultees. Successful consultants do not become confused by means and ends, problems and methods. In short, they are confident, inner-directed, active agents, and their actions communicate their confidence to their consultees.

Motivated by Long-Range Goals and Plans

While successful psychological consultants live in the present, their actions are also guided by long-range goals and plans. They know what they want and where they are going. They manage their time wisely and well. When in a consultation engagement, their consultees' problems take precedence.

Skills of Successful Consultants

In addition to the knowledge and skills of their professional areas of expertise (which are assumed and not covered in this chapter), successful consultants must be in possession of a large repertoire of consultation skills. Their repertoire of skills includes, among others, consultant-consultee relationship skills, communication skills (listening, speaking, and writing), marketing consulting services skills, and management and business skills.

Horton and Brown (1990) explored the empirical research on the importance of interpersonal communication skills in consultation and found that the facilitative characteristics of consultants and their appropriate use of verbal and nonverbal skills were important in the consultation process. However, because the majority of empirical research studies available were conducted in school settings, generalizability of the findings to other settings is limited. Also, much of the research reviewed by Horton and Brown is correlational: showing a correlation of one variable to another is *not* showing cause and should not be interpreted as cause. The need for additional research in this area is evident.

Relationship Skills

While consultants' relationship skills are important throughout the consulting process, they are especially important during initial contact. Consultees have been known to decide whether they think they can work with a consultant after only a few minutes of their first meeting. In short, their decisions are subjective and often intuitive, based on a visceral feeling that they cannot explain rationally. Moreover, their first impressions are often lasting and, once formed, can be difficult to change. Only later can they give explanations such as the following: "The consultant treated me as a professional." "The individual seemed genuinely interested in our problem and sensitive to our needs." "I saw no evidence that the consultant was trying to sell us a prepackaged program or viewed our problem from a skewed or biased perspective." "The person just looked honest—like someone I felt I could trust."

Because most individuals are unaware of the nonverbal messages they send to others at first meetings, consultants may benefit from role-play situations involving three other people—one to play the role of a prospective consultee, and two to serve as objective observers. Videotaping is also helpful, since it permits consultants to observe their own nonverbal messages. What messages are the consultant's posture and gait as he or she enters the room sending to the prospective consultee? How do the consultee and observers rate the consultant's eye contact? What message did the prospective consultee receive from the consultant's handshake? What distance does the consultant keep between himself or herself and the consultee? Is the consultant dressed appropriately for this first meeting? How much time does the consultant spend listening? Talking? When listening, does the consultant seem to hear what is being said? Does the consultee detect any offensive odors—strong perfume, aftershave? Does the consultant's body language and speech patterns indicate that he or she is relaxed? Nervous? Hesitant? Self-conscious? What are the observers' overall ratings and specific recommendations for change? Often awareness alone is enough to change a consultant's nonverbal behaviors that interfere with a positive consultant-consultee relationship.

Doing some homework before the first meeting is also helpful to the consultant. Knowing something about the consultee and the consultee's agency/business/institution before the meeting can also be valuable. For example, in the case of an agency, who are the agency's clients and what services does the agency provide? How many professionals does the agency employ? What are their specialties? Does the agency also employ nonprofessional personnel? What are their duties? Is the agency governed by a local, state, or federal board of directors? Who is the chief administrator? Will this person attend the first meeting? Has anything been in the news about this agency recently that an informed consultant should know? Wise consultants will make it their business to enter an initial interview situation as fully prepared as possible.

Communication Skills: Listening, Speaking, and Writing

The performance of expert consultants in their professional specialties is irrelevant if they are unable to convey their expertise convincingly to their consultees. Effective communication and marketing skills are a must. To succeed in a highly competitive business, consultants must be able to sell themselves and their services. Prospective consultees want to meet the experts offering solutions to their problems, particularly problems they are unable to resolve themselves or cannot fit into the present work flow. They want to know if these are qualified people they can trust and with whom they can work. They are fully aware that anyone today can call himself or herself a consultant, and they are often skeptical, especially if they have had poor experiences with consultants in the past. Their skepticism causes many today to insist on competitive bidding.

Consulting requires the preparation and delivery of numerous oral and written presentations and reports. Without good listening, speaking, and writing skills, consultants have little chance of success.

Listening Skills   Of the three communication skills (listening, speaking, and writing), successful consultants assign highest priority to listening. Skilled listeners hear more than words. They employ attending skills that provide them with other valuable sensory information. For example, successful consultants are open to the nonverbal, physical behaviors of their consultees—posture, eye contact, facial expressions, hand and arm gestures, pace of speech, voice tone, emphasis placed on certain words, silences, and time given to ideas and topics. Paying attention to consultees' perceptions, interpretations, feelings, attitudes, and values gives consultants added information that they can use to understand their consultees and their consultees' problems. This close attention has numerous benefits for both consultants and consultees.

Perhaps one of the greatest benefits for consultants is that, by concentrating on attending skills, they are less prone to accept the consultees' initial statement of the problem and so can avoid offering advice based on too little information. Empathic, nonjudgmental responses from consultants encourage consultees to explore their problem in depth and also set the conditions that enable consultees to become actively involved in working toward solutions. Successful consultants are aware that initial presenting problems are often more likely to be descriptions of symptoms than of root cause. For example, the problem presented to a consultant by an agency department head during their initial meeting was the inability of her staff to learn the skills necessary to integrate new technology into the department's work-flow system. She wanted the consultant to design and conduct a training program to teach these skills. When asked what had been done internally, she said that she had made a number of attempts, but none seemed to work. Suspecting that the consultee was describing symptoms rather than cause, the consultant requested an opportunity to become better acquainted with the new technology and to interview individual staff members. She quickly learned the following:

1. The new technology would, indeed, improve the department's work-flow system. Not only would it eliminate repetitive steps in the present system and reduce errors, it would also speed the work-flow process considerably.

2. The skills necessary to integrate the new technology were not difficult and should be fairly easy to teach in a short period.

3. The department staff had not been involved in the selection of the new technology, nor had they been informed of the rationale for its purchase—a new government regulation that would significantly increase the number of clients using the services the department provided.

4. Lacking this knowledge, the staff concluded that the department head's motivation for purchasing new technology was to reduce department operation costs by reducing the number of staff required to do the work. In short, they were convinced that learning the skills necessary to integrate the new technology would cost many of them their jobs. Only by extending the learning period would they have the time they needed to find other positions.

5. Once the consultant discovered that the cause of the problem was not *inability* but rather *fear and reluctance,* the consulting problem was redefined and its solution became fairly simple: Inform the staff of the new government regulation and the projected increase in clients. Assure them that their jobs were not in jeopardy, and develop a short-term retraining program to teach the skills they needed to develop. Had the consultant not listened as carefully as she did during the initial contact, she might have accepted the consultee's presenting problem and accepted the request to develop a training program.

By giving their full energy, time, and attention, consultants communicate their respect for the consultees, their patience, and their genuine interest in helping. This approach not only helps establish an egalitarian and collaborative consultant-consultee relationship, but it also demonstrates that consultation is a personal service requiring the collaborative effort of all involved.

Metzger (1993) is convinced that consultants with good listening and attending skills learn more than those who lack these skills:

> Frequently, interviews with client principals generate as much or more valuable information and facts for defining problems and developing solutions as any other source of data, including questionnaires and attitudinal surveys. However, the effectiveness of the interview and the robustness of the information surfaced from those interviews are predicated on the consultant's listening skills. (p. 10)

Speaking Skills　To become an effective, dynamic speaker requires a great deal of practice. To this end authorities in the field of consultation, regardless of specialty, recommend that those preparing to become consultants accept every opportunity to hone their speaking skills. For example, Metzger points out that successful consultants do not limit the state, regional, and national conferences they attend to those of the associations in their professional specialties. Rather, they make a point of learning about the associations of targeted consultees and submit applications to present papers, research reports, training workshops, or seminars:

> Because most business people get tired of hearing from their own specialists year after year, conference after conference, if you are able to deliver a solid talk that provides practical new insights and advice to your audience, there is every reason to believe you will get additional offers to speak, not only at future industrial conferences, but also at key meetings held by industrial leaders within their own companies. (Metzger, 1993, p. 25)

Metzger further offers sound advice to consultants making presentations to conference groups:

1. "Never plan to talk for more than 30 or 45 minutes" (p. 26). The remainder of the allotted time should be a question-and-answer period.
2. "The smaller the audience (25–50), the better" (p. 26). Large audiences are less intimate and not conducive to effective marketing of your ideas and consulting practice.
3. "Always be sure to know who is in your audience" (p. 26). Without this knowledge it is impossible to tailor your presentation to their needs.
4. "No matter how much you want to say to your audience, pare it down to a few key information points that you believe your audience should understand, and stick to getting those three or four information points across—no more or you risk losing your audience" (p. 26).
5. "Whether you have been given 30 minutes or 75, your talk should start by telling the audience what you are going to say, say it crisply and practically, and then close by telling your audience what you just said" (p. 26). Forceful repetition is the basis of all marketing and advertising.
6. "Never talk as a scholar to a group of executives. Speak as an executive to other executives. Use the clinical 'we' whenever possible" (p. 26). Identification with your audience is crucial to your credibility as an expert.
7. "Use visuals, preferably overhead transparencies, to make key points or to demonstrate conclusions from your statistics, and have hard copies in case the fifth estate is present, have at least two copies of your complete talk available as a handout" (p. 27).
8. "Contrary to popular myth, do not start or end your business speech with a joke to warm up your audience" (p. 27).
9. "Practice, practice, and practice" (p. 27).
10. "Always try to influence which speaking slot you will be assigned at conferences and conventions" (p. 27). Morning programs are preferable. Avoid the last hour of the last day—few, if any, will attend.

Writing Skills   Though often underrated in the literature of consultation, clear and concise writing is an essential skill of successful consultants (Holtz, 1990; Kahn,

1987; Kelley, 1981; Metzger, 1993). Kahn (1987), who lists the ability to write clearly as "Primary Consulting Skill No. 4," is emphatic about the importance of writing: "If you are comfortable with the three previous skill categories—analyzing, organizing, and speaking—but have some discomfort about writing, don't even think about going into the consulting business until you have improved your writing abilities to a high degree of confidence" (p. 17). Metzger (1993) also views writing as a *critical* consultant skill. In Tuller's (1992) ten "universal areas of knowledge" for tomorrow's consultants, outstanding communication skills hold fifth position. Few writers stress the importance of good writing more than Kelley (1981).

Project Proposals. The project proposal is often the determining factor in whether prospective consultees decide favorably on consultation engagements. Successful consultants, therefore, spend a great deal of time and effort both planning and preparing project proposals. Many develop a complete work plan to be certain all information is accurate before beginning to work on their project reports. Rather than viewing project proposals as tasks that must be performed, they view their proposals as opportunities to demonstrate what they can do for their consultees.

Proposal formats vary, depending on the type, complexity, and cost of the consulting engagement. For small, short-term projects, suitable for the independent consultant, a letter of understanding may be sufficient. Complex, long-term projects that involve greater risks for both consultants and consultees, that are open for competitive bidding, or that require a complete cost/price analysis, call for more formal, written, project proposals that consultees may study, evaluate, and consider at length. The procurement process may take between three and sixteen months. Since proposals are written with the consultees' needs in mind, they should include all elements pertinent to those needs.

Kelley (1981) suggests that consultants choose the report headings they believe are applicable to their specific situations from the headings listed in Box 12.1. Space limitations in a single chapter make it impossible to comment on each of the 17 progress report headings Kelley suggests. However, 10 that should appear in nearly every proposal merit some elaboration:

1. *Introduction.* The purposes of the introduction are, first, to demonstrate to the consultee that the consultant understands the consultee's problem and the facts associated with it (Greenbaum, 1990); second, that the problem is indeed serious enough to merit outside consultation; and third, that the consultant is interested and qualified to give that help. The consultant's competence is mentioned repeatedly throughout this book, but it cannot be overemphasized that consultants should not accept a consulting project for which they lack the necessary capabilities and expertise.

When the consultant realizes the consultee's problem is complex and that there are a number of possible causes, he or she may suggest that it will be necessary to define the consulting project's objectives and scope more clearly. The consultant should then present an approach to do this.

2. *Purpose and Goals of the Proposed Engagement.* The consultant presents the purpose and goals in terms of specific and measurable outcomes. Progress can later be measured against these goal statements, by both the consultant and the consultee.

Box 12.1
Kelley's (1981) suggested progress report headings (See pp. 306–307)

1. Table of Contents
2. Introduction
3. Purpose and Goals of the Proposed Engagement
4. Estimate of Benefits
5. Approach, Scope, and Plan
6. Project Schedule and Management Plan
7. Nature of Final Output
8. Progress Reports the Client Can Expect
9. Pricing Summary
10. Qualifications, Staffing, and Ethics
11. Use of Outside Consultants
12. Role of Consultee's Personnel
13. Support of Top Management
14. Function of Steering Committee, If Any
15. Disclaimers
16. References (Written permission required)
17. Summary

---

3. *Estimate of Benefits.* Under this heading, the consultant describes anticipated benefits of the consulting project to the consultee. The consultee should not interpret the anticipated benefits as promises.

4. *Approach, Scope, and Plan.* Here, the consultant defines, as precisely as possible, the parameters of the proposed consultation services. Procedures and techniques, however, should be presented in general terms. The intent of the proposal is not to present a plan the consultee can use as a blueprint to conduct the consulting project himself or herself (for example, the proposal could mention the use of structured interviews or questionnaires without including the questions; a measurement of personality characteristics but not the specific instrument could be cited).

Later problems may be avoided if the consultant presents his or her policy on the issue of confidentiality in this section of the proposal. It is vital that consultees and the employees and clients of the consultees' organization understand that what they say to the consultant, unless life-threatening to self or someone in the organization, will be considered confidential.

5. *Project Schedule and Management Plan.* Here the consultant outlines, in chronological order, each major stage to be performed, and specifies the timing of each stage of the project and the flow of tasks (time charts and flowcharts are helpful). Here, also, the consultant outlines the management procedures for the consultee to implement. The consultant must then fulfill the project schedule, since the consultant's relia-

bility will be judged in terms of his or her ability to meet these deadlines. In meeting obligations on a timely basis, the consultant models expected consultee behavior.

6. *Progress Reports the Client Can Expect.* The consultant informs the consultee of the frequency and timing of progress reports. Consultees want to be kept informed of the progress of the consulting project, especially if the project is to run for weeks or months. If the progress reports do not appear in the project proposal, cost of preparation may not be billed to the consultee.

7. *Pricing Summary.* The pricing summary is an explanation of *all* fees, type of fee arrangement, billing procedures, and timing of bills. It is important to show a clear relationship between costs and services. Make certain, also, that these are understood to be estimates. If the consultee requests a flat, not-to-exceed fee, consultants must specify that work that adds to the scope of the proposed project or follow-up work, which is unpredictable at the writing of the proposal, is to be billed at additional hourly rates. This is especially true when the consulting project is organizational development, where revisions, changes, user instruction, and other follow-up work may be required. Consultants cannot charge for follow-up work based on a not-to-exceed fee without a follow-up hourly rate agreement.

A **bracket-fee** arrangement (hourly based, but with a fixed limit) also favors consultees by protecting them from cost overruns. New consultants are discouraged from accepting either **fixed-fee contracts** or bracket-fee contracts, especially if the consulting problem is novel or complex. Inexperienced consultants should also avoid **contingent fees** (no fee until the consulting result is judged successful) and **deferred fees** (consultant fee spread over an extended period) except under special circumstances.

8. *Role of Consultee's Personnel.* The consultant outlines the help expected from the consultee's executives and staff. If at all possible, specify people, duties, and time required. Unless an organization's middle managers, supervisors, and staff know that the consultant is there by the mandate of the top administrator or board of directors, the consultant stands little chance of their full involvement in the consulting process, particularly if the consulting process calls for even minor disruptions of the organization's work flow or after-hours work of the organization's employees or clients.

9. *Support of Top Management.* Support of top management is crucial to the project's success. Here is the place to ensure that top managers communicate their support to all concerned. The consultant should be explicit in requesting this support.

10. *Disclaimers.* In this section of the project proposal, spell out in clear language any restrictions on the consultant's responsibility (for example, benefits depend not only on the consultant's efforts but also on the consultee's decisions, actions, and support; success requires the cooperation of all involved in the consulting effort).

Progress or Interim Reports   Regular progress or interim reports throughout the consulting project enhance communication between consultants and consultees. Consultees appreciate being kept informed of the consulting project's progress. In addition, regular reports provide them with a sense of personal involvement in the project, particularly when they are given the opportunity to review the report draft *before* finalization and when significant objections are accommodated (Lippitt & Lippitt, 1973). Progress and interim reports that supply consultees with visible evidence that consultants are working hard on their behalf also increase their acceptance and appreciation (Kelley, 1981). Finally, if these goals are achieved, consultees are more likely to accept the consultant's recommendations in the final report and, more important, assist in their implementation. They are also more likely to seek the consultant's assistance if problems arise in the future.

Progress and interim reports also benefit consultants. They document verbal exchanges that might otherwise be forgotten, "any substantial departures from the initial proposal or contract warrant," and "any new or important event during the project" (Kelley, 1981, p. 187). Finally, progress and interim reports also have legal value should any disputes emerge either during or after the consulting project.

Final Report   Both Kahn (1987) and Kelley (1981) remind their readers that a consultant's image and reputation will be affected (favorably or unfavorably) by that "final report"—the end product of most consultants' work. Kahn states that "long after your assignment has ended, that report will be evidence of your consulting abilities. It is, in many ways, your ultimate 'calling card'" (p. 15). The final report may also generate future consulting business.

The goal of the final report, according to Kelley (1981), is evaluation that, when performed well, "acts as a quality-control mechanism, a learning device, a legal protection, and a marketing tool" (p. 208). The final report serves as documentation that the consultant has completed the consulting project's objectives, including any modified objectives that might have been added and agreed to during the consultation process. The final report should assess and report the consultees' long-term benefits.

As stated above, preparing and writing the final report can be a unique and valuable learning experience for the consultant. It is an opportunity to compare this project with similar projects performed earlier. The comparison can then be used to determine what might be done differently in future projects. For example, was the approach satisfactory? Were the assessment instruments the best available? Were the progress reports timely and informative? Are there ways to improve the recommended innovations? Are there ways to reduce costs? Could the same results be achieved with fewer client expenditures? Were all outcomes of the project proposal or contract met?

The final report should also be a learning tool for the client. Could the client use the report to solve the same problem later, either without or with limited consultant assistance? In brief, the final report should not only document the consultant's efforts on behalf of the client, but also teach the client what he or she might do if the same problem should arise later.

One purpose of the final report is to serve as some protection should later legal issues arise. Not only is the final report evidence of the consultant's professionalism and effectiveness; along with the project proposal, it is evidence that all objectives were in fact met.

Also, the final report can be an effective marketing tool. When pleased with the consultant's final report, the consultee is likely to call on the consultant if he or she requires outside assistance with future problems. Satisfied clients are also more likely to refer business or professional associates to the consultant who has willingly and continually documented his or her consulting efforts.

The final report usually marks the termination of the consulting relationship. Exceptions are consulting projects that call for specific follow-up visits or periodic evaluation reports by the consultant. If the final report is clear and comprehensive to the consultee, it helps pave the way to a smooth ending of a successful consulting experience.

Marketing Skills

Independent consultants addressing the subject of becoming a consultant in their writings *all* stress the importance (indeed, the necessity) of marketing their consulting services (for example, Holtz, 1990; Kelley, 1981; Metzger, 1993; Tuller, 1992; Weinberg, 1985). While possession of current knowledge and skills in the consultant's professional specialty certainly holds top priority from our standpoint, knowledge and skills alone, though necessary, do not guarantee a successful consulting practice. Marketing is also a key factor in the development of a successful, long-term consulting practice. It must, therefore, be granted high priority, whether the consulting practice is full or part time. Without consultees there is no consulting practice.

Unfortunately, few, if any, of the psychological consultants in practice today have had any training or experience in marketing, accounting, finance, management, or taxes. We find it interesting to note how many of the writers we have cited in this chapter included among their reasons for writing the secondary gain of marketing their consulting services (Holtz, 1990; Kelley, 1981; Metzger, 1993; Tuller, 1992). Though their reasons for placing so much emphasis on the importance of marketing varied, there was surprising agreement. For example:

1. They all knew of knowledgeable, skilled, and personable consultants whose businesses failed because they were unaware of or ignored the importance of regular marketing practices.
2. They are all aware that marketing methods, techniques, and tools are seldom included in the graduate programs of the consultants' professional specialties.
3. They are also aware that professionals attracted to psychological consulting are often reluctant to market their services. Indeed, some view active marketing practices as unprofessional.
4. They are personally acquainted with new consultants who became too dependent on a few, first, long-term clients and were totally unprepared and forced out of business when these clients unexpectedly did not renew their contracts.

Business and Managerial Skills

Psychological consultants considering an independent, full-time practice are confronted with a number of difficult questions (many of which call for answers that must come from outside their professional training):

- Should they incorporate?
- Should they retain a lawyer?
- Should they seek the services of an accountant?

- Should they purchase professional liability insurance?
- Should they recruit associates or partners?
- What is the best way to finance their new practice?

While it is not our intention to advise you on decisions you will be required to make, some advantages and disadvantages of certain decisions should be discussed. Before making any final decisions, however, psychological consultants considering a full-time, independent practice should confer with an attorney and tax expert.

Should the New Consultant Incorporate?   As with most of the questions just cited, incorporation has both advantages and disadvantages. The most obvious advantage, according to Holtz (1990), Kelley (1981), and Metzger (1993), is that incorporation limits the consultant's liability: "If someone sues your corporation, and even gets a judgment against it, your personal property is normally immune to that judgment" (Holtz, 1990, p. 76). Incorporation will require additional bookkeeping and accounting tasks and a few extra taxes. These disadvantages may be balanced, however, by the tax shelter advantage of incorporation.

Second, the costs of incorporation are not prohibitive. The forms are simple for an uncomplicated **close corporation** (one held "closely" with limited participation—stocks cannot be sold to the public).

Should the New Consultant Retain a Lawyer?   This question should probably be reworded. There are numerous reasons for retaining a good lawyer. Holtz (1990) cites the following: to do things for you that require legal expertise and/or familiarity with the system, to advise you as a legal expert, to advise you as an objective observer, and to represent you and your interests (p. 78). A better question might be: How do I find a lawyer who will not attempt to make my business decisions, and who will not only give advice but also explain the rationale for that advice in language I can understand? While most independent consultants may want the assistance of a lawyer to set up and organize the consulting practice, once these tasks are completed, the lawyer's services will only be needed if legal problems arise.

Does the New Consultant Need an Accountant?   We do not intend to teach even the rudiments of accounting in this chapter. We also do not intend to recommend specific record and bookkeeping systems for psychological consultants starting an independent practice. First, we are not qualified. Second, as Holtz (1990) so clearly points out, although every business, including the small, independent consulting practice, is required to keep records,

> the actual functions and elements of the system may vary widely from one organization to another, depending on several variables, chief of which are the size of the organization, the nature of the organization's activities, and the nature of the accounting system itself. (p. 80)

Third, the space allotted to a single subheading of a chapter makes even a superficial introduction to records and bookkeeping a formidable task. What, then, are our purposes? Since most counselors, psychologists, and social workers will require the assistance of an accountant to design or select and set up their record and bookkeeping systems and to complete their quarterly local, state, and federal tax reports, we recommend that they conduct a careful search for the "right" person. It is assumed that consultants want an accountant who can explain the system they design or select in a language they can understand, one who will listen carefully and patiently to their questions and give the time necessary to answer them, and one whose advice is worth serious consideration but who also leaves the final decisions to them. To find these qualities in an accountant, ask other consultants who retain an accountant who they use and whether or not they are satisfied and why. Ask them, also, how satisfied they are with the record and bookkeeping systems they currently employ. Check accounting software programs on the market and discuss those that you think might appeal to you with a computer expert to be certain they will work with your present hardware and memory capacity. He or she may also be able to refer you to small business owners who use the program.

While most psychological consultants starting a consulting practice are aware that an accounting system is necessary for tax purposes, few understand that the true purpose of an accounting system is to furnish them with the information they need to make sound management decisions. Ledger figures on overhead costs, sales figures, costs of sales, markup, and profit enable the manager of a consulting practice "to discover almost immediately any increases in cost, decline in sales, slippage in profitability, and relative profitability of one type or sale of product [consulting engagements] over another" (Holtz, 1990, p. 83). When starting their consulting practice, independent consultants can easily become so involved in the activities of a consulting project that they are unaware that costs are higher than their practice can bear for more than a short period, and neglect to take timely action to correct the problem.

The New Consultant's Office   It should be evident at this point that consultants, whether or not it is their intention, are continually projecting personal and professional images to their prospective and contracted consultees. We have attempted to demonstrate how a consultant's personality characteristics; relationship skills; listening, speaking, writing, and marketing skills; and business and management skills may influence the image of the consultant perceived by a prospective or contracted consultee. At least part of the consultee's image of the consultant is also shaped by physical and material factors: the location of the consultant's office, parking facilities, office decor and furniture, office space (for example, reception area, conference room), and quality of the corporation's brochures, logo, stationery, letterhead, and business card.

Depending on the emphasis consultees place on these factors, each contributes (favorably or unfavorably) to their views of the consultant's image. While it can be rationally argued that the physical and material factors listed have little to do with a consultant's area of expertise or capabilities as a consultant, consultees' perceptions of a consultant's image are seldom rational. Yet to ignore their perceptions could be costly, especially to the new consultant embarking on a highly competitive business venture.

Writers in the field (Greenbaum, 1990; Kelley, 1981; Metzger, 1993; Tuller, 1992) agree that many new consultants begin their consulting businesses from an office in their homes. For most who do, it is a simple matter of economics. A home office reduces considerably the start-up costs of a new business. By converting a room in their home to an office, they avoid the rent and utilities of outside office space. They eliminate the costs of commuting and parking. They can hold equipment costs to a minimum: desk chair, lamp, typewriter, bookshelves, briefcase, filing cabinet, appointment book, stationery, brochures, and business cards. Indeed, if they already own most of the furniture and equipment, initial purchases may be limited to reference materials (books, journals, newspapers), the installation cost of a second telephone line, and the cost of an answering machine or answering service. They may consider hiring a secretary on an as-needed basis, provided they can find an agency that offers satisfactory lead and turnaround time. Finally, they would be well advised to carry additional insurance: professional liability, automobile, property and casualty, health and life.

Tuller (1992) recommends, and we agree, that consultants who can afford it should consider investing in a high-quality computer, letter-quality printer, fax machine, and business software. Also, "every office today should have basic software for accounting, word processing, financial forecasting and analysis, data base storage, desktop publishing, and telecommunications" (Tuller, 1992, p. 55). Not only will this help keep administrative work to a minimum, but it will also increase the speed and accuracy of records management, communications, marketing and report generation, data retrieval, and travel arrangements.

In addition to reduced start-up costs and the ability to deduct the percentage of the home space used for an office from certain household expenses (utilities, house payments, property taxes, and telephone bills) for tax purposes, working at home has other advantages. These advantages include being closer to family; being away from office gossip, politics, and power struggles; no longer being subject to the whims of a supervisor; and the freedom to manage one's own time and schedules.

Consultants working from their homes are also likely to experience some disadvantages. Those who enjoy close relationships with their fellow workers, or who are stimulated by sharing ideas with others, may find the isolation of working at home distracting or even depressing. Some find concentration difficult with the normal family activities at home (for example, the sounds of television and stereo, a barking dog, a baby crying). They may also find it too easy to go to the kitchen for a cup of coffee or a snack. Their children may not be able to understand that Mom or Dad are at work when they can hear them in their office at home. Consultees visiting the consultant at his or her home office may form an entirely different image from the image formed during a presentation in a conference room. From their viewpoint, the consultant may seem less professional, less impressive, less competent outside the formal trappings of a business setting. They are accustomed to perceiving an invitation to a business associate's home as a social event, not a place to conduct serious business, review a project proposal, negotiate a contract, or reveal their business concerns and needs.

Education and Training of Successful Consultants

As we pointed out throughout this book, there is a growing need for graduate education programs in consultation, and the educational institutions and professional associations of the mental health specialties are responding to this need by adding consultation theories, strategies, methods, and techniques to their curricula. In addition, national, regional, and state professional associations in the fields of counseling, psychology, and social work are offering seminars and workshops for members considering a career in consultation. Professional associations are also encouraging their members to submit articles on consultation for publication in their journals, newsletters, monographs, and handbooks.

In 1986, the American School Counselor Association (ASCA) listed competencies in consultation in its professional development guidelines for secondary school counselors. In 1988, theories on applications of consultation became a program accreditation requirement of the Council for Accreditation of Counseling and Related Programs (CACREP). That year, the Association for Counselor Education and Supervision (ACES) also published two handbooks on consultation (Brown, Kurpius, & Morris, 1988).

Numerous surveys indicate that school psychologists rate consultation either very important or most important of all the functions they perform (for example, Martin & Meyers, 1980; Smith & Lyon, 1985). Further, school psychologists typically express a desire to spend more time consulting with school administrators, teachers, and parents (Cook & Patterson, 1977; Hughes & Falk, 1981). The interest of school psychologists in consultation is manifest also in the increased quantity and quality of articles published in their journals in the past two decades.

Unfortunately, the gap today between consultation practice and training remains wide. Furthermore, a number of serious obstacles block any significant closure of this gap in the near future. The graduate programs of the psychological specialties from which consultants are recruited (psychology, counseling, social work), while endorsing the consulting role of their specialty, offer only minimal explicit preparation of consultants. The reasons for this vary but include, among others:

1. Their established programs are tightly scheduled and largely inflexible.
2. The majority of present faculty possess only limited training and experience in the consultation process.
3. The budgets of many higher education systems have been cut to the point where only specialty requirements are being met.
4. Difficult professional and political decisions are required before systematic and sequenced training in consultation can be developed and incorporated into existing graduate programs.

According to Conyne and O'Neil (1992), the greatest shortcomings of present programs are: (1) the expansion beyond mental health consultation to organization consultation, and (2) the development of quality supervised practice similar to the supervised practice now present in most counseling and psychotherapy graduate programs.

Although consultation is not new, relatively few of today's consultants received their training in formal graduate courses. Rather, they learned through trial and error while on the job. Some of the more fortunate may have served an informal apprenticeship under a mentor. Informal training has its shortcomings, such as a credibility problem due to lack of credentials and lack of supervision.

The education program typically recommended for consultants is divided into three areas, patterned after the graduate programs for counselors and clinical psychologists:

1. Didactic classes to provide the needed knowledge bases
2. Laboratory experiences or practica to provide behavioral skills
3. Supervised field experiences or internships to provide judgmental competencies

Brown (1985) and Brown, Pryzwansky, and Schulte (1987) believe that unless research contradicts these recommendations, the effective training program will involve all three of the training modalities just listed. Didactic courses alone are inadequate, for it is in the practicum that trainees gain feedback from their consultees, and where the level of the trainee's consultation skills are determined.

Before a formal graduate training program for consultants can receive wide acceptance, specific competencies must be carefully and clearly identified and defined. Brown, Pryzwansky, and Schulte (1987) believe the trend may be toward two separate specialties—organizational and human services consultation. However, they point out that until there is empirical evidence for key competencies, we will have to settle for the recommendations of professional groups.

Summary

Although empirical research on the personality characteristics of effective and successful psychological consultants is sparse, there is nonetheless a high degree of general agreement among the writers in the field, whose opinions admittedly are based on informal interviews, questionnaires, and personal observations. For example, successful consultants are reported as having interpersonal and communication skills similar to those found in research to be facilitative in the therapeutic relationship: they are trusting and growth-oriented, accepting and nonjudgmental, genuine and spontaneous, caring and respectful, and skilled in empathic listening and responding. In addition, successful psychological consultants are self-motivated and efficient time managers; indeed, they possess many of the personal characteristics of entrepreneurs.

While professionals with expertise in psychology, counseling, and social work have many of the personality characteristics mentioned above, few have the necessary knowledge, training, and experience to manage a successful business enterprise today, including an independent consulting business. Unless they join an established consulting firm or team, or work for an extensive period with a mentor, psychological consultants will need to acquire business knowledge and skills: marketing skills, information on setting and collecting fees, accounting and bookkeeping skills, and knowledge of tax laws, liability needs, and the advantages and disadvantages of incorporation. In short, while they need not be experts in every area, they must know when and where to seek expert assistance in areas where they lack knowledge and experience (for instance, an accountant to set up an adequate bookkeeping system, a tax expert, a reliable attorney, an interested banker).

Glossary

Bracket-fee   A consulting fee based on an hourly rate but held to a fixed limit.

Chance encounters   Unintended meetings with previously unknown persons.

Close corporation   A corporation held "closely" with limited participation—stocks cannot be sold to the public.

Contingent fee   No fee until the consulting result is judged successful.

Deferred-fee   A consulting fee spread through installments over an extended period.

Empathic understanding   Understanding another person by attempting to sense that person's inner world and feelings—in a sense becoming that person without losing one's self and objectivity in the process.

Fixed-fee contract   A consulting fee that is not to exceed a fixed limit.

ANNOTATED BIBLIOGRAPHY

A comprehensive resource for anyone contemplating a career as a psychological consultant, Herman Holtz's book *How to Succeed as an Independent Consultant* (2nd ed., 1990) should be required reading. Holtz's definition of consulting is unique but worth considering. He does not view consulting as a profession in itself; rather, he defines consulting as "a way of practicing a profession." Professionals who turn to psychological consulting "change only the arrangements under which they offer their services and often the kind of individuals and organizations for whom they render their services" (p. vi). Psychological consulting, then, is a specialty within a profession—the profession in which they consult is the prime identifier of what consultants do and is of critical importance in marketing their services.

In *How to Succeed as an Independent Consultant,* Holtz (1990) grants special emphasis to the skills of marketing and sales—skills he considers absolutely necessary for survival in a highly competitive business. He also stresses the importance of communication skills, both speaking and writing. Chapter 8, "Proposal Writing: A Vital Art," is the best discussion of this topic that we have found in the consulting literature. Readers who wish to pursue this subject in even greater depth may want to read Holtz's other books.

Robert Kelley, consultant, teacher, and recipient of the Consulting Psychology Award, addresses his book *Consulting: A Complete Guide to a Profitable Career* (1981) to both consultants and consultees. As mentioned earlier in this chapter, those considering whether to leave their primary specialty area to begin an independent consulting practice will find the self-assessment exercises in Chapter 2 of Kelley's book well worth reading. Chapters 2 through 7 focus on establishing an independent consulting practice. In Chapters 8 through 15, Kelley instructs his readers on how to conduct a consulting assignment. Readers will discover that Kelley not only tells them *what* to do, but also *how* to do it. It is worth noting that he does both without resorting to jargon, a plus for the inexperienced consultant or the consultant in training.

Both experienced and inexperienced consultants will find answers to many of their questions in this book. For example: How do I identify and contact target clients? How should I set fees? What is the best way to formulate recommendations? And how do I implement them?

We found Kelley's book clearly written, interesting, and comprehensive. While Kelley is naturally positive about consulting as a challenging career, the self-assessment exercises and his words of caution throughout the book present a realistic view of the difficulties and hazards of starting any new business.

Lawrence W. Tuller's book *Cutting Edge Consultants: Succeeding in Today's Explosive Markets* (1992) is an excellent source for psychological consultants, particularly those who think they may want to work as management consultants in business and industrial settings. Tuller, a management consultant for over 15 years when writing this book, discusses in some depth 8 general areas of knowledge vital to doing a quality job, regardless of which market niches a consultant chooses. His own market areas include banking and finance, communication skills, and personal computers. Independent practitioners, new consultants, consultants in preparation, and consulting firms doing business with smaller clients will find Tuller's suggestions and strategies informative and helpful.

Cutting Edge Consultants also describes a business increasingly dominated by global competition, new technology, cross-border financing, and multinational mergers. In addition, the book discusses the skills required to take advantage of the 14 "hottest markets" and the "most important trends" for consultants. Other topics of interest include recommended marketing techniques, organization and staffing structures, and billing methods—areas not usually included in the curricula of graduate programs in psychology, counseling, and social work.

REFERENCES AND SUGGESTED READINGS

Allport, G. W. (1955). *Becoming: Basic considerations for a psychology of personality.* New Haven, CT: Yale University Press.

Bandura, A. (1986). *Social foundations of thought and action: A social cognitive theory.* Englewood Cliffs, NJ: Prentice-Hall.

Brown, D. (1985). The pre-service training or supervision of consultants. *Counseling Psychologist, 13,* 410–425.

Brown, D., Kurpius, D. J., & Morris, J. R. (1988). *Handbook of consultation with individuals and small groups.* Alexandria, VA: Association for Counselor Education and Supervision.

Brown, D., Pryzwansky, W. B., & Schulte, A. C. (1987). *Psychological consultation: Introduction to theory and practice.* Boston: Allyn & Bacon.

Brown, D., Spano, D. B., & Schulte, A. C. (1988, June). Consultation training in master's level counselor education programs. *Counselor Education and Supervision, 27,* 323–330.

Burrus, D., with Gittines, R. (1993). *Technotrends: How to use technology to go beyond your competition.* New York: HarperCollins.

Conoley, J. C. (1981). Emergent training issues in consultation. In J. C. Conoley (Ed.), *Consultation in schools: Theory and research procedures.* New York: Academic Press.

Conyne, R. K., & O'Neil, J. M. (Eds.). (1992). *Organizational consultation: A casebook.* Newbury Park, CA: Sage.

Cook, V., & Patterson, J. C. (1977). Psychologists in the schools of Nebraska: Professional functions. *Psychology in the Schools, 14,* 371–376.

Dougherty, A. M. (1990). *Consultation: Practice and perspectives.* Pacific Grove, CA: Brooks/Cole.

Gazda, G. M., Asbury, F. R., Balzer, F. J., Childers, W. C., & Walters, R. P. (1991). *Human relations development: A manual for educators* (4th ed.). Boston: Allyn & Bacon.

Greenbaum, T. L. (1990). *The consultant's manual: A complete guide to building a successful consulting practice.* New York: Wiley.

Hall, D., & Barker, L. W. (1988, Spring). Pursuing private practice in consultation. In *Consultation Network: Newsletter of the Association for Counselor Education, 1*(12), 1, 3–4.

Holtz, H. (1990). *How to succeed as an independent consultant* (2nd ed.). New York: Wiley.

Horton, G. E., & Brown, D. (1990, March/April). The importance of interpersonal skills in con-sultee-centered consultation: A review. *Journal of Counseling and Development, 68*(4), 423–426.

Hughes, H. N., & Falk, R. S. (1981). Resistance, reactance, and consultation. *Journal of School Psychology, 19*(2), 134–142.

Hughes, J. N. (1979). Consistency of administrators' and psychologists' actual and ideal percep-tions of school psychologists' activities. *Psychology in the Schools, 16,* 234–239.

Kahn, S. (1987). *Getting into the consulting business.* Stamford, CT: Longmeadow Press.

Kelley, R. E. (1981). *Consulting: A complete guide to a profitable career.* New York: Charles Scribner's Sons.

Lippitt, G., & Lippitt, R. (1973). *The consulting process in action.* La Jolla, CA: University Associates.

Martin, R., & Meyers, J. (1980). School psychologist and the practice of consultation. *Psychology in the Schools, 17*(4), 478–484.

Maslow, A. H. (1970). *Motivation and personality* (3rd ed.). New York: Harper & Row.

Metzger, R. O. (1993). *Developing a consulting practice: Survival skills for scholars* (Vol. 3). Newbury Park, CA: Sage.

Parsons, R. D., & Meyers, J. (1984). *Developing consultation skills.* San Francisco: Jossey-Bass.

Pressman, R. M., & Sieger, R. (1983). *The independent practitioner: Practice management for the allied health professional.* Homewood, IL: Dorsey.

Rogers, C. R. (1980). *A way of being.* Boston: Houghton Mifflin.

Smith, D. K., & Lyon, M. A. (1985). Consultation in school psychology: Changes from 1981–1984. *Psychology in the Schools, 22,* 404–409.

Tuller, L. W. (1992). *Cutting edge consultants: Succeeding in today's explosive markets.* Engle-wood Cliffs, NJ: Prentice-Hall.

Vaux, A., Stockdale, M. S., & Schwerin, M. J. (Eds.). (1992). *Independent consulting for evalua-tors.* Newbury Park, CA: Sage.

Wallace, W. A. (1993). *Theories of personality.* Needham Heights, MA: Allyn & Bacon.

Weinberg, G. M. (1985). *The secrets of consulting: A guide to giving and getting advice success-fully.* New York: Dorset House.

CHAPTER THIRTEEN

Trends in Psychological Consultation

Chapter Overview

Current Trends and the Future of Psychological Consultation
Information Technology
Computer Technology
Globalization
Demographics
Educational Reform
Biotechnology
Industrial Modernization and Robotics

Trends in Certification and Licensure

Opportunities Awaiting Psychological Consultants

Summary

Glossary

Annotated Bibliography

References and Suggested Readings

◆ It is not the purpose of this chapter to predict the long-term future of psychological consultation or to present possible alternative scenarios for psychological consultation in the 21st century. Past and current attempts at prediction by futurists have only resulted in diverse and conflicting views. Part of the difficulty is that readers can find confirming evidence for whatever view they hold of the future. Those who fear the destruction of the planet and the annihilation of humanity can find writers who present convincing evidence to confirm their fear. Those who believe that new technology of the 21st century will bring resolution to the many complex problems they face today can find substantive evidence, often accompanied by presentations of utopian scenarios, to support their beliefs.

Why, then, include a chapter on trends?

1. We are convinced that psychological consultants *must* be forward thinkers.
2. We can, with some degree of safety, predict that psychological consultation will change in the next ten years.
3. We can predict, also with some confidence, that those changes will often be unanticipated and will emerge in unexpected ways.
4. By focusing on current decisions and trends that we believe hold high potential for the future of psychological consultation, we can examine an array of alternative directions.
5. If present decisions and trends do contribute to the shape of the future, psychological consultants are already well into it. In short, to quote Margaret Mead (in Toffler, 1972): " 'The Future is Now' " (p. 50).

Current Trends and the Future of Psychological Consultation

Futurists have identified current global, interrelated trends that they believe may profoundly alter the future of individuals, institutions, businesses, industries, nations, and even current views of reality. While futurists recognize that the permanence of the trends they identify is always in doubt and that the accuracy of their forecasts depends on variables that are unknown and, in many instances, unknowable (for example, human fallibility and politics and new scientific discoveries and technological advances), they insist that today's consultants need to understand the impact of present trends on the next generation. From among the many trends that could be included, we have selected seven that we believe are of the most immediate concern to psychological consultants. Change in any one of the trends listed below will almost certainly bring change to others:

1. Information technology
2. Computer technology
3. Globalization
4. Demographics
5. Educational reform
6. Biotechnology
7. Industrial modernization and robotics

Information Technology

It is impossible to look at the current trends in information processing and not grant information technology high futurity value. The trend in information technology has been evident for some time, at least in industrialized countries, where information is recognized as a valuable strategic resource. Naisbitt (1982), for example, traced the beginning of "the information society" to the late 1950s. Toffler (1970), in one of his earlier works, refers to the years that followed as the "Second Wave" or the movement toward a postindustrial society. This was a period when a mass of information (not to be interpreted as knowledge) was collected and the electronic nets for storage and dissemination of that information were developed.

Originally created as a communications network for universities and military research sites, the **Internet** today is described by Allman, Sussman, and Pollack (1993) as "the worldwide web of thousands of computer networks linking research institutions, academia, individuals, businesses" (p. 71). Further, the Internet is a major gateway to cyberspace and is accessible to anyone with a computer, a phone line, and a **modem** (MOdulator-DEModulator to transfer acoustical or computer data). Navigating the nternet can be difficult for neophyte consultants, particularly if they want to tap all four levels: the direct-route approach, which requires the ability to operate the UNIX operating system; the dial-in direct account, through a company called an Internet service provider; a dial-in terminal, which limits the services available; and the E-mail account, which limits services to the exchange of messages. Three of the most popular and less expensive commercial, online service providers—CompuServe, Prodigy, and America Online—offer entry to the E-mail system of the Internet but as yet are not true Internet services. There is "a trend for cities to establish *free nets,* for no-cost or low-cost public access through libraries" (Lewis, 1994, p. 4), and colleges and universities often permit enrolled students and faculty to use their Internet facilities at no cost.

Today's information networks are not only offering more complex services to more people, but they are also "integrating and evaluating data, drawing automatic inferences, and running input through sophisticated models" (Toffler, 1990, p. 116). In short, the trend toward information technology has not hit a plateau. The ultimate impact of information technology on world cultures remains in question. But "this 'leap' to a higher level of diversity, speed, and complexity requires a corresponding leap to higher, more sophisticated forms of integration. In turn, this demands radically higher levels of knowledge processing" (Toffler, 1990, p. 81).

Because the trends presented in this chapter are interrelated, we will elaborate on the information technology trend—particularly its dependence on advances in computer technology (voice commands, parallel processing, artificial intelligence, completion of the installation of fiber optics, and so on)—in discussing the other trends. Rapid access to information also enhances the consultant's potential to solve problems. Specialized information and innovative ideologies, for example, are only seconds away.

Networks are egalitarian. They are no longer reserved for a small group of computer-elite practitioners. Information, today, is as accessible to the independent consultant as it is to the large consulting firms. Indeed, any individual who possesses the computer hardware and is willing to put forth the effort to learn a few skills can tap the information networks. According to Cook et al. (1994), search languages—which will soon accommodate voice requests for information in English—will make obtaining information easier for consultants.

Perhaps most important, networks also give independent consultants instant contacts and the opportunity for dialogue with others in their field around the globe, a distinct advantage for those who feel the isolation of working alone or who wish to benefit from the advice and experience of other consultants in their own and related specialty areas. In addition, consultants can learn from and participate in ongoing practice and research efforts. Future psychological consultants may not choose to wait for published research data. From the submission of a final manuscript to publication, many of today's professional journals are at least a year (and sometimes as many as three) behind in publishing final reports of research.

Computer Technology

The history of computer technology is one of rapid and continuous advancement. During the past decade, especially, the speed, functions, and memory of computers increased significantly while the cost of these advances declined. Applications of computer technology during the same period resulted in a broad range of labor- and cost-saving effects. Business, industry, and more recently, service organizations have all profited from the introduction of computer technology. Further, more and more families are purchasing computers for the home, and, as Naisbitt (1982) predicted, this will "soon be followed by a software implosion to fuel it" (p. 26). Add to this their interconnection in ramified networks and there will be a profound effect on the way families relate to each other and organize their lives (Shane, 1987).

The demands and implications of computer technology for psychological consultants cannot be overestimated. Computers are a strategic resource for consultants who must master the tools and stay informed of recent advances in their profession, or they will be left behind by those who do. It is crucial that psychological consultants continually upgrade their knowledge and skills through retraining and continuing education. They must stay informed of the latest software (management, scheduling, accounting, recordkeeping, tax, statistics, personnel testing, word processing, and database programs), not only for themselves but also because they are working with consultees and organizations who expect consultants to be familiar with current technology. Almost all psychological consultants could benefit from one of the more sophisticated portable computers in their briefcases, along with software designed to assist in problem-solving tactics and methodologies for common consultation problems, a database for storing forms and proposals, and a word processing program for preparing memorandums, letters, and reports.

Human-computer interaction is already recognized as an area in great need of research:

> As more and more offices, factories, hospitals, and small businesses are using micros, word processors, and the like, the more important the relationship between the person and the machine becomes, in terms of productivity, health, career development, and work roles. (Hollway, 1991, p. 159)

Most futurists and psychological consultants are optimistic about the impact of microcomputers. They point to the many present and possible ways that people can benefit from becoming electronic collaborators. Burrus (1993), however, warns: "In the end, it is not as important to know what to do with technology as it is to know what technology does with us" (p. 18).

Shane (1987) is also convinced that psychological consultants should explore unexpected patterns in the human-computer relationship. He advocates the expansion of

ergonomics (the science of improving the physical relations between people and their machines) to encompass "**psycho**ergonomics"—the study of psychological stress resulting from the "interaction of mind and machine" imposed by human-computer relationships (p. 19). As an educational consultant, Shane (1987) reports that when children age four to six are introduced to computers, they carry on a dialogue with the computers as if they were human, much the way they talk to a doll or a pet. While he does not consider this phenomenon harmful, he also reports that adolescents, both male and female, who become intensely involved in computer and video games for prolonged periods may develop attacks similar to epilepsy. This phenomenon he views with greater concern. Shane is also concerned that the overuse of computers at an early age could impoverish the imagination and creativity of some users.

Until longitudinal research studies reveal more about the human-computer relationship, parents will have to assume responsibility for preventing their younger children from becoming completely attached to the computer. Looking back at the profound influence of television on family life, it is evident that this will be no small accomplishment. Again, psychological consultants may be called on to assist parent and teacher groups concerned about the impact of human-computer relationships on children.

Toffler (1980) is more optimistic about the impact of these relationships on children. He is convinced that, as more and more children develop close relationships with computers, they "will begin to use computers with a grace and naturalness that is hard for us to imagine today" (p. 189). He also speculates that, in time, computers "can be expected to deepen the entire culture's view of causality, heightening our understanding of the interrelatedness of things, and helping us to synthesize meaningful 'wholes' out of the disconnected data whirling around us" (p. 191). Indeed, Toffler (1980), an intuitive forecaster, goes even further: "The intelligent environment may eventually begin to change not merely the way we analyze problems and integrate information, but *even the chemistry of our brains*" (p. 191; emphasis added).

Government officials, educators, and women's groups are also expressing their concern that present computer education programs are contributing to the separation of the "haves" and "have-nots" and are widening the gender gap in computer literacy. Children in wealthy families and boys in general enter school more comfortable with computers, and Ellen Hale (1995a) reports: "The gap is only magnified from there" (p. D-1). While comprehensive, long-range studies of the gender gap in computer literacy are sparse, there is evidence that it exists. Hale (1995a) cites the following as examples:

> Nationwide, women's pursuit of computer science degrees has declined nearly 20 percent since 1984. . . . Even in cyberspace, women are in short supply. Only 10 percent to 15 percent of users of on-line services are women, although the medium ideally would seem blind to gender. (p. D-1)

With their knowledge of child development and learning, psychological consultants are being called on by school administrators, teachers, and parents to help resolve the inequity in computer education. Some of the changes they recommend are:

1. Parents should hold boys and girls to the same expectations—for instance, while they often insist that their son stick with computer science courses, they permit their daughter to withdraw without objection or argument.

2. Parents should place the home computer in a neutral place (as opposed to the boy's bedroom or the father's study, for example), and instruct the children on its use and the careers that call for computer literacy. Further, children should see *both* parents using the computer. Modeling is an excellent learning strategy.

3. Schools are encouraged to offer single-gender classes in mathematics and computer sciences. If this is not possible, the Girl Scouts should be encouraged to do something in this area. Girls should have an opportunity to enroll in computer camps, clubs, and summer classes. Presently boys outnumber girls three to one in these areas (Hale, 1995a).

4. Parents and teachers should make girls aware of the subtle messages aimed at them by the media, particularly computer magazines, which often exclude women or show them performing only in clerical roles. Supportive adults should be alert for articles and pictures of professional women using the computer.

While the deadly, adversarial human-computer relationship of Dave Bowman and HAL, presented by A. C. Clarke in his book *2001: A Space Odyssey* (1968), remains consigned to fiction, some futurists do see reason to research the impact of the extensive use of computers on people, particular on young users. Does computer competency at a young age increase the use of computers to play pranks or commit crimes (for example, break codes to gain access to confidential or security files and protected software programs, introduce a new destructive virus, and steal **automated teller machine** (**ATM**) codes and cellular telephone numbers—either for personal use or to sell to others)? Who is more qualified than psychological consultants to address and research the problems arising from the human-computer relationship?

Globalization

International marketing (marketing between countries) has been a fact for many businesses and industries for some time. Montana and Charnov (1987) point out that visible proof of this is readily available: "Raise the hood of any late-model U.S. automobile" (p. 407), or visit almost any large foreign city. Engine parts bear a multiplicity of foreign manufacturing labels. U.S. products (automobiles, films, recordings, blue jeans, to name a few) are evident in the major cities of most countries. **Multinational companies** (establishing a company and doing business in a foreign host country) are also increasingly evident. Just a few examples of U.S. businesses and industries that have established branches in foreign countries are IBM, numerous fast-food chains, major automobile companies, banks, and investment firms. Global marketing and advanced technology are perhaps the two greatest reasons for this trend. The homogenization of worldwide tastes and preferences for certain products and services opens national borders and fosters opportunities for businesses and industries that want to take advantage of an expanding market. Economic reasons also contribute. Two are presented by Montana and Charnov (1987): **absolute advantage** (a country that can produce exclusively, or nonexclusively but with less cost than other countries) and **comparative advantage** (producing a product or service that other countries are unable to match in quality or price). Other reasons include: (1) a need for natural resources not available in a home country, (2) proximity to the consumer to minimize transportation costs, and (3) a significant reduction in labor costs.

Tuller (1992) is convinced that tomorrow's consultants must, as their consultees must, become globally oriented as the consulting industry matures or face oblivion. He strongly recommends that both independent consultants and consulting firms begin immediately to establish a worldwide databank of political, professional, and financial contacts.

Just as businesses and industries are opening new markets in other countries, so too must consultants look for global marketing opportunities for their consulting specialties. Those who do will soon discover that global consultation requires new knowledge and skills and appropriate licenses and registration. They recognize also that they must become familiar with the legal, political, financial, and tax anomalies of the country and region in which they plan to do business. They will often need a partner or associate in the host country. And they learn that religion, prejudice, and political connections can exert a significant impact on most international transactions; indeed, some require a synergistic blending of all three. Finally they learn that the very nature of consultation in a host country requires certain lifestyle and personality characteristics. For example, global consultants must enjoy traveling and seeing new places. They must be able to forgo the convenience of working out of the home office and work entirely on the consultee's premises. They must be flexible enough to spend lengthy periods away from family, friends, and their normal support systems. Global consultation also requires access to sophisticated methods of communicating with their home office.

Most part-time or sole practitioners, such as academics with regular teaching and research assignments, are not flexible enough to meet the requirements of global consultation. Moreover, they cannot afford extended periods in remote areas away from their home office. Even those who may be able to accept consultation assignments during summer months or a sabbatical risk losing their consultee base in their home country. Unless they have partners or an extremely competent administrative assistant to cover the home office while they are gone (for instance, marketing for new consultation projects, taking care of administrative matters, and keeping in contact with prospective and former consultees), they may find it necessary to build an entirely new consultee base when they return. Marketing is a continual process and cannot be ignored for long periods. Even long-term consulting relationships can disappear overnight.

Demographics

A current trend, not only certain but also measurable, is the surge in the world's population and the rising demographic imbalances between first- and third-world countries. As first-world countries continue to gain in wealth, technology, and good health, third-world countries see little gain in these areas. Present and evolving **demographic** trends (vital and social statistics of populations—births, deaths, immigration, and so on) will create new and exacerbate present needs and problems in practically every work setting of psychological consultants.

MacFarquhar (1994) warns that future demographic problems depend on whether stabilization of birth rates occurs in certain heavily populated countries, particularly

China, India, Pakistan, Indonesia, Brazil, and Nigeria. The population of China presently numbers 1.2 billion and is growing at about 14 million annually, despite an active program aimed at zero population growth.

> If China had grown at the same rate as India over the past decade, the world would have 70 million more people today. India is due to add 500 million people and overtake China as the world's most populated country by 2040. (MacFarquhar, 1994, p. 57)

Regardless of what actions nations take to curb population growth, the population of this planet will almost certainly double in the next century. Thus, "humanitarian disasters . . . are a herald of the new era of resource limits" (Budiansky, 1994, p. 58). Demographers concur that population must be recognized as a global problem rather than a problem of any single nation. Moreover, so long as the gap continues to widen between the "have" and "have-not" societies of the world, "have-not" families will continue to stream to the "have" societies, not only in search of food but also to share the improved living standards found there.

The United States, which has the most lenient immigration policies of the developed countries, will continue to be viewed by immigrants from less fortunate countries as the most desirable and most accessible destination. While there are rival and often different forecasts on demographic trends in the United States (usually due to differences in their estimation of illegal migrants and faulty census methods), Naisbitt's (1982) references to California as the "Ellis Island of the 1980s" and Miami as the "Gateway to the Caribbean and to all of South America," though dated, seem an accurate summation of most current demographic reports and forecasts for the United States. The enormous influx of Spanish-speaking immigrants during the 1980s gave the term *diversity* a new dimension for the cities of Los Angeles, New York, Miami, Chicago, and San Antonio, and they may be joined by other cities. Indeed, according to Naisbitt (1984), "By the 1980s, the U.S. had the fourth largest Spanish speaking population in the world" (p. 246). There has also been a significant increase in the Asian population in the United States, in particular from Vietnam and China.

Kennedy (1993) points to significant changes *within* the present population of the United States. For example, by the early 21st century there will be many more people 60 years of age or older. This group "is forecast to leap to 52 million in 2020 and 65.5 million in 2030" (p. 311). As members of this group retire in increasing numbers, their replacements will become more and more difficult to find, particularly in areas that require a high degree of education and technical knowledge and skill.

Any sudden shift in demographics (whether caused by migration or immigration, loss or gain in businesses or industries, or decrease or increase in a particular age group) will almost certainly create a number of serious, complex, and interrelated problems in the city or state affected. Because city and state officials often lack the knowledge and problem-solving skills necessary to resolve these problems, they will be forced to look to consultants for assistance. For example, a sudden significant increase in immigration can create an equally sudden increase in the number of unemployed, a rapid drain on financial resources that, in turn, affects the budgets of the city's and state's human service agencies (for example, employment, social work, health, housing). The city's and state's infrastructure—education system, highway system, water purification system, trash disposal system, police and fire departments—may also swiftly become inadequate. With high unemployment, city and state taxes are diminished. Youth, particularly the more educated, migrate to other states where there are employment opportunities for jobs at the level of their preparation. With a significant loss of this age group, new businesses and industries that require educated and skilled workers are far more difficult to attract. Crime is also likely to increase during high levels of unemployment. The unemployed are less likely to have medical insurance.

As demographic transitions exert pressures on cities, states, and geographic regions to either resolve or accept the consequences of inaction, the need for consultants should intensify. Indeed, there are tremendous opportunities for consultants with expertise in such crucial areas as the following: attracting new businesses and industries, developing education and training programs to upgrade the technical skills of the unemployed, and developing opportunities for entrepreneurs desiring to start new business ventures. In short, consultants will be needed in all strategic planning and development activities.

Educational Reform

Psychological consultants working in educational settings (see Chapter 6) need to be aware *now* of the current perceptions of trends in education if they are to anticipate and plan for the changes they and their consultees may face in the future. Educators at every level (early childhood education through graduate school) are being pressured to improve not only their academic standards and programs but also their social service offerings.

It is already evident that some current trends for change in education are in conflict. Evident, as well, are the many demands for change in education being legislated by federal and state government bodies—often without additional funding. One of the greatest challenges facing psychological consultants in educational settings may well be helping their consultees arrive at a consensus on which of the current trends have the greatest potential for reaching into the future and then, in collaboration with their consultees, determining the order in which these first-intensity trends should be articulated and addressed.

Funding the many changes that educators will have to confront in the next decade poses an equally great challenge, particularly if the present trend of declining federal and state funding for education continues. Educational systems at all levels are being forced to do more with less. Restraints are being placed on new programs, and funding for present programs is being cut. Special education programs are being reduced by integrating the students of these programs into regular classes. Many student personnel programs have undergone restructuring while simultaneously being charged with meeting the needs of an ever-increasing diversity in the student population, greater retention of enrolled students, and educational programs in substance abuse, career planning and placement. Indeed, schools are being asked to address the many ills of society.

Practically all colleges and universities are seeking alternative funding resources. Grant writing has become an art form and a major topic of faculty development programs. Contracts with businesses, government agencies, and industries for special research projects, once limited to the major research institutions, are now being actively sought by graduate schools in the sciences, medicine, and business across the country, despite the problems introduced by this action (for instance, ethics, outside control of participants, and publication of research; see Chapter 6).

Biotechnology

Kennedy (1995) defines **biotechnology** as "any technique that uses living organisms or processes to make or modify products, to improve plants or animals, or to develop microorganisms for specific use" (p. 70). Barker (1992; see also Naisbitt & Aburdene, 1990) forecasts universal applications for biotechnology, not only in medicine and agriculture but also in such areas as polymer manufacture, computer chip design, education, and energy. Despite biotechnology's potential for abuse and the questions about its ethical, legal, and social implications that will no doubt increasingly arise as the millennium approaches, there seems little reason to believe the trends in biotechnology will either slow or reverse. Indeed, it is far more likely that advances in the field will increase at an even more rapid pace.

The global imbalances in food supplies and health, already great, promise to get worse (Kennedy, 1993). Because overpopulation in second-world countries has already produced resource wars, exacerbated ethnic tension, contributed to social instabilities, fueled external expansionism, and created mass migrations to first-world countries, the potential of biotechnology to feed hungry nations and solve many health problems increases the funding of research in these areas (Naisbitt & Aburdene, 1990; Kennedy, 1993).

Biotechnical applications on growing food in the field and creating synthetic products in vitro can both speed and increase the production of food (Naisbitt & Aburdene, 1990). They can also create a revolution in food production and, in doing so, affect farmers with redundancy and eliminate the jobs of truckers and food store companies. In short, biotechnology offers both to ease and to complicate a global food problem. While psychological consultants are not directly involved in biotechnology, they can play a vital role in assisting individuals, communities, and industries to adopt biotechnical applications.

Industrial Modernization and Robotics

The accuracy of the predictions made by some futurists (Boyette & Conn, 1992; Clarke, 1968; Naisbitt, 1982; Naisbitt & Aburdene, 1985, 1990; Toffler, 1970, 1972, 1980; Williams, 1983) is astounding. Many are realized, some surpassed, and a few, such as robotics, err in timing and await fulfillment. **Multisensory robots** (computers that are mobile, programmed to perform a variety of jobs, and reactive to their environment) are not yet a reality, or at least not yet in use and functioning in the numbers predicted. Smart robots are not likely to displace "50 to 75 percent of all factory workers" before the end of the century (Naisbitt, 1982, p. 23), nor are they likely in the same period to perform all the complex tasks predicted in the farming, mining, lumber, and space industries. However, with the development of sophisticated sensors and input devices, it is only a matter of time before they do this and more.

The reasons that advances in robotics have been slower than anticipated are not limited to technology or even cost, which is great. Indeed, today's newest computers have adequate memory capacity and processing speed. One of the greatest obstacles is the perceived high risk of negative human reaction and rejection, not only of those displaced by the robots but also of society in general. Many business and industrial managers have, therefore, limited the application of robotics to ways that do not threaten people (such as jobs considered too hazardous or too demeaning, repetitive, or dirty for humans).

In the future, robots will be applied beyond the dangerous jobs. Their use will erode employment opportunities for both unskilled and skilled workers: "Britain's national trade unions have demanded that no new technology be introduced unilaterally by management" (Naisbitt, 1982, p. 23). Where the adversarial relationship between management and organized labor exists, union leaders view robotics not only as management's way to control labor as the application of robotics becomes more widespread, but also as a way of dehumanizing workers. Here again, psychological consultants are in position to help managers deal with the highly controversial issues raised by extensive applications of robotics. Replaced workers will need the help of experts as they assess their career options, seek new jobs, or look for training opportunities to acquire new job skills (see Chapter 9).

Trends in Certification and Licensure

As indicated earlier in this book (see Chapters 1 and 11), psychological consultants are usually professional specialists (for example, psychologists, counselors, and social workers) who chose either to practice consultation as a career or to augment the practice of their professional specialty by working part time as consultants. As we pointed out in Chapter 11, most are members of professional associations and societies in their specialty areas and are, therefore, obligated to adhere to the ethical codes of their particular professional affiliation. Many are also licensed or certified to practice in their professional specialty and so are regulated by the laws of the states in which they practice.

While the licensing and/or certification of psychological consultants is often a topic of debate, not only for consultants and their consultees but also for legislators and government officials, Kelley (1981) reminds readers interested in this topic that "currently, no government laws regulate consulting. Some consulting associations award certificates to consultants who meet certain minimum standards. These certificates carry no legal meaning, nor do they indicate that consultants without them are inferior in training or competence" (p. 234).

Just as the differences in the ethical codes of the psychological consultants' primary or related professional affiliations create dilemmas in a consulting practice, problems in dual licensing or credentialing are almost certain to arise. One of the first questions asked in a discussion of licensure is, "If I already possess a license to practice as a psychologist/counselor/social worker in this state, why must I obtain another license to consult in that field?" Many successful independent consultants have no desire and see no reason to give up their freedom. Others argue that licensing in psychological consultation is premature at this time, that psychological consultants should wait until consulting competencies, training, and standards are more clearly defined, or until psychological consultants can establish commonly accepted principles or procedures for the practice of consultation in this area. Still others point out that, because psychological consultation is fragmented into a number of specializations, psychological consultants must form a corporate group (a professional association or society) to establish commonly accepted principles or procedures for the practice of psychological consultation. Gallessich (1982) strongly recommends interassociation exploration of a generic code of ethics and regulations by professional organizations whose members practice consultation. Opponents to the views just cited argue that psychological consultants have waited far too long, and warn that if they do not act soon, others (state and federal governing bodies, for example), whose members know little about psychological consultation, will act for them.

Opportunities Awaiting Psychological Consultants

In his forecast of opportunities in consulting covering the first half of the 21st century, Kelley (1981) envisions three developmental stages for the life cycle of consultation. During the present or infancy stage, he sees the formation of numerous new consulting firms that will capitalize on a rapidly increasing need for nearly all consultation specialties. The second or adolescent stage, which begins at the turn of the century, will be marked by the rapid growth and expanding markets of the largest and strongest consulting firms. The stage of maturity, which Kelley (1981) believes will occur between 2020 and 2030, is a period when three to ten firms in each consulting specialty will dominate the world markets. Even if his forecast is correct and the domination by large consulting firms becomes a reality, Kelley (1981) assures the small consulting firms and independent consultants that technology will give them opportunities and sufficient market niches for successful practices, particularly individual consultants who lack the capital to call on the large consulting firms for assistance.

Although Tuller (1992) addresses management consultants as his primary readers, he also believes that the future holds substantial growth opportunities for all types of consultants. Further, he agrees with Kelley that the more successful, large firms will become "superpowers," forcing small and mid-sized firms to adjust, either by merging into the large forms or by downsizing to limited specialties.

As mentioned earlier in this chapter, information has become a strategic resource for decision makers at all levels in all areas. They know they must rely on consultants to provide them with the information they need to make wise decisions, and they are willing to pay for that service. The consultant who can gather, analyze, synthesize, and package available information into useful societal applications is, and for the foreseeable future will continue to be, in great demand.

SUMMARY

Numerous methods, ranging from reasoned intuition to complex mathematical formulas, are employed in attempts to forecast what changes might occur in the near and distant future of psychological consultation. The method most commonly employed by experienced consultants is based on current decisions and trends. From the many trends identified in the literature as likely to generate the greatest impact on the future, we selected seven first-intensity trends that we find most relevant to psychological consultation. These are: (1) information technology, (2) computer technology, (3) globalization, (4) demographics, (5) educational reform, (6) biotechnology, and (7) industrial modernization and robotics. In addition to the seven trends, opportunities awaiting psychological consultants and the future issues of certification and licensure are also discussed in this chapter.

GLOSSARY

Absolute advantage   In marketing, a country that can produce a product exclusively or nonexclusively but with less cost than other countries.

Automated Teller Machine (ATM)   A machine that provides automated banking services.

Biotechnology   "Any technique that uses living organisms or processes to make or modify products, to improve plants or animals, or to develop microorganisms for specific use" (Kennedy, 1993, p. 70).

Comparative advantage   Producing a product or service that other countries are unable to match in quality or price.

Demographics   Vital and social statistics of populations—births, deaths, immigrants, and so on.

E-Mail account   Limits services on the Internet to the exchange of messages.

Ergonomics   The science of improving the physical relations between people and machines. Because computers require a more intimate association than usual between people and machines, Shane (1987) refined and expanded this definition to encompass **psycho**ergonomic elements—that is, reducing *psychological* as well as physical stress created by the human-computer relationship.

Fiber optics   The use of hairlike glass fibers to replace more costly, bulky, and far less efficient copper wires. Data are received at the speed of light.

Free nets   A provider system established by some cities for no-cost or low-cost public access to the Internet through public libraries.

Global marketing   A convergence of consumer taste and value in certain product characteristics, permitting the use of universal marketing techniques.

International marketing   Marketing between countries.

Internet   The worldwide web of thousands of computer networks linking research institutions, academia, individuals, and businesses.

Megatrends   Large social, economic, and technological changes that, though slow to form, exert influence for some time. According to Naisbitt (1982), Megatrends have the scope and feel of a decade's worth of change.

Modem   MOdulator-DEModulator, a device used to transform acoustical or computer data.

Multinational company   Establishing a company and doing business in a foreign host country.

Multisensory robots   Computers that are mobile, programmable to perform a variety of jobs, and able to react to their environment.

Terminal phobia   The fear some people experience when first seated in front of a computer terminal.

ANNOTATED BIBLIOGRAPHY

Psychological consultants who want to become aware of current trends and unresolved problems that they may face in the next decade or longer cannot overlook the works of the futurists. For example, they could benefit from becoming familiar with the writings of Alvin Toffler (*The Futurists*, 1972; *Learning for Tomorrow: The Role of the Future in Education*, 1974; *Power Shift*, 1990; *The Third Wave*, 1980), John Naisbitt (*Megatrends: Ten New Directions Transforming Our Lives*, 1982), and Naisbitt and Patricia Aburdene (*Re-inventing the Corporation: Transforming Your Job and Your Company for the New Information Society*, 1985; *Megatrends 2000: Ten New Directions for the 1990s*, 1990). Though these works were published some years ago, many of the trends and problems they address are still with us and promise to remain with us well into the future. This fact alone is a tribute to the accuracy of these authors' analyses and forecasts and evidence that they were ahead of their time.

Nearly a decade since the publication of *Megatrends*, Naisbitt and Aburdene give their readers 10 new directions for the 1990s in their book *Megatrends 2000*. They help their readers understand megachanges in the areas of the arts, nationalism, women's rights, privatization, and religious revival. *Megatrends 2000* is thoughtful, analytic, and optimistic. Naisbitt and Aburdene's faith in the individual is manifest throughout their book. Psychological consultants will find the authors' structure of the 10 new megatrends valuable as they measure and revise their own worldviews, career and job decisions, and individual life goals and lifestyles.

Naisbitt and Aburdene believe technological changes will challenge and empower individuals rather than oppress or control them. Further, they present a view of the future that offers far greater opportunities for women, minorities, people with disabilities, and retirees as companies adjust to an information economy that demands intelligence and skills over brawn.

After reading Toffler's and Naisbitt's optimistic views of the future, readers will benefit from Hughes's *World Futures: A Critical Analysis of Alternatives* (1985). While Hughes agrees that the trends Toffler and Naisbitt identify are of interest and recommends that attempts "to mine these selected future studies for some generalizations" could prove beneficial, he also questions their methodology for selecting trend categories and their exclusion of certain areas of major concern (that is, food, energy, violent and other types of asocial behavior from terrorism to rape and drug abuse, and civil rights). Hughes also expresses concern that these works may reflect "the fashion of press and public attention." Hughes then outlines competing views of the future of the global development system, and the values and political structures that "provide controlling, directing, or steering mechanisms for determining which of the future alternatives we want to see evolve."

Psychological consultants, particularly those practicing or preparing to practice in educational settings, will find Harold G. Shane's 1987 monograph on future studies, *Teaching and Learning in a Microelectronic Age,* both interesting and informative. Though written especially for educators, it is an excellent resource for psychological consultants, whether they are seeking to increase their background knowledge or attempting to keep informed about how microtechnologies are entering their personal and professional lives. Shane also explores current and future developments in the use of robots, some uses and opportunities of the silicon chip, and the multilevel education and training necessary for children and adults if they are to function effectively in the microelectronic age of the future, both where they work and in their homes.

Shane's monograph includes a bibliography selected from some 1,400 references that he consulted between 1983 and 1986. In addition, he presents digests of 18 education reform reports, published during this same period, many of which continue to cause debate.

Though Lawrence W. Tuller's 1992 book *Cutting Edge Consultants: Succeeding in Today's Explosive Markets* is written primarily for business and industrial consultants— he examines such topics as new realities every consulting firm must face and focuses on a global market, new technology, cross-border financing, and multinational mergers— psychological consultants will also profit from reading this book. Of particular interest to psychological consultants are Tuller's first and last chapters, "Winds of Change" and "The Future of Consulting in a Changing World."

REFERENCES AND SUGGESTED READINGS

Allman, W. F., Sussman, V., & Pollack, K. (1993, December 6). A Baedeker for the first electronic tourist: How to begin exploring the world online. *U.S. News & World Report,* 71–72.

Axelson, J. A. (1985). *Counseling and development in a multicultural society.* Monterey, CA: Brooks/Cole.

Bardon, J. I. (1985, July). On the verge of a breakthrough. *Counseling Psychologist, 13*(3), 355–362.

Barker, J. A. (1992). *Paradigms: The business of discovering the future.* New York: Harper-Collins.

Barrow, C. W. (1993, Fall). Will the fiscal crisis force higher education to restructure? *Thoughts and Action, ix*(1), 7–24.

Boyett, J. H., & Conn, H. P. (1992). *Workplace 2000: The revolution reshaping American business.* New York: Plume/Penguin Books.

Budiansky, S. (1994, September 12). 10 billion for dinner, please. *U.S. News & World Report,* 57–58, 60, 62.

Burrus, D. (1993). *Technotrends.* New York: Harper Business.

Carnegie Council on Policy Studies in Higher Education. (1980). *Three thousand futures.* San Francisco: Jossey-Bass.

Clark, J. (Ed.). (1993). *Human resource management and technical change.* Newbury Park, CA: Sage.

Clarke, A. C. (1968). *2001: A space odyssey.* New York: New American Library.

Cohen, W. (1993, August 30–September 6). Exporting know-how: Service companies are keeping the U.S. competitive in foreign markets. *U.S. News & World Report, 53,* 56–57.

Cook, W. J., Collins, S., Flynn, M. K., Gutman, M., Cohen, C., & Budiansky, S. (1994, March). Technology: 25 breakthroughs that are changing the way we live and work. *U.S. News & World Report, 116*(17), 46–47, 48, 50–52, 56, 58–60.

Cook, W. J., Egan, J., & Cohan, W. (1993, August-September). The levitation of a giant: A bold move into cellular communication signals new direction. *U.S. News & World Report, 115*(9), 58–59.

Darling-Hammond, L. (1988). The futures of teaching. *Educational Leadership, 46*(3), 4–10.

Dougherty, A. M. (1995). *Consultation: Practice and perspectives in school and community settings.* Pacific Grove, CA: Brooks/Cole.

Drucker, P. F. (1974). *Management: Tasks, responsibilities, practices.* New York: Harper Colophon Books.

Duncan, C. F., & Pryzwansky, W. B. (1988). Consultation research: Trends in doctoral dissertations 1978–1985. *Journal of School Psychology, 26,* 107–119.

Earley, T. M., & Hulse, D. (1986, January). Humanizing a technological society: Ethical implications for the counselor. *Journal of Counseling and Development, 64,* 334–336.

Etzioni, A. (1983). *An immodest agenda: Rebuilding America before the 21st century.* New York: McGraw-Hill.

Ferguson, C. H. (1993). *Computer wars: The fall of IBM and the future of global technology.* New York: Times Books.

Flynn, M. K. (1994). Software to simplify your life. *U.S. News & World Report, 116*(1), 62.

Gallessich, J. (1982). *The profession and practice of consultation: A handbook for consultants, trainers of consultants, and consumers of consultation services.* San Francisco: Jossey-Bass.

Gallessich, J. (1985, July). Toward a meta-theory of consultation. *Counseling Psychologist, 13*(3), 336–354.

Gardner, J. W. (1984). *Excellence* (Rev. ed.). New York: Norton.

Gray, H. H. (1987). Demography as destiny. In R. M. Kidder (Ed.), *An agenda for the 21st century* (pp. 61–68). Cambridge, MA: MIT Press.

Hale, E. (1995a, February 26). Gender gap in computer literacy troubles educators, women's groups. *Herald Dispatch* (Huntington, WV), p. D-1.

Hale, E. (1995b, February 26). Is computer education kid friendly? *Herald Dispatch* (Huntington, WV), p. D-1.

Hayes, L. (1992, December). An interview with Jonathan Kozol: A simple matter of humanity. *Phi Delta Kappan, 74*(4), 334–337.

Helmer, O. (1983). *Looking forward: A guide to futures research.* Beverly Hills, CA: Sage.

Hencley, S. P., & Yates, J. R. (1974). *Futurism in education: Methodologies.* Berkeley, CA: McCutchan.

Hollway, W. (1991). *Work psychology and organizational behavior: Managing the individual at work.* Newbury Park, CA: Sage.

Hot tracks in 20 professions. (1993, November). *U.S. News & World Report, 106,* 109–112.

Howard, A. (1991). New directions for human resources practice. In D. W. Braw & Associates, *Working with organizations and their people* (pp. 219–251). New York: Guilford Press.

Hughes, B. B. (1985). *World futures: A critical analysis of alternatives.* Baltimore, MD: Johns Hopkins University Press.

Jennings, C. L. (1992). The growing importance of multiculturalism for independent consulting. In A. Vaux, M. S. Stockdale, & M. J. Schwerin (Eds.), *Independent consulting for evaluators.* Newbury Park, CA: Sage.

Johnston, W. B., & Packer, A. H. (with contributors). (1987, June). *Workforce 2000: Work and workers for the 21st century.* Indianapolis, IN: Hudson Institute.

Kelley, R. E. (1981). *Consulting: The complete guide to a profitable career.* New York: Charles Scribner's Sons.

Kennedy, P. (1993). *Preparing for the twenty-first century.* New York: Random House.

Kent, P. (1994). *The complete idiot's guide to the Internet.* Indianapolis, IN: Prentice-Hall Computer Publishing.

Kidder, R. M. (1987). *An agenda for the 21st century.* Cambridge, MA: MIT Press.

Klein, D. C. (1983). Future directions for consultation by mental health systems. In S. Cooper & W. Hodges (Eds.), *The mental health consultation field.* New York: Human Sciences Press, 221–229.

Lewis, P. H. (1994, August 15). First-time tourist guide to the Internet. *Bottom Line,* 13–14.

MacFarquhar, E. (1994, September 12). Population wars. *U.S. News & World Report,* 54–57.

Masini, E. (Ed.). (1983). *Visions of desirable societies.* New York: Pergamon Press.

Mazade, N. A. (1983). Past, present, and future. In S. Cooper & W. Hodges (Eds.), *The mental health consultation field* (pp. 233–242). New York: Human Sciences Press.

McNichol, T. (1994, January 21–23). Fellow travelers on the info highway. *USA Weekend,* 4–6.

Mead, M. (1972). The future: Prefigured cultures and unknown children. In A. Toffler (Ed.), *The futurists,* 27–50.

Milstein, M. M. (1986, July). The future of consultation in public education. *Urban Education, 21*(2), 149–168.

Montana, P., & Charnov, B. (1987). *Management.* New York: Barron's Educational Series.

Naisbitt, J. (1982). *Megatrends: Ten new directions transforming our lives.* New York: Warner Books.

Naisbitt, J., & Aburdene, P. (1985). *Re-inventing the corporation: Transforming your job and your company for the new information society.* New York: Warner Books.

Naisbitt, J., & Aburdene, P. (1990). *Megatrends 2000: Ten new directions for the 1990s.* New York: Avon Books.

Newman, D. (1992, December). Technology as support for school structure and school restructuring. *Phi Delta Kappan, 74*(4), 308–315.

Ogilvy, J. (1993, Fall). Three scenarios for higher education: The California case. *Thought and Action, ix*(1), 69–124.

Parsons, R. D., & Meyers, J. (1984). *Developing consultation skills.* San Francisco: Jossey-Bass.

Schoonmaker, D. (1994, May). Hitchhiking on the electronic highway: Want to see the world without leaving your chair? *Writer's Digest, 58,* 60–61.

Shane, H. G. (1987). *Teaching and learning in a microelectronic age.* Bloomington, IN: Phi Delta Kappa Educational Foundation.

Shane, H. G., & Shane, J. G. (1974). Educating the youngest for tomorrow. In A. Toffler (Ed.), *Learning for tomorrow: The role of the future in education* (pp. 186–196). New York: Vintage Books.

Toffler, A. (1970). *Future shock.* New York: Bantam.

Toffler, A. (Ed.). (1972). *The futurists.* New York: Random House.

Toffler, A. (Ed.). (1974). *Learning for tomorrow: The role of the future in education.* New York: Vintage Books.

Toffler, A. (1980). *The third wave.* New York: William Morrow.

Toffler, A. (1990). *Power shift: Knowledge, wealth, and violence at the edge of the 21st century.* New York: Bantam Books.

Tuller, L. W. (1992). *Cutting edge consultants: Succeeding in today's explosive markets.* Englewood Cliffs, NJ: Prentice-Hall.

Weil, R., & Bova, B. (Eds.). (1983). *The Omni future almanac.* New York: World Almanac Publications.

Williams, R. (1983). *The year 2000: A radical look at the future—and what we can do to change it.* New York: Pantheon Books.

Witmer, J. M., & Sweeney, T. J. (1992, November/December). A holistic model for wellness and prevention over the life span. *Journal of Counseling and Development, 71,* 140–148.

◆ GLOSSARY

Absolute advantage   In marketing, a country that can produce a product exclusively or non-exclusively but with less cost than other countries.

Accountability   In the consultation field, the obligation of consultants to be answerable and responsible with respect to professional commitments.

Adhocracy   Defined by Waterman (1992) as "any form of organization that cuts across normal bureaucratic lines to capture opportunities, solve problems, and get results." In an adhocracy, "the boss" is defined as the individual who has the most knowledge and skills *at the moment*. In short, knowledge is granted authority at the time it is needed.

Advocacy   An activity in which one individual supports or speaks on behalf of another. Advocates assume the role of supporters to help those who cannot help themselves.

American Association of Higher Education (AAHE)   A national professional association for both administrators and faculty in higher education. The AAHE hosts a national conference and publishes a journal, in addition to providing other services.

American Counseling Association (ACA)   The major organization of counseling professionals who work in educational, health care, residential, private practice, community agency, government, and business and industry settings. The ACA's mission is to enhance human development throughout the life span and to promote the counseling profession.

American Psychological Association (APA)   The major professional association for psychologists in the United States.

American School Counselors Association (ASCA)   One of the divisions of the ACA. The ASCA publishes two journals, one for elementary and another for secondary school counselors.

Anecdotal records   Often handwritten, informal records maintained at the discretion of a child care staff member to document a child's behavior.

Antecedents   In behavioral theory, a term describing the conditions that occur immediately before a specific behavior.

Assessment   In consultation, the multilevel process of collecting information specific to the consultation problem.

Automated Teller Machine (ATM)   A machine that provides automated banking services.

Behavioral consultation   An approach to consultation that integrates behavioral psychology and research into consultation practices.

Behavioral medicine   A broad field of health care in which psychological professionals apply principles of behaviorism in treating the behavioral elements that contribute to medical disorders. Behavioral medicine is rooted in the belief that physical illness and behavior are intimately connected.

Behavioral norms   In an organizational context, the implicit or explicit boundaries of acceptable group or organizational behavior.

Behavioral plan   In behavioral consultation, a framework through which consultees implement changes within the client's environment that eliminate problem behaviors.

Biomedical model   In medical and health care settings, a model that conceptualizes illness as a biological development in which disease is caused by the natural processes of the body or invasive external agents (bacteria, viruses, or microorganisms).

Biotechnology   "Any technique that uses living organisms or processes to make or modify products, to improve plants or animals, or to develop microorganisms for specific use" (Kennedy, 1993, p. 70).

Bracket fee   A consulting fee based on an hourly rate but held to a fixed limit.

Case-oriented consultation   A consultation practice in which consultants and consultees engage in collaboration relative to the needs and characteristics of a specific child.

Chance encounters   Unintended meetings with previously unknown persons.

Characterological distortions   In Caplan's (1970) mental health consultation model, a source of consultee–client impasse in which the consultee's psychiatric disturbances distort perceptions of the client's behavior.

Checklists   Formal or informal lists of items on which consultees and other participants identify their perceptions or other items.

Chief executive officer (CEO)   The top executive officer, responsible to a board of directors or a board of trustees.

Child development   The range of physical, cognitive, and emotional factors that make up a child's sequential growth.

Child development program   A broad description of child care programs that target the child's cognitive, physical, and emotional growth.

Client   An individual, program, or system in the care of the consultee. Clients and consultees usually have direct, formal relationships.

Client-centered case consultation   A type of mental health consultation in which a professional consultant extends specialized knowledge to help a consultee with an existing client-related issue.

Client history   A collection of information, facts, and observations that provide a developmental account of the past.

Close corporation   A corporation held "closely" with limited participation—stocks cannot be sold to the public.

Cognitive-behavior theory   A learning theory that posits that human learning integrates cognitive (thoughts, interpretations, images) and behavioral (emotions, actions) factors.

Collaboration   Cooperation between consultant and consultee in working toward consultation goals. The process of collaboration requires both parties to share information, responsibilities, and commitment to problem solving.

Collaborative team consultation   Consultation in which a variety of psychological, technological, and management specialists work together to resolve complex human resource problems or issues in order to facilitate organizational change.

Comparative advantage   Producing a product or service that other countries are unable to match in quality or price.

Compromise   A conflict resolution strategy that requires parties in conflict to agree to terms somewhere in the middle of their two positions.

Conflict   A clash in values, attitudes, or behaviors resulting from natural and expected human differences.

Conflict resolution   Planned and organized consultation applications aimed at the mediation, resolution, or management of conflicts and the enrichment of interpersonal relationships.

Consensus   A decision-making technique particularly useful when groups experience conflict over a course of action or a decision. Consensus requires all members to consent to the final disposition of the decision.

Consequences   In behavioral theory, a term that describes the conditions that occur immediately following a specific behavior.

Consultant   An individual—usually a psychological professional—who provides consultation to consultees. The consultant is assumed to have the expertise and methodological understanding necessary to help consultees resolve psychological concerns of their clients or others.

Consultation constituents   Those who participate in the planning and implementation of consultation.

Consultation evaluation   Determination of the extent to which the consultation problems have been resolved or eliminated and of the usefulness of processes and decisions contributing to such outcomes.

Consultation fit   The degree to which a consultant is matched (in terms of competencies, interests, and values) to a consultation assignment.

Consultation goals   The specific outcomes that will resolve or eliminate the problems addressed in the consultation process.

Consultation in child development settings   Refers to a broad helping process in which a psychological consultant provides assistance to an adult (teacher, aide, social services staff, parent) who has explicit child care responsibilities.

Consultation stage   An identifiable interval—consisting of specific tasks and dynamics—in the consultation process. Consultation stages tend to be loosely structured and sequenced along a developmental continuum.

Consultee   An individual, such as a human service provider, business manager, or supervisor, who requests help from a consultant. The consultee has a work-related concern regarding a client or client-related program or system.

Consultee-centered administrative consultation   A type of mental health consultation in which a professional consultant extends specialized knowledge to address a consultee's deficient administrative or program skills (Caplan, 1970).

Consultee-centered case consultation   A type of mental health consultation in which a professional consultant draws on specialized knowledge to address consultee characteristics that inhibit a client's treatment (Caplan, 1970).

Content expert   A consultant who primarily shares expertise or provides information in the problem-solving process. In this role, the problems of consultees stem more from the need for specialized information and less from deficient organizational or human processes.

Contingent fee   A fee for consultation services that is paid only when specific outcomes are realized.

Contracting   The process through which a consultant and consultee negotiate and agree on terms for working together. The contract may be a formal document, an informal agreement, or a letter of understanding.

Cost-benefit evaluation   Within the framework of consultation, comparing the value of outcomes with consultation costs (for example, fiscal, time, materials, and effort).

Council for Accreditation of Counseling and Related Educational Programs (CACREP)   An accrediting body for graduate counselor education programs. Graduate counselor education programs seeking professional program accreditation are required to perform a lengthy self-study, submit a report of the study for review, and arrange for an on-site visit of an accreditation team.

Cultural norms   Behavior based on shared philosophies, ideologies, values, and assumptions, especially about the "proper" ways to solve problems and arrive at decisions.

Deferred fee   A consulting fee spread through installments over an extended period.

Demographics   Vital and social statistics of populations—births, deaths, immigrants, and so on.

Demonstration   An experiential training method in which trainers or participants model desired interactions, skills, and other behaviors.

Diagnosis   In consultation, the act of identifying or classifying the consultation problem and its probable cause.

Direct personal involvement   In Caplan's (1970) mental health consultation model, a source of consultee–client impasse where the consultee replaces the professional relationship with a personal relationship.

Displaced discussions   Consultant-consultee interactions that avoid confrontation. A consultee's biases or stereotypes are displaced onto or approached through parables, anecdotes, or dramatic portrayals (Caplan, 1970).

Downsizing   A reduction of an organization's workforce as a method of coping with worsening economic conditions. The impact of downsizing is greatest for employees engaged in staff-oriented work or secondary production processes (staff as opposed to line positions).

Ecological factors   Within the context of child assessment, the physical, social, and psychological dynamics that surround the child.

Egalitarian   A term used to describe consultation relationships in which the consultant and consultee are considered equals. Egalitarian relationships are commonly described as "person-to-person" relationships; they are nonhierarchical.

Elicitor   A term proposed by Bergan (1977) to describe the direct and information-specific questions used by behavioral consultants to control the consultee's responses. Elicitor questions direct the content of consultant-consultee interaction.

E-mail account   Limits services on the Internet to the exchange of messages.

Emitter   A term proposed by Bergan (1977) to describe open-ended, noncontrolling questions or statements used by behavioral consultants to acquire information from consultees about a client's behavior. Emitter statements encourage consultees to respond with autonomy and spontaneity.

Empathic understanding   Understanding another person by attempting to sense that person's inner world and feelings—in a sense becoming that person without losing one's self and objectivity in the process.

Employee assistance programs (EAPs)   Programs originally designed to provide individual and group counseling to alcohol-abusing employees in business and industrial settings. Many EAPs today offer a broader range of remedial and preventive counseling services to troubled employees. Counseling may, for example, pertain to substance abuse, marriage and family problems, career planning and placement, stress, termination, and retirement.

Employee stock options (ESOs)   Stock option plans created as an incentive by companies and industries operating on the assumption that employees who own stock in the business or industry in which they are employed take greater interest in its success. Once vested, employees become "financial partners," and the success of the company or industry is in their financial interest.

Empowerment   In consultation, increasing the client's or consultee's sense of personal power. Empowered consultees are able and motivated to resolve consultation problems.

Entry stage   The period during which a consultant comes into the consultation relationship and assumes a formal helping role. Consultants enter organizations physically, psychologically, and socially.

Equifinality   A principle that emphasizes that there are no single solutions to organization systems problems and that organizational revitalization can occur through many alternative actions. The principle was defined by Katz and Kahn (1966).

Ergonomics   The science of improving the physical relations between people and machines. Because computers require a more intimate association than usual between people and machines, Shane (1987) refined and expanded this definition to encompass **psycho**ergonomic elements—that is, reducing *psychological* as well as physical stress created by the human-computer relationship.

Evaluation   Systematic and coordinated inquiries and processes that attempt to determine the positive or negative worth of activities, variables, procedures, or changes.

Evaluation design   The nature or structure of the plan for collecting data about the consultation process. The design reflects critical decisions and establishes practices relative to data collection.

Exit interview   A planned meeting, conducted during the termination stage of consultation, signaling the end of the consultation relationship.

Experiential   A term that describes a style of learning emphasizing a "learning-by-doing" format. Participants are active in the training process as they realize opportunities for interaction, rehearsal, participation, and performance evaluation.

External consultant   An independent, professional, outside consultant contracted by an organization for a specified period to assist with the resolution of a particular problem. The external consultant is separated financially, socially, and emotionally from the consultee's system.

Faculty development centers (FDCs)   Centers on college and university campuses whose goal is to make both administrators and faculty more aware of their roles in the development and support of both new and experienced faculty. FDC personnel are involved in research, program development, and follow-up evaluations.

Faculty wellness programs   Institutional programs to promote and maintain the health and overall well-being of faculty.

Family therapy   A direct service to the entire family in which parents and children participate simultaneously with a therapist to correct problems in the family.

Feasibility   Suitability and practicality of data for a particular situation and setting.

Fiber optics   The use of hairlike glass fibers to replace more costly, bulky, and far less efficient copper wires. Data are received at the speed of light.

Fixed-fee contract   A consulting fee that is not to exceed a fixed limit.

Formative evaluation   In consultation, a form of evaluation that examines the ongoing decisions, actions, and processes of consultation while they are occurring.

Free nets   A provider system established by some cities for no-cost or low-cost public access to the Internet through public libraries.

Gainsharing   An incentive based on key indicators, such as cost reduction, value added, profits produced, time saved, sales increased, services delivered, or receptivity to innovative change.

Global marketing   A convergence of consumer taste and value in certain product characteristics, permitting the use of universal marketing techniques.

Goal attainment scaling   A process of evaluating goal accomplishment in consultation in which each objective is measured with respect to the degree of accomplishment rather than in an all-or-nothing manner.

Goal setting   A stage of the consultation process during which realistic goals are devised. Goal setting presupposes the accurate assessment and diagnosis of consultation problems.

Health psychology   The area of psychology that specializes in health maintenance and disease prevention. Health psychologists are professionals who help individuals develop wellness practices, apply behavioral and psychological strategies to health promotion, and treat health disturbances with psychology as a frame of reference.

Hidden clients   The employees and clients of an organization who were not involved in the decision to seek consultation services, who may be expected to participate in a study of the organization, and who may be affected by the outcome of the consultation process.

Holistic interventions   Within the context of health and wellness, interventions that perceive the individual as a "whole" person made up of dynamic divisions or subsystems (including behavioral, psychological, and lifestyle components) capable of exerting significant influences on that organism.

Human resource planning and development (HRPD) programs   Any single definition of HRPD programs at this time would have to be so general as to be meaningless (for example, programs to enhance human resource management). First, no one program works in every business or industrial setting. Second, there are successful human resource systems at all stages of development. Third, human resource specialists and psychological consultants in business and industrial settings conceptualize their roles in HRPD programs in terms of an organization's specific needs (see **Organizational development**, below).

Informal constraints   Extensions, elaborations, and modifications of formal rules, socially sanctioned norms of behavior, and internally enforced standards of conduct.

Interface   A point of connection, overlap, or interchange where competitive groups cross boundaries to accomplish their desired result.

Internal consultant   A consultant employed within the same general setting or organization as the consultee.

International Society for Technology (ITSE)   Now an affiliate of NCATE.

Internet   The worldwide web of thousands of computer networks linking research institutions, academia, individuals, and businesses.

Intervention   In consultation, a planned method or strategy of addressing consultation problems.

Interviews   Purposeful and directed meetings, usually conversational, with one person in the interview having the responsibility for their progress and development.

Intrasystem variables   Formal and informal power structures, normative structure, role clarity, decision patterns, and formal and informal communication systems.

Jargon   Favorite terms and phrases unique to the organization that must be learned by the external consultant if much of the data gathered during the assessment stage is to be accurately interpreted.

Latent content   Hidden intent or meaning.

Learning style   A unique blend of receiving, processing, and responding to information.

Lump-sum bonus plans   Set bonus figure awards for outstanding performance that benefits the company. A lump-sum bonus may be awarded to an individual or a team.

Marketing   The total effort of consultants to convince consultees that their needs and wants can be satisfied through the consultant's services (Kelley, 1981). Emphasis in marketing is on needs rather than on services or products.

Marriage counseling   A therapeutic approach to work through marital problems. The counselor or therapist may work with either husband or wife or both.

Mediation   A process of conflict resolution in which a third party serves as an agent in conveying information or communication between parties.

Megatrends   Large social, economic, and technological changes that, though slow to form, exert influence for some time. According to Naisbitt (1982), megatrends have the scope and feel of a decade's worth of change.

Mental health consultation   A model of consultation in which professional consultants work directly with consultees to address the mental health needs of clients and consumers.

Mentoring programs   Programs that provide new faculty with mentors—experienced faculty committed to helping them through their first year(s) on the job. Programs vary from one educational setting to another.

Modem   MOdulator-DEModulator, a device used to transform acoustical or computer data.

Multidisciplinary team   With respect to medical settings, includes health care professionals and paraprofessionals, all with similar patient treatment goals. Team members make various contributions depending on their background and training.

Multinational company   Establishing a company and doing business in a foreign host country.

Multisensory robots   Computers that are mobile, programmable to perform a variety of jobs, and able to react to their environment.

National Council for Accreditation of Teacher Education NCATE   The only body officially sanctioned by the U.S. Department of Education to accredit schools of education.

Negotiation   A practice that entails bargaining where parties that wish to come to an agreement dispute the nature and terms of the agreement.

New-generation managers   Managers convinced that traditional hierarchical organizations and management strategies are no longer appropriate for today's conditions, and who are, therefore, breaking with tradition by experimenting with innovative organizational structures, a variety of work units, and continuing education and training programs.

Nontraditional compensation   Examples are gainsharing, pay-for-knowledge, lump-sum bonus plans, and employee stock options. Nontraditional compensation is offered to motivate and reward employees.

Observation   A popular method of gathering consultation information through the deliberate viewing of events.

Obtrusive data collection   Methods of gathering important consultation information that require some disruption of the consultee's schedule and flow of activities.

Open system   An organization dependent on its external environment for survival. Such systems are open to the influences of the external world.

Organization   A group of people working together to achieve some goal or purpose; an organization requires cooperation among people to perform work activities prescribed by established policies and procedures.

Organizational changes   Alterations in any of the various organizational conditions and processes that emerge from consultation.

Organizational culture   The pattern of behaviors, norms, and values that prevails in an organization and shapes employee performance.

Organizational development (OD)   The application of knowledge from the behavioral sciences to organizational problems.

Organizational diagnosis   The process through which consultants and consultees assess organizational problem areas, isolate causal elements, and conceptualize organizational needs.

Organizational structure   The arrangement of individuals, groups, and programs (subsystems) that make up the whole organization. The primary purpose of an organization's structure is to arrange work processes and jobs to accomplish organizational goals.

Paradigm   Within an organizational context, a pattern of thinking that defines the practices, principles, and rules leading to success.

Paradigm shift   An alteration in the fundamental, conceptual thinking that organizations apply to explain their work and their future.

Paradoxical injunction   A theme reduction technique where the consultant persuades the consultee anticipating a disastrous outcome to behave as if the disaster were not inevitable and, by so doing, helps reduce or invalidate the strength of the theme (see **Theme interference**).

Parent conference   A face-to-face meeting or interview between a psychological consultant and parents that focuses on the problems or needs of a child or family.

Parent consultation   A consultation format in which consultants interact with parents as consultees regarding the needs and problems of children.

Parent education   A multifaceted intervention that has an instructional focus. Parent education has the implicit purpose of improving parents' childrearing competencies while enhancing certain personal attributes associated with parenting.

Parent teacher association (PTA)   A volunteer organization founded in Washington, D.C., in 1897 that is devoted to the education, welfare, and protection of children and youth. Membership in a local unit includes membership in the state branch and in the National Congress of Parents and Teachers.

Pay-for-knowledge   A series of knowledge and skill modules to qualify employees for other positions. Completion of a new module adds an increment to the employee's salary base.

Power   The ability of one party to influence others to behave in ways that satisfy the individual exerting the power.

Presenting consultation problem   The problematic issue or need identified by the consultee during the preliminary contact stage of consultation.

Prevention-oriented consultation   Consultation interventions designed to prevent the recurrence of undesirable conditions affecting children.

Problem diagnosis sessions   Assessment meetings in which various constituents can exchange information integral to client, program, or organizational problems.

Problem statement   A succinct statement resulting from assessment and diagnosis of the consultation problem. Problem statements are an outgrowth of collaboration between the consultant and consultee.

Process   In consultation, an organized and planned approach that proceeds through a series of action steps or stages. The consultation process proceeds from a beginning point to an end point. The process nature of consultation implies a systems approach in which success during one stage can affect success in other stages.

Process facilitator   A consultant who engages in process-oriented problem solving. The consultant, as a process-minded professional, helps consultees identify and correct deficient processes or activities that create organizational problems.

Processing   In training, an experiential method that allows participants to clarify, interpret, and analyze their participation in training activities.

Program-centered administrative consultation   A type of mental health consultation in which a professional consultant addresses program, rather than human, deficits (Caplan, 1970).

Project teams   Adaptive, problem-solving, temporary systems of diverse specialists working as a team to make change happen.

Psychoeducation   A term that refers to the cumulative processes used to teach individuals psychological skills and knowledge so that they can cope efficiently with existing illnesses or prevent future illnesses.

Psychological consultation   A broad helping approach in which qualified psychological consultants help consultees (1) resolve work-related issues pertaining to individuals, clients, or programs that they are responsible for, (2) become active agents in achieving solutions to problems, or (3) strengthen consultees' work-related competencies to address similar issues in the future.

Psychological consultation in child development settings   A broad helping process in which child- and family-oriented consultants provide help to consultees (teachers, aides, social services staff, parents) relative to the psychological and developmental needs of young children.

Psychological consultation in health care settings   Consultation processes and actions, delivered from the perspective of psychology and mental health, that supplement the efforts of medical personnel in rendering comprehensive care to patients.

Psychological education   The cumulative processes in which child development programs implement curricula that educate children in the areas of emotional development, self-esteem, and psychosocial competence.

Psychological liaison-consultation   An underdeveloped form of consultation in which psychological specialists play a key role in medical settings. They provide assistance with medical problems that cannot be resolved by traditional means.

Psychological professional   A psychological or mental health provider who has formal training, background, and related experience in the psychological sciences. He or she provides assistance to patients who present complex psychological disturbances (often in addition to health problems).

Psychosomatic medicine   A broad field within the health care arena that views physical illness as the product of interactions between psychological and physical processes.

Qualitative data   A type of subjective data that provide important generalizations or estimates of quality. Qualitative data are often informal estimates expressed in nonnumerical form.

Quantitative data   Observable, objective, and measurable information that can be synthesized and expressed numerically. Quantitative results often yield important factual information about a hypothesis or variable.

Rapport   In consultation, agreement, cooperation, and harmony between constituents.

Reactance   Action in response to another action (for example, the threat of change).

Reactions   Consultees' and other participants' thoughts, feelings, attitudes, and opinions about the consultation process.

Reciprocal determinism   Bandura's (1978) term that describes the dynamic and reciprocal interactions among an individual's behavior, interpersonal processes, and environment.

Records   Documented, chronological accounts of the actions or behavior of the consultee or organization in reference to the consultation client, program, or individual.

Rehearsal   A practical and powerful experiential exercise in training programs in which participants practice targeted relational or behavioral skills.

Reliability   The dependability of information over time. Data are reliable when they are consistent, stable, and trustworthy.

Research   Investigation or experimentation that attempts to explain particular phenomena or issues. Research contributes to the knowledge in a particular field.

Resistance   Active or passive opposition to the real or anticipated changes accompanying consultation.

Resources   In educational settings, people, money, facilities, equipment, energy, and time.

Returning students   Older, life-experienced adults who return to the college environment to begin a college career or to "retool" to meet career or occupational demands.

Role playing   A common experiential training method in which participants, in groups of two or more, practice or rehearse interactions pertinent to training goals.

Sanctioned authority   Authority granted the consultant by a senior administrator in the organization. Unlike line authority (authority of position), sanctioned authority requests staff cooperation and clearly specifies personnel and records that are to be available to the consultant in the assessment and diagnostic stages of the consultation process.

Satisfaction measures   Indications of the contentment consultees and other participants experience with the consultation process and its outcomes.

Scanning   Linked to assessment in consultation, scanning is the practice of observing or considering the various environments surrounding a consultation setting and problem.

Self-efficacy   In a social learning context, the belief in one's ability to succeed or accomplish something (Bandura, 1989).

Semiautonomous work units   Often organized to reduce the complexity of managing product diversification in conglomerate organizations, ultimately creating change in both the structure and function of the organization. The establishment of semiautonomous work units can lead to interunit conflict and confrontation if not handled properly.

Seminars   Workshops or classes that present current information, useful strategies, or innovative practices to help participants stay abreast of developments in their work.

Sequential conditions   In the behavioral consultation model, a term that describes the pattern of times or days in which a specific behavior occurs.

Simple identification   In Caplan's (1970) mental health consultation model, a source of consultee-client impasse where the consultee identifies rather than empathizes with the client.

Simulation   An experiential training method that involves the application of games, exercises, or situations that mimic real circumstances or project participants into contrived roles.

Social interest   For Alfred Adler, social interest was synonymous with psychological health.

Social learning theory The process of learning in which people learn by observing, construing, and evaluating the behaviors of others (Bandura, 1989).

Strategic planning The process through which organizational leaders scan existing realities and envision impending trends to help the organization plan for and achieve its future.

Subgroups An experiential training method in which larger groups are divided into smaller groups to increase participants' interactions and involvement.

Subsystem In systems organizations, a term that describes the smaller divisions or elements making up the total system.

Summative evaluation In consultation, a form of evaluation that focuses on consultation outcomes and goal attainment.

Supervision The process in which supervisors, with specialized training and experience, have authority over the work of others. Supervision implies a hierarchy of power in a relationship, along with the evaluation and monitoring of supervisee performance.

Surveys Written statements or questions designed to elicit valuable information or perceptions about particular consultation issues or problems.

Syllogism In Caplan's (1970) mental health consultation model, the form that themes assume when consultees believe that if a specific condition exists, then an inevitable result is linked to the condition (if A exists, B must be true).

Synchronizing Implies that one party's initiative to enter a conflict meeting matches the other party's readiness.

Synergistic teams Teams propelled by a collective, unidirectional, and motivating energy.

Systems theory A widely held philosophy that depicts the organization as a whole as consisting of smaller, interactive subsystems.

Team A group that shares a common purpose and employs cooperative problem-solving techniques.

Team building A collection of diverse methods that encourage groups to function as teams. Team building encourages groups to learn the fundamental skills of effective teamwork.

Team spirit An intangible, collective sense of unity and commitment to the group among team members.

Team systems Systems including a variety of work teams, project teams, quality-control circles, and semiautonomous work units.

Teamwork The process or state of working as a team.

Technical assistance (TA) A consultation approach in which consultants help child development programs assess their services, identify weaknesses, and propose remedial strategies that conform to published operating standards.

Terminal phobia The fear some people experience when first seated in front of a computer terminal.

Termination stage The end of the consultation process.

Theme In Caplan's (1970) mental health consultation model, a term that describes an unrealistic, emotionally laden belief or perception that potentially impairs therapy and other relationships.

Theme interference A term coined by Caplan (1970) to describe a consultee who anticipates a disastrous outcome because of an unresolved personal past defeat or failure.

Theme interference reduction Persuading the consultee that the disastrous outcome of theme interference is *not* inevitable (see also **Paradoxical injunction**, a technique employed by the consultant to reduce theme interference).

Therapy A formalized, psychological helping process, usually involving two parties. The therapist is a psychological professional who helps a client resolve direct, personal issues. Client issues usually involve behavioral or emotional disorders that inhibit growth and adaptation.

Third-party consultation An approach to conflict resolution that requires the active participation of an objective consultant, skilled in conflict resolution practices.

Training A structured, planned instructional process in which learners acquire information or skills intended to enhance their ability to perform their work. Inherent in these activities is an evaluation process assessing the learning accomplishments of students or trainees.

Training design An account of how a proposed training intervention is to occur; the design includes the training program's purpose, method, and format.

Training proposal Usually a written document that presents the consultant's credentials and training ideas. A training proposal outlines relevant information about a proposed training program.

Transference A source of consultee-client impasse where consultees project feelings (of past relationships or fantasies) onto the client.

Tripartite relationship A triadic or three-party relationship consisting of the consultant, consultee, and client. The tripartite relationship is a reciprocal relationship in which the interaction among the three parties varies with each consultation situation.

Unobtrusive data collection Methods of gathering important consultation information without significantly disrupting the consultee's schedule or flow of activities.

Usability The degree of helpfulness and practicality of evaluation data. Data are useful when they are presented in ways that translate into viable decisions or judgments.

Validity With respect to evaluation, the degree to which data measure what they are intended to measure.

Win-win solutions In conflict resolution, an approach founded on the philosophy that each faction has a vested interest and that a creative solution can be achieved where both parties benefit.

Work-unit teams Teams (appointed by managers) whose responsibilities and objectives are clearly defined. Team members meet regularly with their managers to discuss team performance and develop action plans to improve productivity and raise quality levels.

◆ Subject Index

◆ Name Index

TO THE OWNER OF THIS BOOK:

We hope that you have enjoyed *Psychological Consultation* as much as we have enjoyed writing it. We'd like to know as much about your experiences with the book as you care to offer. Only through your comments and the comments of others can we learn how to make *Psychological Consultation* a better book for future readers.

School: _____

Your instructor's name: _____

1. For what course was this book assigned? _____

_____

2. What did you like most about *Psychological Consultation*? _____

_____

_____

3. What did you like least about the book? _____

_____

_____

4. Were all of the chapters assigned for you to read? _____

   If not, which ones weren't? _____

5. If you used the Glossary, how helpful was it as an aid in understanding psychological concepts and terms?

_____

_____

6. In the space below, or in a separate letter, please let us know what other comments abouts the book you'd like to make. (For example, were any chapters or concepts particularly difficult?) We'd be delighted to hear from you!

_____

_____

_____

_____

Optional:

Your name: _____ Date: _____

May Brooks/Cole quote you, either in promotion for *Psychological Consultation* or in future publishing ventures?

Yes: _____   No: _____

Sincerely,

William Wallace
Donald Hall

Brooks/Cole is dedicated to publishing quality publications for education in the human services fields. If you are interested in learning more about our publications, please fill in your name and address and request our latest catalogue, using this prepaid mailer.

Name: _____

Street Address: _____

City, State, and Zip _____